EPIDEMIOLOGY OF DISEASES

EPIDEMIOLOGY OF DISEASES

EDITED BY

D. L. MILLER
MD, FRCP, FFCM
Professor, Department of Community Medicine
The Middlesex Hospital
Medical School, London

R D T FARMER
MB, MFCM, MRCGP
Senior Lecturer in Community Medicine
Westminster Medical School, London

FOREWORD BY

SIR RICHARD DOLL
Regius Professor of Medicine
University of Oxford

BLACKWELL SCIENTIFIC PUBLICATIONS
OXFORD LONDON EDINBURGH
BOSTON MELBOURNE

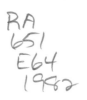

© 1982 by
Blackwell Scientific Publications
Editorial offices:
Osney Mead, Oxford, OX2 OEL
8 John Street, London, WC1N 2ES
9 Forrest Road, Edinburgh, EH1 2QH
52 Beacon Street, Boston
  Massachusetts 02108, USA
99 Barry Street, Carlton
  Victoria 3053, Australia

First published 1982

Set by Macmillan India Ltd
Bangalore and
Printed in Great Britain at
The Alden Press, Oxford

DISTRIBUTORS

USA
  Blackwell Mosby Book Distributors
  11830 Westline Industrial Drive
  St Louis, Missouri 63141

Canada
  Blackwell Mosby Book Distributors
  120 Melford Drive, Scarborough
  Ontario, M1B 2X4

Australia
  Blackwell Scientific Book Distributors
  214 Berkeley Street, Carlton
  Victoria 3053

British Library
Cataloguing in Publication Data

Epidemiology of diseases.
  1. Epidemiology
  I. Miller, D. L.   II. Farmer, R. D. T.
  614.4   RA651

  ISBN 0-632-00686-2

Contents

SECTION 5 · DISEASES OF THE GENITO-URINARY SYSTEM AND BREAST

SECTION 6 · ENDOCRINE DISEASES

SECTION 7 · LOCOMOTOR AND NEUROLOGICAL DISEASES

SECTION 8 · ACCIDENTS AND SUICIDE

Contents

List of Contributors

M W ADLER MD, MRCP, MFCM *Professor, Academic Department of Genito-urinary Medicine, The Middlesex Hospital Medical School, London*

ELIZABETH M BADLEY DPhil, *Deputy Director, ARC Epidemiology Research Unit, The University of Manchester*

R J BERRY MA, DPhil, MD, FRCP, FRCR *Professor, Department of Oncology, The Middlesex Hospital Medical School, London*

J CHAMBERLAIN MB, FFCM *Senior Lecturer in Epidemiology, Institute of Cancer Research, London*

J R T COLLEY MD, FFCM *Professor, Department of Community Health, The University of Bristol*

J CONNOLLY MB, MPhil, MRCP, MRCPsych *Senior Lecturer in Psychiatry, Westminster Medical School, London*

G DEAN MD, FRCP(I), FFCM(I) *Director, The Medico-Social Research Board, Dublin*

C DU V FLOREY MD, FFCM, MPH *Deputy Head, Department of Community Medicine, St Thomas's Hospital Medical School, London*

P C ELWOOD MD, FRCP, FFCM *Director, MRC Epidemiology Unit, Cardiff*

R D T FARMER MB, MFCM, MRCGP *Senior Lecturer in Community Medicine, Westminster Medical School, London*

N S GALBRAITH MRCP, FFCM *Director, Communicable Disease Surveillance Centre, London*

B G GAZZARD MD, MRCP *Consultant Physician, The Westminster and St Stephen's Hospitals, London*

D R JONES BA, MSc, PhD *Senior Lecturer in Medical Statistics, Westminster Medical School, London*

G KAZANTZIS PhD, FRCP, FRCS, FFCM, FFOM *Senior Lecturer in Occupational Medicine, The London School of Hygiene and Tropical Medicine*

P LANCE MB, MRCP *Senior Medical Registrar, The Westminster Hospital, London*

M W McNICOL FRCP *Consultant Physician, Cardiothoracic Department, The Central Middlesex Hospital, London*

D L MILLER MD, FRCP, FFCM *Professor, Department of Community Medicine, The Middlesex Hospital Medical School, London*

A NIXON FRCS, FRCS(C), DIH *Senior Occupational Medicine Adviser Shell UK Ltd, London*

CATHERINE PECKHAM MD, FFCM *Reader in Community Medicine, The Charing Cross Hospital Medical School, London*

P O D PHAROAH MD, MSc, FFCM *Professor, Department of Community Health, The University of Liverpool*

E M ROSS MD, FRCP, DCH *Senior Lecturer in Child Health and Community Medicine, Department of Community Medicine, The Middlesex Hospital Medical School, London*

EMER SHELLEY MB, MRCPI, MSc *Senior Registrar in Epidemiology, Medico-Social Research Board, Dublin*

H TUNSTALL PEDOE MA, MD, FRCP, FFCM *Professor, Cardiovascular Epidemiology Unit, Ninewells Hospital and Medical School, The University of Dundee*

M P VESSEY MD, FRCP(E), FFCM *Professor of Social and Community Medicine, Department of Community Medicine and General Practice, The University of Oxford*

W E WATERS MBBS, FFCM, DIH *Professor of Community Medicine, Faculty of Medicine, The University of Southampton*

PHILIP H N WOOD FRCP, FFCM *Director, ARC Epidemiology Research Unit, The University of Manchester*

A J ZUCKERMAN MD, DSc, FRCPath, MRCP *Professor of Microbiology, Director, WHO Collaborating Centre, The London School of Hygiene and Tropical Medicine*

Foreword

RICHARD DOLL

Doctors, like Molière's Bourgeois Gentilhomme who had been talking prose for 40 years without knowing it, had practiced epidemiology for centuries before it began to be recognized as a special branch of medical science. This recognition happened only a little more than a hundred years ago, with the establishment of the Epidemiological Society of London in 1850 and the publication in 1873 of John Parkin's book *Epidemiology; or the Remote Cause of Epidemic Disease in the Animal and in the Vegetable Creation.* At the time, epidemiologists were solely concerned with infectious diseases which occurred in easily recognizable epidemics and, it was hoped, could be controlled if the conditions in which the epidemics appeared could be defined. The methods of epidemiology, however, had never been limited to the study of such diseases and had been used intuitively in the two preceding centuries –by Lind to describe the conditions that led to scurvy in seamen, by Ramazzini to describe lead poisoning in artist painters, and by Pott to describe cancer of the scrotum in chimney sweeps.

That the study of the incidence of disease and its variation in different groups, characterized by constitutional, behavioural, or environmental differences, was concentrated on infectious disease, is easy to understand when the crudity of the tools available to the would-be epidemiologist is borne in mind. Epidemiologists must count and counting makes sense only if the units counted can be defined with sufficient precision to be reasonably alike. Until the latter half of the 19th century it was, by and large, only the infectious diseases that were sufficiently distinctive and sufficiently common for any but the most exceptional physician to be able to count cases and compare the numbers observed under different sets of conditions. This limitation was indeed so severe that even Hirsch (1864), whose three-volume text on geographical and historical pathology covered in meticulous detail all existing epidemiological knowledge, devoted only 20 of his 58 chapters to what we would now describe as noninfectious disease.

It did not follow, however, that epidemiologists necessarily raised their sights when it became possible to do so. The advances in microscopy, biochemistry, and the experimental study of animals were so impressive that they carried all before them and epidemiology, instead of developing, was dismissed as a soft subject limited to correlations of observational data that could not be tested by experiment and were inevitably hard to interpret. The triumphs of laboratory medicine and biology in general that culminated in the discovery of the genetic code have, indeed, been great; but they have not solved all the problems of clinical medicine and the prospects of their doing so in the near future seem, if anything, to have receded. In some cases, too, the paths that have been followed have led a long way from the practical problems of daily life. It is questionable, for example, how far the *in vitro* diagnosis of mutagenicity of many of the chemicals that can be discovered in minute amounts in the environment is relevant to the development of cancer in men and women. This, at least, epidemiology avoids; for it has the great advantage that it starts not from the 10 000 chemicals that pollute a particular area, but from the 10 000 deaths that occur in that area each year. It may be more likely to overlook the many small effects of these chemicals than laboratory studies; but it is much less likely to overlook the large determinants of contemporary morbidity rates and trends, irrespective of whether they are chemical or infectious in origin.

With the growth of laboratory facilities, automated analysis, and the potential for storing biological specimens, epidemiologists now have the possibility of collaborating with laboratory scientists in the detailed investigation of biological phenomena on a much larger scale than ever before. They need no longer confine themselves to armchair analyses of statistical data, clinical and social records, and replies to questionnaires, but can test collaboratively in the field ideas that have been developed in the laboratory and, in the laboratory, ideas that have been thrown up by the vagaries of human behaviour in the wild.

Gradually, over the last 30 years, it has come to be realized that the whole of medicine is the epidemiologist's field and that all types of medical specialist may gain something from knowledge of the epidemiological aspects of their subject. It is, therefore, appropriate that David Miller and Richard Farmer should now for the first time bring together in a single volume for the non-specialist the epidemiological features of the main morbid conditions that characterize the developed world. Not quite all of them, however, as mental disease is represented only by successful and attempted suicide – perhaps for the good reason that this alone of the common mental diseases can as yet be counted with reasonable reliability.

Acknowledgements

This book aims to provide a compact account of the epidemiology of some of the common and more important contemporary diseases and medical conditions. The emphasis is on those aspects of epidemiological knowledge that are relevant to the practising clinician as well as those responsible for preventive health programmes. We have been fortunate in enlisting the help of a large number of distinguished contributors and we are grateful to them for their work and support. We are particularly grateful to Professor Sir Richard Doll for writing the foreword.

The task of producing the manuscript was greatly eased by the painstaking assistance of Mrs Sylvia Cook for which we are most grateful. We are also pleased to acknowledge the help of Mrs Jane Katjavivi of Blackwell Scientific Publications.

Professor D L Miller
Dr R D T Farmer

SECTION 1 · INFECTIOUS DISEASES

Chapter 1 · Acute Respiratory Infections

D L MILLER

Acute respiratory infections (ARI) give rise to much misery, inconvenience and loss of working time even though, in economically advanced communities, they usually cause only relatively minor illness in most people. In poorer communities they are a major cause of death as well as morbidity, especially in infants and young children. Recent advances in microbiology, particularly in virology, have greatly increased knowledge of the agents responsible for acute respiratory infections and of the ways in which they spread. Some bacterial respiratory infections, such as whooping cough, diphtheria and pneumococcal pneumonia, can now be prevented by immunization or can be treated with antibiotics. Consequently death from these infections in developed countries is rare. However, most minor and many of the more serious respiratory infections are caused by viruses; these are more difficult to manage. Thus, although a great deal is known about the causes and epidemiology of acute respiratory infections, doctors are still unable to prevent or to cure the great majority of them.

The problem

Study of the epidemiology of acute respiratory infections is complicated by a number of problems. These can be grouped under four headings: variations in clinical definitions, the diversity of the pathology of acute respiratory disease, the difficulty of identifying the agents involved, and uncertainty over the interpretation of microbiological findings.

Variations in definition

The diagnostic labels used by doctors can be classified into those which refer to the aetiology of the disease, those that reflect specific pathology or morbid condition, and those that describe symptom complexes. In the case of acute respiratory infections there is no consistent taxonomic convention. For example, the term 'pneumonia' describes a particular pathological condition for which there are many causal agents. 'Pharyngitis' identifies a site of inflammation. 'Influenza' refers to a condition caused by a specific agent, although the label is often used without seeking confirmation from virological investigations. The term 'common cold' reflects traditional beliefs about the cause of a familiar

3

symptom complex. The confused taxonomy is reflected in the lack of consistent diagnostic criteria for the classification of acute respiratory infections. This has relatively minor importance in the clinical management of individuals, but it makes mortality and morbidity data from different sources difficult to interpret. Many attempts have been made to arrive at generally acceptable diagnostic criteria and conventions which will overcome this problem[1,2,3] but none is yet firmly established.

Pathological diversity

Acute respiratory infections may cause inflammation of the respiratory tract anywhere from the nose to the alveoli, with a wide range of combinations of symptoms and signs which do not correlate closely with any particular aetiological agents[4]. On the one hand, the same syndrome can be caused by a number of different agents. On the other hand, although infection with the same agent tends to be characterized by a similar pattern of features in epidemics, it can cause a variety of syndromes in different individuals, or infect without causing any symptoms. Little is known about what determines the variability of the clinical response to infection in different people. Consequently aetiological agents cannot be predicted with confidence from clinical features alone, unless there is an epidemic in the population. Therefore general recommendations for treatment based on clinical findings in the individual patient must be framed with caution and strategies for prevention cannot be based on epidemiological analysis of clinical records alone. They must be supported by the results of laboratory investigations.

Identification of respiratory agents

A large number of different agents – bacteria, viruses and other microbes – can cause acute respiratory infections[4]. This means that a range of culture systems, serological and other techniques, must be used to identify possible infecting agents. Many of these require considerable skill and experience for reliable use. Moreover, the laboratory procedures are generally expensive in time and materials, particularly those used in virology. Some respiratory viruses are very labile and this makes it essential to have the laboratory close to the patient. For these reasons the sensitivity of tests in routine use is often disappointing and isolation rates tend to be low. All this has seriously impeded research into their epidemiology. However, new techniques such immunofluorescence, radio-immune assay and enzyme-linked immunosorbent assay (ELISA)[5] promise to simplify routine diagnostic work and improve prospects for large scale population studies.

Pathological significance of infection

Many potentially pathogenic respiratory agents, particularly bacteria such as the haemophilus, pneumococci and streptococci, are frequently found among the normal commensal organisms carried in the healthy upper respiratory tract. Other agents such as influenza and other viruses, frequently cause asymptomatic infections. Thus, neither the isolation of an agent from the upper respiratory secretions or sputum (which may be contaminated by upper respiratory organisms), nor the demonstration of serological evidence of infection concomitant with an acute respiratory illness, can be regarded as proof that the agent identified was the cause of the illness. Isolation of the agent directly from the site of involvement (e.g. by lung aspirate) or blood culture is regarded by some as essential before aetiological conclusions can be drawn. Such specimens are rarely available and great care must be exercised in interpreting the results of laboratory investigations on other types of specimen.

Infecting agents

The microbial agents that cause acute respiratory infection are numerous and they include bacteria, viruses and biologically intermediate agents[6]. Even within species they can show a wide diversity of antigenic types.

Bacteria

The bacteria involved (Table 1.1) can all be isolated with varying frequency from carriers and cause illness in only a minority of infected persons. Their most serious effects are usually found in persons whose resistance is already impaired by general debility resulting from malnutrition, chronic systemic disease, chronic lower respiratory tract disease, or a concomitant primary virus infection, such as influenza. In this respect elderly persons are particularly vulnerable. Some bacterial species, for example *Streptococcus pneumoniae* and *Bordetella pertussis*, can be divided into a number of serotypes which are antigenically distinct. The various types tend to follow different patterns of epidemiological behaviour affecting different groups of the population and having different geographical distributions. This has particular practical importance for the manufacturers of polyvalent vaccines, who must take account of locally prevalent antigenic types of the relevant species when compounding their products.

Viruses and other agents

The viruses that have been found in association with acute respiratory disease are numerous. They are the primary cause of the great majority of acute respiratory

Table 1.1. Bacterial species associated with acute respiratory disease.

Bacteria	Age group(s) most frequently affected	Characteristic clinical features
Bordetella pertussis	Infants and young children	Paroxysmal cough
Corynebacterium diphtheriae	Children	Nasal/tonsillar/pharyngeal membranous exudate ±severe toxaemia
Haemophilus influenzae	Adults	Acute exacerbations of chronic bronchitis pneumonia
	Children	Acute epiglottitis (*H. influenzae* type B)
Klebsiella pneumoniae	Adults	Lobar pneumonia ±lung abscess
Legionella pneumophila	Adults	Pneumonia
Staphylococcus pyogenes	All ages	Lobar and broncho-pneumonia (esp. secondary to influenza) ±lung abscess
Streptococcus pneumoniae	All ages	Pneumonia (lobar or multilobular) Acute exacerbations of chronic bronchitis
Streptococcus pyogenes	All ages	Acute pharyngitis and tonsillitis

illnesses. However, the severity of the illness is often determined by whether or not secondary bacterial infection occurs, particularly in the case of lower respiratory tract infections. The evidence on the role of these viruses as causes of respiratory disease has been painstakingly accumulated, partly from epidemiological studies of patients with or without respiratory illness in whom there is laboratory evidence of infection, and partly from controlled experiments in human volunteers. Unfortunately most laboratory animals are not susceptible to the majority of respiratory viruses that are pathogenic in man. This means that they cannot be used to assist in these studies.

The agents currently considered to be capable of causing acute respiratory disease are shown in Table 1.2. The list includes some non-viral agents. These are listed with viruses for convenience because it is usual to carry out tests for infection with them in virology laboratories. All these agents are normally spread by the airborne route, but as most viruses do not survive for long outside the respiratory tract, the chains of transmission are maintained by direct person-to-person contact. Nevertheless, it is often hard to trace these chains, sometimes because of transmission by asymptomatic individuals, but also because of the ubiquity of the numerous agents involved and the lack of any clinical distinction between the illnesses most of them cause.

Although some species of respiratory viruses include many antigenically distinct variants, the majority are antigenically stable and stimulate a good

Table 1.2. Viruses and other agents associated with acute respiratory disease.

Agents	Age group(s) most frequently affected	Characteristic clinical features
Viruses		
Adenoviruses – endemic types (1, 2, 5)	Young children	Lower respiratory
– epidemic types (3, 4, 7)	Older children and young adults	Febrile pharyngitis and influenza-like illness
Enteroviruses (ECHO and Coxsackie)	All ages	Variable respiratory
Influenza A	All ages	Fever, aching, malaise, variable respiratory
B	School children	Occasional primary pneumonia / Secondary bacterial pneumonia in elderly
C	Rare	Mild upper respiratory
Measles	Young children	Variable respiratory with characteristic rash
Parainfluenza 1	Young children	Croup } re-infection in later life: mild upper respiratory
2		
3	Infants	Bronchiolitis and pneumonia
Respiratory syncytial virus	Infants and young children	Severe bronchiolitis and pneumonia
Rhinoviruses (multiple serotypes)	All ages	Common cold
Coronaviruses		
Other agents		
Chlamydia type B (Psittacosis)	Adults exposed to infected birds	Influenza-like illness and atypical pneumonia
Coxiella burnetii (Q fever)	Adults exposed to sheep and cattle	Atypical pneumonia
Mycoplasma pneumoniae	School children and young adults	Febrile bronchitis and atypical pneumonia

antibody response. Thus infection with any particular variant is likely to confer reasonably long-lasting specific immunity against that virus although, of course, the individual remains susceptible to any one of the other hundred or more respiratory viruses. The one exception to this rule is the influenza virus. This requires special explanation in order to understand its epidemiology.

There are three distinct antigenic types of influenza virus – A, B and C. They comprise a stable core nucleoprotein with surface 'spikes', the haemagglutinin (H) and neuraminidase (N) components. Immunity to influenza is related to the production of specific antibody to the surface antigens. Both the H and N components are antigenically labile and the classification of influenza viruses into subtypes is based on the characterization of these two antigens. From time to time, at intervals of 10–20 years, a major 'shift' in one or the other or both of these antigens occurs leading to the birth of a new subtype. Minor antigenic changes within subtypes, known as 'drift', occur more frequently. Both types of change are of great epidemiological significance because whenever an antigenic 'shift' occurs, previously acquired antibody gives no protection and herd immunity to the new subtype is negligible. Consequently there is a risk of a major epidemic or a pandemic. The effects of 'drift' are similar but less dramatic because of partial protection from antibodies to earlier variants. They are nevertheless important in determining the pattern of influenza epidemics, which in the present state of knowledge are as unpredictable as they are inevitable.

Sources of data

Mortality

Mortality rates for acute respiratory infection derived from routine death certification statistics are exceptionally precarious as indices of mortality from this group of diseases, for three reasons. Firstly, there are diagnostic problems; these have already been described. Secondly, acute respiratory infection is frequently a complication of another lethal condition, such as cancer or chronic cardiac, renal or lung disease which, according to coding rules, will usually be selected as the 'underlying cause' of death rather than the respiratory infection itself. Thirdly, knowledge of the existence of an epidemic may influence the certifying doctor's diagnostic preference. For these reasons the full contribution of acute respiratory infections to total mortality will be revealed only by multiple cause analyses. Even then doubts will remain about variations in diagnostic accuracy and how this may affect the data on the relative importance of the different diagnostic categories and supposed aetiological agents.

Morbidity

It is even more difficult to obtain reliable data on morbidity caused by acute respiratory infections. Few sources exist except in countries with well-developed health information services.

The main routine sources used in the United Kingdom are admissions to hosptial (Hospital Activity Analysis), sickness records in industry, schools and institutions, and consultations with general practitioners. In some countries, for example the United Kingdom and the Netherlands, a series of 'Sentinel' surveillance units has been established, based on primary care services, which are supported by the laboratory investigation[8] of specimens from a sample of patients. Additional information is available from special surveys such as the General Household Survey or the Morbidity Surveys in General Practice carried out by the Royal College of General Practitioners (RCGP) and the Office of Population Censuses and Surveys (OPCS)[7]. Hospital admissions are not a very satisfactory source of information because the criteria for admission for this group of diseases in different localities vary independently of the nature of the clinical illness and its severity. Sickness absence records have the disadvantage that they refer only to the working population which usually comprises people in those age groups least at risk from acute respiratory infections. General practitioner consultation rates are routinely available for a small number of practices only and these may not be representative of all practices.

Laboratory data

The collation of laboratory reports of positive results on specimens submitted from patients with symptoms of acute respiratory infections, has proved valuable both for monitoring changes in the incidence of infections due to particular organisms, and for detecting changes in the antigenic types of prevalent agents. This procedure has been particularly useful in influenza virus surveillance. In Britain, reports from laboratories have been collated by the Public Health Laboratory Service (PHLS) for more than 30 years and figures are published each week in the PHLS Communicable Disease Report (CDR). Summary analyses of these and other indices of the incidence of influenza and other respiratory infections are also published at intervals in the CDR, particularly during the epidemic season.

The World Health Organization (WHO) has been collecting and disseminating information on prevailing influenza viruses and the extent of epidemics since 1947[8]. To assist in this monitoring programme the WHO established a network of 101 national influenza centres in 71 countries. These act as watch stations for the collection of laboratory and epidemiological information. There are also 2

WHO Collaborating Centres for reference and research on influenza, where newly isolated virus strains can be fully characterized and advice given on strains to be included in vaccines. The collated information is published in the WHO Weekly Epidemiological Record.

In 1963 WHO established a system for the routine collection and distribution of information on all virus infections detected by laboratory tests. By 1973 laboratories in 45 countries were participating in the scheme[9]. The bulk of the reports still come from a small number of countries with well-developed virus diagnostic laboratory services. Nevertheless, despite the small numbers involved, they provide an indication of the relative importance of different agents, the types of clinical illness they produce, the population groups most affected, and of general trends in their incidence. The results are published in quarterly and annual summary reports.

Incidence

Mortality

In all countries acute respiratory infections are among the principal causes of death. Bulla and Hitze[6] in a global review based on data from 88 countries in 5 continents, with a total population of nearly 1200 million people, reported that deaths attributed to acute respiratory infections in these countries in 1972 totalled over 666 000. These accounted for nearly two-thirds of all respiratory deaths and for 6.3 % of deaths from all causes. About 75 % of the deaths were ascribed to pneumonia (bacterial or viral) and another 9 % were diagnosed as influenza.

Rates vary between countries and they tend to be 2 or 3 times higher in the least developed countries than in the most developed. The reasons for these differences are probably multiple. They include not only differences in climatic conditions but also differences in housing, in the general level of industrialization and socio-economic development. Poor nutrition, especially in children, is particularly important in determining susceptibility to infections. However, there can be considerable variations even within areas of similar socio-economic development, where such factors as the level of air pollution may influence the outcome of acute infections in those with pre-existing lung disease. Local mortality rates are particularly affected by the extent of influenza epidemics. These epidemics tend to have a relatively greater impact on acute respiratory infection mortality rates in developed countries where, when influenza is not epidemic, the rates are usually low.

Age-specific mortality rates show wide differences between countries. In general, rates tend to be high in infants and young children and in the elderly in all countries, although the age groups with the highest rates can differ. In developing countries, where malnutrition is often a major problem, the rates in children tend to be the highest. In some of these countries infant mortality rates from acute respiratory infections may exceed 20 per 1000 live births. By contrast, in developed countries, where respiratory infections are only exceptionally fatal in infants but are commonly terminal in the elderly, rates in the older age groups are the highest. The size of the discrepancies in mortality rates between countries is much greater in infants than in the elderly. For example, in 1970–73 the infant mortality rate from acute respiratory infections in a group of Middle American countries was 10 times that in North American countries[6]. During the same period a group of developing countries in Asia experienced 3 times the European rate. By contrast, at ages of 75 years and over the Middle American mortality rate from acute respiratory infections was only twice the North American rate, and the developing countries of Asia had a lower rate than European countries. From the age of 5 years onwards the reported mortality rates declined sharply, but in African and Asian countries they still accounted for one-fifth of all deaths between the ages of 5 and 14 years. Thus the age structure of the population in different countries critically affects the nature of the problem attributable to acute respiratory infections and the extent of mortality due to this cause. It must be stressed that the foregoing analysis is based on published mortality figures and that these are likely to be much less reliable in developing countries than elsewhere. Therefore, they must be interpreted with caution.

Morbidity

Since data on morbidity due to acute respiratory infections do not exist in most countries, geographical comparisons are not possible. Almost all existing information comes from a few developed countries, all with rather similar socio-economic and climatic conditions. A study in England during the 1960s[10] showed that in General Practice the mean annual consultation rate for all acute respiratory infections was about 34 per 100 person-years, nearly two-thirds of this being accounted for by cases of common cold and pharyngitis. Rates in children were several times higher than in adults, particularly for upper respiratory tract infections (Fig. 1.1). Rates of pharyngitis and primary otitis media increased from infancy to a peak at the age of 5 years. Middle respiratory tract infections (laryngitis, croup and tracheitis) were commoner up to the age of 5 years than they were thereafter. Lower respiratory tract infections, after declining to a minimum rate in young adults, increased in incidence again in those over 45 years of age. The changing relative significance of different diagnostic categories of acute respiratory illness through the age groups is shown in Fig. 1.2. This reinforces the observation that it is in people over the age of 65 years that lower respiratory tract infections assume particular significance, accounting for about 40 % of all consultations.

Infectious Diseases

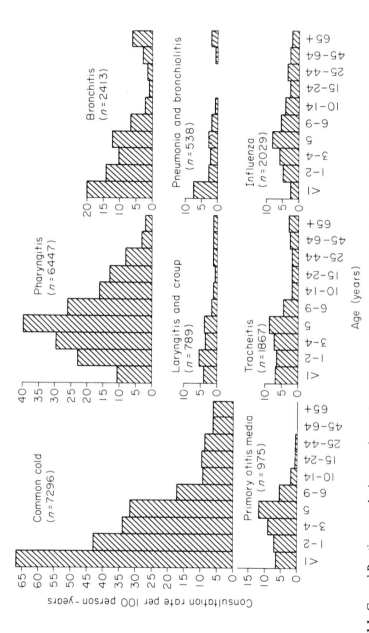

Fig. 1.1. General Practice: consultation rates by age for each diagnosis, England. Total number in sample as follows.[10]

Age (years)								
<1	1–2	3–4	5	6–9	10–14	15–24	25–44	45–64	65 +
969	2175	2091	1109	3968	4445	8458	17015	14973	6690

n Total number of cases observed for each infection.

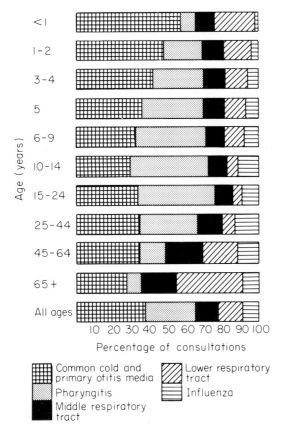

Fig. 1.2. General Practice: percentage distribution of consultations by diagnosis for each age group, England[10].

In temperate zones respiratory infections occur more often in the winter than in the summer months, possibly due to a tendency for people to spend time inside poorly ventilated buildings in the winter, conditions which favour the spread of infections that are transmitted directly from person to person by the airborne route. Seasonal variations in incidence in the English study, however, were less marked than might have been expected (Fig. 1.3) except in the case of influenza which was almost confined to the mid-winter months. At the other extreme, pharyngitis showed little seasonal variation.

The incidence of bronchitis and pneumonia in infancy is associated with several factors, particularly a history of such illness in a sibling and parental respiratory symptoms and parental smoking. The latter may be amenable to change. Lower respiratory illnesses in infancy may affect respiratory function and liability to develop respiratory symptoms in later life.

Infectious Diseases

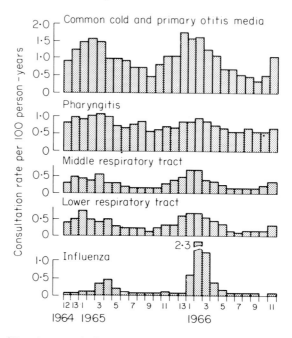

Fig. 1.3. General Practice: consultation rates by 4 week periods, England[10].

In a survey of children admitted to hospital with acute respiratory infections in England[10] during 1965–66, nearly 60% had lower respiratory tract illnesses (Table 1.3). The proportion with lower respiratory tract illness was greater in children living in conurbations than amongst those living in small towns. More than half of those admitted from conurbations were under 1 year old compared with only one-third of those from small towns (Table 1.4). More than one-third of the admissions of infants aged under 3 months were for bronchiolitis (Fig. 1.4). Older children were more likely to have bronchitis or pneumonia. About 11% of cases in the 2–4 year age group had croup; cases of tonsillitis and pharyngitis accounted for about a quarter of those in all age groups over 2 years. There was a substantial winter increase in numbers of admissions for lower respiratory tract illnesses, especially for bronchiolitis, but less variation in the remainder.

Analysis of certificates of incapacity for work in the United Kingdom shows that about one-fifth of all days lost from work due to sickness are certified as being due to respiratory disease, and at least half of this is due to acute respiratory infections. The figure may be higher during influenza epidemics. The causes of sickness absence from school show a similar pattern. The data from the United Kingdom are probably typical of the rates that would be found in many developed countries in temperate climates. Fragmentary information from

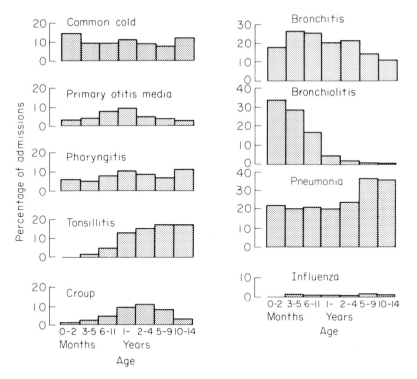

Fig. 1.4. Children in hospital: percentage distribution of admissions by diagnosis for each age group. Total number in sample as follows[10].

Age (months)			Age (years)			
0–2	3–5	6–11	1–2	2–4	5–9	10–14
1108	1064	1293	1430	1664	847	179

developing countries suggests that acute respiratory infections there may account for between one-quarter and one-half of all illness episodes and that rates are particularly high in young children.

WHO programme

The high mortality and massive morbidity rates attributable to acute respiratory infections have long been a matter of serious concern in all countries. The complexity of the problems they present and the lack of specific treatment or effective preventive measures have imposed serious constraints on programmes aimed at reducing their incidence. However, the discrepancies that exist between the mortality rates in developed and in developing countries and between specific

Infectious Diseases

Table 1.3. Children in hospital: percentage distribution of admissions by diagnosis and size of town.

Diagnosis	Size of town			All hospitals
	Conurbations	Large towns	Small towns*	
Common cold & primary otitis media	13.4	24.5	12.7	15.8
Pharyngitis & tonsillitis	16.3	17.7	20.5	17.9
Croup	4.2	5.0	12.5	6.8
Bronchitis, bronchiolitis & pneumonia	65.4	52.6	53.5	59.0
Influenza 0.7	0.2	0.7	0.6	
Total admissions	3608(100 %)	1784(100 %)	2198(100 %)	7590(100 %)

* Population less than 150 000.

Table 1.4. Children admitted to hospital: percentage distribution of admissions by age and size of town.

Age	Size of town			All hospitals
	Conurbations	Large towns	Small towns*	
Months				
0–2	17.0	13.6	11.5	14.6
3–5	16.6	12.8	10.7	14.0
6–11	18.9	16.3	14.8	17.1
Years				
1	19.1	18.2	19.0	18.8
2–4	19.3	21.4	26.7	21.9
5–14	9.1	17.8	17.4	13.5
All ages	3608(100 %)	1784(100 %)	2198(100 %)	7590(100 %)

* Population less than 150 000.

groups within the same countries, suggest that fatality rates could be reduced if fuller use were made of existing treatment and control procedures. For this reason the WHO Assembly in 1976 decided that, in its Sixth General Programme of Work for 1978–83, the existing long-established programme directed to the control of tuberculosis should be extended to other 'communicable diseases of the respiratory system'. The priority to be given to the problem was further endorsed by the 1979 Assembly which urged member states to intensify their efforts in this direction. This will involve both improving the primary medical care services and developing better methods for early detection, treatment, and where possible prevention of acute respiratory infections.

Specific bacterial infections

Pertussis (whooping cough)

Whooping cough (see also Chapters 3 & 12) is mainly a disease of infancy and early childhood. It is highly infectious and thus infants and young children exposed in the home to siblings with the disease experience high attack rates. Infection is rarely, if ever, subclinical and immunity after a clinical attack is usually lifelong. Most deaths occur in infants, those under the age of 3 months being particularly vulnerable.

Death rates in the 19th century were very high. These have declined steadily throughout this century but in the 1940s in Britian they still amounted to about 1000 annually[12]. There was a further dramatic fall in mortality rates from about 1945 onwards. This was a reflection more of a decline in case fatality rates than of a decline in incidence, which followed about 10 years later with the introduction of an effective pertussis vaccine. The contribution that the vaccine has made to the control of the disease has been widely debated. It has certainly not been as effective as some other vaccines. Despite acceptance rates in Britain of 75–80 %, epidemics continued to occur every 3 to 4 years throughout the 1960s and 1970s. Changes in the prevalent serotypes causing disease and suboptimal potency of the vaccines may have been responsible for these epidemics. Vaccine composition has been adjusted accordingly. Some cases of coughing diseases notified as whooping cough may be caused by viruses (notably respiratory syncytial virus, parainfluenza viruses and adenoviruses) and not by *Bordetella pertussis*, but the proportion is probably small. The fall in vaccine acceptance rates following the public alarm generated by reports of brain damage caused by the vaccine was followed by a major new epidemic starting in 1977–78 when numbers of notifications reached levels similar to those in the 1950s. The question of vaccine safety has not been totally resolved, but the balance of risk from the disease and possible risk from the vaccine seems to favour continued vaccination.

Diptheria

Like whooping cough, diphtheria was one of the most frequently fatal childhood infections in the 19th century. Now, in the United Kingdom and most developed countries, it is a rare disease. During the decade 1968–77 notifications in England and Wales averaged 9 per annum. There was total of 6 deaths from the disease during that period. Most cases now arise from importation of the infection by unimmunized travellers. The death rate from diphtheria was first reduced following the development of an antioxin for treatment of the disease around the turn of the century. Even so, up until 1940 when the vaccine was introduced, there was an average of about 50 000 cases which caused 2500 deaths each year. The success of diphtheria immunization in virtually eliminating the disease is remarkable, particularly since the vaccine, being a toxoid, is not directed against the organism itself. For this reason at first there were fears that although the clinical disease might be controlled, immunization would not reduce carrier rates, but in fact carriers are rare. However, the risk of introduction of infection from countries where the disease is still rife means that immunization rates must be maintained at a high level.

Pneumococcal pneumonia

Many bacteria may cause pneumonia (Table 1.1). However, the most frequent is the pneumococcus and the most important cause of death is pneumococcal pneumonia. Before the introduction of antibiotics fatality rates were between 20 and 40 %. The disease occurs in all climates and seasons of the year, although it is commoner in the winter. In developed countries it is now a relatively rare disease compared with 30–40 years ago. It is now principally seen in occasional outbreaks in residential institutions. However, it remains common in some poorer and more remote communities, for example in the Highlands of New Guinea where it is by far the most important respiratory pathogen and a common cause of death[11].

Pneumococci are often found in the upper respiratory tract of healthy persons; they are spread by droplet infection from person to person but, except in individuals whose resistance to infection is impaired, transmission rarely leads to disease in contacts. Of the many serotypes of pneumococcus only relatively few cause pneumonia, though the types prevalent in different communities may vary. This fact and the recent emergence of strains of pneumococci resistant to penicillin, has encouraged attempts to produce polyvalent polysaccharide vaccines. The results of trials in high risk communities have been encouraging[11].

Legionnaire's disease

This disease takes its name from an outbreak of a serious pneumonia with high death rate in persons attending a convention of the American Legion in Philadelphia in the USA in 1976[13]. The organism, isolated with difficulty from the lungs of some of the fatal cases, was a previously unrecognized Gram-negative bacillus with fastidious growth requirements which has been named *Legionella pneumophila*. Epidemiological reappraisal of several earlier unexplained outbreaks of pneumonia and examination of stored sera from some of those affected in these outbreaks, has shown that this was not a new infection.

In the original outbreak 182 cases of acute respiratory disease occurred and

29 (16 %) of the patients died. This has been about the average case fatality rate in other outbreaks. Investigations suggested a common source of infection, probably airborne rather than case-to-case spread, although this can sometimes occur. The organism has been isolated from water storage tanks and, in particular, from the evaporative condensers that form part of air-conditioning systems[14]. Contaminated dust has also been suspected as a source of infection.

All age groups may be affected but reported cases have tended to be mainly in middle-aged adults. Subclinical infection appears to be quite frequent among exposed individuals and the incidence is greatest in the warmer months of the year, possibly because air-conditioners are most often used at this time of year.

There is much to be learned about the epidemiology of this condition before effective preventive measures can be devised and implemented. Meanwhile, it has caught the public imagination as a 'new' disease and, with justification, has created some alarm.

Specific viral infections

Influenza

Influenza has probably afflicted man for centuries. History records many epidemics of respiratory disease which, from the descriptions given, were almost certainly influenza. Unlike most infections, which tend to be associated with poor standards of personal and public hygiene and poor physical health, influenza is no respecter of persons. Attack rates can be very high in all types of community. The disease can have devastating consequences on the maintenance of normal social and working life and imposes heavy burdens on medical and welfare services. It is usually relatively mild and most deaths occur in the very young, the elderly and in those with chronic disease. Occasionally, however, as in the 1918–19 pandemic, when about 20 million people died, young adults also suffer high fatality rates. In most epidemics the increased mortality and morbidity is much greater than may appear from deaths and illnesses ascribed to influenza, because the infection often hastens death due to other causes[15]. It also gives rise to illnesses that are not diagnosed as influenza or do not reach medical attention.

Influenza occurs mainly in epidemics or pandemics and less often as localized outbreaks, particularly in residential institutions. Attack rates in epidemics can vary from less than 10 % in the general population to 40 % or more in closed communities. For reasons that have been explained earlier, when a new subtype appears a pandemic is almost inevitable. However, although everyone is theoretically susceptible, not everyone is necessarily infected when first exposed. With successive epidemics more people acquire immunity to the new variant and consequently the size of epidemics tends to diminish. The appearance of a new subtype is usually accompanied by disappearance of the old subtype although it may reappear some years later. The origin of new subtypes is obscure. Direct mutation from the antecedent virus seems unlikely and recombination or hybridization between human and animal or bird strains in which a man-adapted virus acquires H and N antigens from an animal virus has been proposed as a possible explanation[16]. This would be consistent with evidence that the same H and N antigens may 'recycle', reappearing after many years absence. When this happens people who were alive at the time the antigen was last circulating remain immune[17]. This type of antigenic change cannot be predicted, but by careful monitoring of influenza viruses prevalent in all parts of the world[18] it is often possible to detect new variants before they become widespread. This allows manufacturers time to prepare appropriate vaccines in sufficient quantities to offer protection at least to the most vulnerable groups of the population, though not to all.

The size of epidemics between pandemics depends on the interval since the last subtype appeared and the degree to which antigenic drift has taken place. By monitoring both the antigenic changes in the virus and the proportion of population samples with matching or closely similar serum antibodies, it is often possible to predict the likelihood of epidemics in particular communities[19]. The variable pattern of epidemics and their impact on the community as reflected by a number of different indices can be illustrated from the surveillance data routinely collected in Britain (Fig. 1.5).

Most influenza epidemics are due to influenza A virus. These tend to affect people of all ages except when an antigenic variant that has previously circulated reappears. For example, in 1977 the strain H1N1, which had not been in circulation since the 'Asian' virus H2N2 first appeared in 1957, reappeared and caused widespread epidemics. These were almost entirely confined to people under the age of 25 years, most of whom had not previously encountered this antigenic type (Fig. 1.6). Older persons for the most part escaped because they already had antibody to this virus. Since influenza viruses A and B are antigenically distinct and there is no cross immunity between them, epidemics due to each of them occur independently, sometimes simultaneously (Fig. 1.7). As virus B antigens do not change to the same extent or as frequently as those of virus A, pandemics due to the former do not occur. Virus B epidemics tend to affect children more than adults, because they are least likely to have had previous exposure and to possess relevant antibodies (Fig. 1.8).

Influenza epidemics in temperate zones usually occur in the winter months but may occur at other times particularly when a new variant first circulates. The reason for this seasonality is not clear but may be due to the fact that in cold weather people more often crowd together in poorly ventilated buildings. The same may be true in warm-climate countries during the rainy season. Survival of the virus is certainly favoured by low relative humidity and low ambient temperature, but it is less clear whether or not individual susceptibility is enhanced by cold and damp weather.

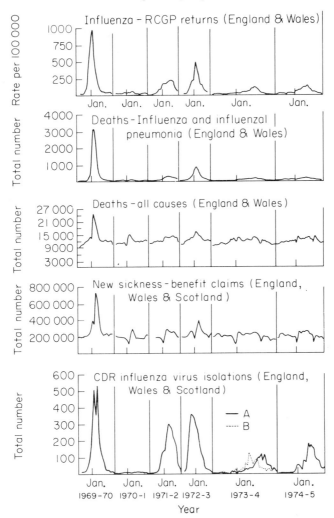

Fig. 1.5. Variable pattern of epidemics and their impact on the community. British influenza surveillance data 1969–75. (Public Health Laboratory Service Standing Committee on Influenza. *Journal of Hygiene, Cambridge* 1977; **78**: 223.)

Another unexplained feature of many influenza epidemics is that they appear to break out more or less simultaneously in many separate locations, unlike the pattern found with most infectious diseases, the spread of which can be traced from person to person and from one locality to another. Even within households where contact is close, secondary attack rates of influenza appear to be low despite the presence of susceptible contacts (Fig. 1.9). Hope-Simpson has suggested that this phenomenon could be explained by the hypothesis that some

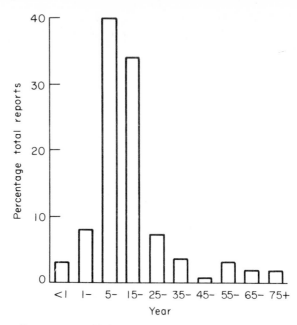

Fig. 1.6. Age-specific occurrence of influenza A, United Kingdom. Total reports = 251 (excluding 5 – age not known). (Public Health Laboratory Service, Communicable Disease Surveillance Centre. Influenza in the United Kingdom 1978–79. *British Medical Journal* 1979; **ii**: 1299.)

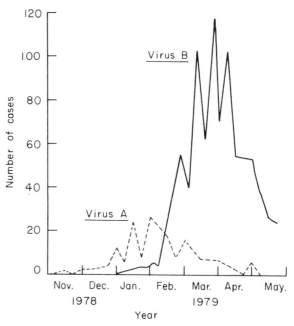

Fig. 1.7. Laboratory reports of occurrence of influenza viruses A and B, United Kingdom, Nov. 1978 – May 1979. (Public Health Laboratory Service, Communicable Disease Surveillance Centre. Influenza in the United Kingdom 1978–79. *British Medical Journal* 1979; **ii**: 1299.)

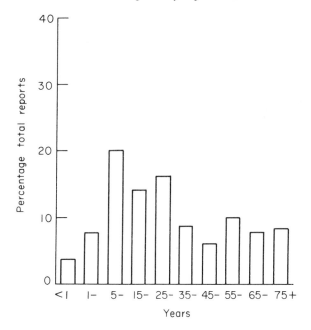

Fig. 1.8. Age-specific occurrence of influenza B, United Kingdom. Total reports = 864 (excluding 69 – age not known). (Public Health Laboratory Service, Communicable Disease Surveillance Centre. Influenza in the United Kingdom, 1978–79. *British Medical Journal* 1979; **ii**: 1299.)

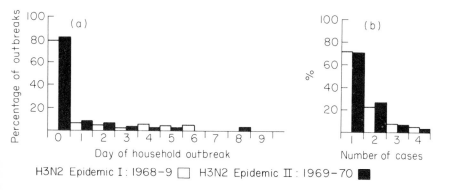

Fig. 1.9. Household outbreaks of type A (H3N2) influenza in a mild epidemic, 1968–69 (total number of households = 53) and in a severe epidemic, 1969–70 (total number of households = 81). (a) Proportion of cases falling each day of household outbreaks, showing similar distribution in the 2 epidemics, with about 80% falling on day 0. (b) Distribution of households by number of persons attacked in them, showing almost identical distribution in the 2 epidemics, with 70% of households in both epidemics having only 1 case of influenza.[20]

infected persons become symptomless carriers and transmit the virus only when a seasonally mediated stimulus reactivates the latent virus[20].

All attempts to control influenza epidemics have so far met with little success and the prospects of achieving control remain poor. Elimination of the virus from its animal and bird reservoirs is impracticable. Attempts to interrupt the spread of the virus by air disinfection have had disappointing results. However, good ventilation of public buildings, the avoidance of crowded places during epidemics and encouraging sufferers to cover their faces with a handkerchief when coughing and sneezing and to stay at home at the first signs of influenza, all seem to be sensible precautions. Vaccines, which have achieved spectacular success in the control of some other infections that spread directly from person to person are in theory the best prospect of controlling influenza. Trials of killed virus vaccines have shown that they can give useful protection, though the degree of efficacy varies. They sometimes give rise to local and systemic reactions, but this is less of a problem with the new subunit vaccines. Live-attenuated virus vaccines have been extensively used in the USSR where they are reported to give good protection. However, the results of trials with these vaccines elsewhere have been less satisfactory. The difficulty is to produce a vaccine in which the virus is sufficiently attenuated to avoid unacceptably frequent reactions, while still stimulating protective immunity in most recipients. The major problem remains the capricious antigenic behaviour of the virus which ensures that there can never be any certainty that the vaccines in current use will be protective against the virus likely to cause the next epidemic.

Current recommendations are that the vaccine should be offered to individuals most likely to suffer complications from the infection such as people with chronic cardiac or respiratory disease or diabetes, and also to the elderly, particularly those in residential institutions where outbreaks can be severe and cause some premature deaths[21]. The vaccine is not recommended to control spread in the general population although it is sometimes given to key workers in public services and industry. A large-scale study of employees in the British Post Office showed little benefit from annual vaccination campaigns, possibly because attack rates are relatively low in most winters, the vaccine is incompletely protective and acceptance rates are low[22].

The versatility of the influenza virus, its potential virulence and its ubiquity, seem likely to present an unremitting threat to man, particularly to those who do not enjoy robust health, and a formidable challenge to preventive medicine for some time to come.

Respiratory syncytial virus (RSV)

RS virus is the most important respiratory pathogen of infants and very young children. It is associated with severe bronchiolitis and pneumonia for which there is no specific treatment and which can be lethal. The infection has been found worldwide, but the incidence is usually higher in industrial than in rural communities[23]. In Britain epidemics due to RSV occur during the winter months each year, with a peak usually in February or March[24]. The majority of reported cases occur in infants. Older children and adults may be infected but in them the illness is usually relatively mild and confined to the upper respiratory tract. Serological studies show that most infants have detectable antibodies at birth but these are lost in the first few months of life. They then begin to acquire antibodies by natural infection, often without apparent illness. Thus by the age of 1 year, about 25 % of children have antibodies, by 2 years of age the proportion has risen to 50 % and by 4 or 5 years of age, nearly all children have antibodies. Breast feeding appears to confer some protection against clinical infection in infants. Natural infection, however, does not appear to protect against later reinfection, often accompanied by illness of equal severity to the first episode. This does not auger well for the success of vaccines and attempts to immunize young children with the vaccines so far produced have failed to protect them. Indeed vaccinated children suffered more severe illnesses in response to subsequent natural infection than unvaccinated controls.

Measles

Unlike most respiratory virus infections, measles (see also Chapter 3) is usually diagnosed with ease because of its characteristic respiratory signs and symptoms and the typical rash. It is endemic in all but the most isolated populations of the world. Outbreaks occur mainly in the late winter and early spring. In most populations prior to introduction of measles vaccine, they recurred regularly at intervals of 2 to 3 years (Fig. 1.10). This epidemic periodicity is probably due to fluctuations in the proportion of immune children in the population. Epidemics occur when the proportion who are immune falls below a critical level and end when susceptibles have been exhausted or are too few to maintain successful chains of transmission. As new susceptible children are added to the population the conditions required for epidemic spread build up again and the cycle recurs.

The incidence usually reaches a peak in children soon after they begin to mix in kindergartens or at school in the age group 3 to 5 years. In urban communities children tend to contract measles earlier in life and in such situations epidemics recur more regularly than in smaller and more isolated communities. Almost everyone acquires the infection during childhood and, since immunity is lifelong, measles is rarely seen in adults.

The disease is usually mild and is regarded by most parents and doctors as a mere nuisance, not to be taken too seriously. However, where poor socio-economic conditions lead to infection very early in life or children are malnourished, particularly where there is a protein deficiency, as in West Africa,

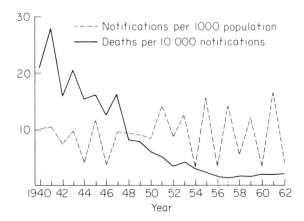

Fig. 1.10. Measles notifications and deaths, England and Wales, 1940–62. (From the Registrar General's Statistical Reviews[25].)

the disease tends to be much more severe and case fatality rates are high. This is also the case when the infection is introduced into 'virgin soil' communities where the infection has not been seen for perhaps a generation or more. There it can sweep through the whole population causing high mortality at all ages. However, the assumption that measles is a trivial illness in countries such as Britain is not entirely justified[25]. It is true that mortality rates have declined steeply since the 19th century and by the 1950s had settled to a very low level (Fig. 1.10). But the frequency of complications which may have serious consequences remains significant. It has been estimated[26] that in Britain in an average epidemic before measles vaccine was introduced, over 6000 children would be admitted to hospital, there would be 2000 cases of neurological complications (including 600 cases of encephalitis) 20 000 with serious respiratory complications and 13 000 with otitis media. Recent studies have confirmed that these rates still apply in Britain in unvaccinated children.

Live-attenuated measles virus vaccine has been shown in controlled trials to have high levels of protective efficacy[27]. However, febrile reactions, sometimes with rash and occasionally with convulsions, occur sufficiently often to be unacceptable to some parents and doctors. Wherever vaccine has been used on a substantial scale the incidence of measles has declined (Fig. 1.11). It is now recommended routine practice in the United Kingdom to offer the vaccine to children between the ages of 12 and 18 months. When given earlier it may not produce a satisfactory antibody response because of the presence of maternal antibody. Measles vaccine acceptance rates in Britain in recent years have been only about 50%. This is unsatisfactory and may mean that the disease will become more common in teenagers and adults in whom it can be more severe than in young children. The duration of immunity after vaccination is uncertain.

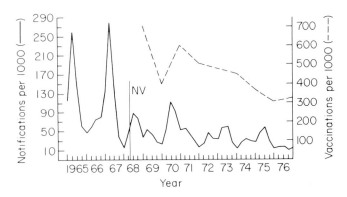

Fig. 1.11. Notification of measles in quarterly periods, Oct. 1964–Dec. 1976, and measles vaccinations 1968–76, England and Wales. NV: National vaccination scheme started. (Fourth Report to the Medical Research Council by the Measles Sub-Committee of the Committee on Development of Vaccines and Immunization Procedures. *Lancet* 1977; **ii**: 571–5.)

The disease has been reported in adults vaccinated in childhood. Revaccination in adults carries a risk of severe side-effects. In the USA it has been decided to embark on an eradication programme. This may be feasible but it has yet to be shown whether it can be sustained indefinitely and whether it will succeed against the twin problems of waning immunity in vaccinated individuals and the risk of reintroduction of the virus from other countries into groups who remain unimmunized or are susceptible for any other reason. An alternative strategy would be the selective use of the vaccine in high risk groups[28].

Other respiratory virus infections

A number of other viruses may cause respiratory infections. Those most frequently responsible are rhinoviruses, parainfluenza viruses, adenoviruses and some enteroviruses. All may cause disease in any part of the respiratory tract and the illness can vary in severity from the trivial to the lethal. All have a worldwide distribution and most of them are more prevalent in the winter than in the summer.

The parainfluenza viruses are important mainly as causes of lower respiratory tract disease in infants and small children. There are 4 types of which type 4 appears to be of little importance. Parainfluenza viruses types 1 and 2 are associated mainly with croup in small children and tend to occur in epidemics about every other year in mid-winter. Type 3 causes mainly bronchiolitis and pneumonia of infants and tends to be endemic with increased incidence in the summer. Infection with these viruses is widespread and most children have serological evidence of past infection by the age of 5 years.

The adenoviruses causing respiratory infection can be divided into the endemic serotypes and the epidemic types. The former are found most often in young children and the latter in young adults, especially those living in residential institutions (e.g. military bases and boarding schools). They cause lower respiratory tract disease in infants, but in older children and adults the typical illness is acute febrile pharyngitis.

Rhinoviruses are usually associated with the common cold, but can cause more serious illnesses, especially in infants. There is a very large number of different serotypes which can cause respiratory illness, and infection with these viruses is found in all age groups, sometimes in the absence of symptoms.

The role of enteroviruses in respiratory infection is uncertain, though some probably are responsible for mainly minor and occasional serious respiratory illnesses.

Vaccines have been developed against some of these respiratory infections. Clinical trials have shown them to be potentially effective, but none is in routine use.

Other respiratory agents

There are 3 other groups of microbial agents which sometimes cause severe pneumonia, usually in sporadic cases.

Q fever, due to *Rickettsia burnetii*, is usually acquired from cattle or from handling the products of conception of sheep. The organism can survive in the dry state and outbreaks have been recorded where contaminated dust has been disturbed. The infection can also be milk-borne.

Psittacosis, due to *Chlamydia* type B, is acquired by inhalation of dust from the desiccated droppings of infected birds or by direct contact with them. This is mainly an occupational hazard of pet bird dealers and of bird fanciers.

Pneumonia due to *Mycoplasma pneumoniae* is more common than Q fever and psittacosis. It occasionally occurs in epidemics in residential institutions and may give rise to severe illness, although some infected persons have only mild symptoms. It can occur at any age, but is most frequent in older children and young adults.

References

1. Hope-Simpson RE, Miller DL. The definition of acute respiratory illness in General Practice. *Postgraduate Medical Journal* 1973; **49**: 763–70.
2. Court SDM. The definition of acute respiratory illness in children. *Postgraduate Medical Journal* 1973; **49**: 771–6.
3. World Health Organization. *Viral respiratory diseases. Report of a WHO scientific group.* Technical report series. No 642. Geneva: WHO, 1980.
4. Poole Pauline M, Tobin J. O'H. Viral and epidemiological findings in the MRC/PHLS survey of respiratory disease in hospital and General Practice. *Postgraduate Medical Journal* 1973; **49**: 778–87.

5. Almeida June D, *et al. Manual for rapid laboratory viral diagnosis.* WHO offset publication. No 47. Geneva: WHO, 1979.
6. Bulla A, Hitze K. Acute respiratory infections: a review. *Bulletin of the World Health Organization* 1978; **56**(3): 481–98.
7. Office of Population Censuses and Surveys. Royal College of General Practitioners and Department of Health and Social Security. *Morbidity Statistics from General Practice. Second National Study, 1970–71.* Studies on medical population subjects. No 26. London: HMSO, 1974.
8. World Health Organization. Influenza: the WHO programme. *WHO Chronicle* 1979; **33**: 7–8.
9. Assaad F, Cockburn WC. A seven-year study of WHO virus laboratory reports on respiratory viruses. *Bulletin of the World Health Organization* 1974; **51**: 437–45.
10. Miller DL. Collaborative studies of acute respiratory disease in patients seen in General Practice and in children admitted to hospital. *Postgraduate Medical Journal* 1973; **49**: 749–62.
11. Riley ID, Andrews M, *et al.* Immunization with a polyvalent pneumococcal vaccine. *Lancet* 1977; **i**: 1338.
12. Joint Committee on Vaccination and Immunization. *Review of the evidence on whooping cough vaccination.* London: HMSO, 1977.
13. Fraser DW, Tsai TR, *et al.* Legionnaire's disease. Description of an epidemic of pneumonia. *New England Journal of Medicine* 1977; **297**: 1189.
14. Leading Article. Legionnaire's disease. *British Medical Journal* 1979; **iii**: 81.
15. Clifford RE, Smith JWG, *et al.* Excess mortality associated with influenza in England and Wales. *International Journal of Epidemiology* 1977; **6**: 115–28.
16. Kilbourne ED. The molecular epidemiology influenza. *Journal of Infectious Diseases* 1973; **127**: 478–87.
17. Schoenbaum SC, Coleman MT, *et al.* Epidemiology of influenza in the elderly: evidence of virus recycling. *American Journal of Epidemiology* 1976; **103**: 166–73.
18. Pereira MS, Assaad FA, Delon PJ. Influenza surveillance. *Bulletin of the World Health Organization* 1978; **56**: 193–203.
19. Pereira MS, Chakraverty P, Dane AR. The influence of antigenic variation on influenza A2 epidemics. *Journal of Hygiene, Cambridge* 1969; **67**: 551–7.
20. Hope-Simpson RE. Epidemic mechanisms of type A influenza. *Journal of Hygiene, Cambridge* 1979; **83**: 11–26.
21. Tyrrell DAJ, Smith JWG. Vaccination against influenza A. *British Medical Bulletin* 1979; **35**: 77–85.
22. Smith JWG, Pollard R. Vaccination against influenza: a five year study in the Post Office. *Journal of Hygiene, Cambridge* 1979; **83**: 157–70.
23. Medical Research Council Committee on Respiratory Virus Vaccines. Respiratory syncytial virus infections: admissions to hospital in industrial, urban and rural areas. *British Medical Journal* 1978; **iii**: 796–8.
24. Editorial. Respiratory syncytial virus: a community problem. *British Medical Journal* 1979; **iii**: 457.
25. Miller DL. The public health importance of measles in Britain today. *Royal Society of Medicine. Proceedings* 1964; **57**: 843–6.
26. Miller DL. Frequency of complications of measles, 1963. *British Medical Journal* 1964; **ii**: 75–8.
27. Medical Research Council Measles Vaccines Committee. Vaccination against measles: a clinical trial of live measles vaccine given alone and live vaccine preceded by killed vaccine. *British Medical Journal* 1966; **i**: 441–6.
28. Smith H. Measles again. *British Medical Journal* 1980; **i**: 766–7.

Further Reading

Christie AB. *Infectious diseases: epidemiology and clinical practice.* 2nd ed. London: Churchill Livingstone, 1974.

Dick GWA. *Immunization*. London: Update Publications Ltd, 1978.

Miller DL, ed. Acute respiratory virus diseases. *Postgraduate Medical Journal* 1973; **49** (577).

Schild GC, ed. Influenza. *British Medical Bulletin* 1979; **35** (1).

Selby P, ed. *Influenza: virus, vaccines and strategy. Proceedings of a working group on pandemic influenza, Rougemont 26–28 January, 1976.* Sandoz Institute publication. No 5. London: Academic Press Inc, 1976.

Stuart-Harris Sir Charles H, Schild GC. *Influenza. The virus and the disease.* London: Edward Arnold, 1976.

World Health Organization Scientific Group. *Viral respiratory diseases.* Technical report series, No 642. Geneva, 1980.

Chapter 2 · Tuberculosis

M W McNICOL

Tuberculosis is a disease caused by infection with mycobacteria. There are several species of the organism which vary in the clinical picture they produce and their method of spread. The 2 most important species affecting man are *Mycobacterium tuberculosis* (the 'human' strain) and *Mycobacterium bovis*. Of these, the former is overwhelmingly the more important. The latter species is now rare in the United Kingdom and in other countries where it has been eradicated from milking herds, or where milk for human consumption is pasteurized. The mycobacteria are unusual organisms, they multiply slowly and have a high resistance to adverse conditions. They are capable of persisting in a dormant but viable phase for many years both within and outside the body.

Natural history of infection

The main route of infection of *M. tuberculosis* is through the respiratory tract, by inhalation of droplets of sputum from people with active cavitating pulmonary tuberculosis, which contain large numbers of bacilli. In the initial stage of infection a small lesion develops, usually in the mid or lower zone of the lungs, associated with a marked reaction in the regional lymph nodes in the hilum of the lungs. This combination is called the *primary complex*. During this initial infection the host can offer only non-specific resistance, and haematogenous dissemination of tubercle bacilli is frequent with lodgement of bacilli in a wide range of organs. In the stage of haematogenous spread, the more acute forms of tuberculosis, tuberculous meningitis and miliary tuberculosis, have their highest incidence. However, in the majority of individuals the primary infection is self-limiting.

Allergy to the tubercle bacillus is acquired during the primary infection and with it some specific resistance. The lesions of the primary complex heal slowly, often without apparent disease either at the site of the primary lesion or other sites of lodgement of bacilli. However, bacilli in all of these sites remain viable and, if at some later date the patient's resistance is lowered, they may multiply, reactivating lesions and producing the more commonly recognized clinical forms of disease.

Reactivation does not usually occur at the site of the primary complex. It most often occurs at one of the other sites of lodgement of bacilli. The lung, which is the main circulatory filter, is the site most commonly affected

31

(approximately two-thirds of cases). Other sites for post-primary disease are lymph nodes (about one-quarter of cases) and, less commonly, bone and kidney. Tuberculosis also occurs in the abdomen, either directly from ingestion of tubercle bacilli, or secondarily by haematogenous spread, as in other forms of post-primary disease.

The post-primary lesions in the lung are usually found in one of the upper lobes or the apex of one of the lower lobes. These sites are the most favourable for multiplication of the organism. The lung lesions can eventually break down, leading to abscess formation and tuberculous cavities. Conditions in the cavity walls are ideal for multiplication of tubercle bacilli. The heavily contaminated sputum from these lesions generates the infected aerosol which perpetuates the cycle of infection.

The outcome of the initial infection depends on the intensity of exposure and the non-specific resistance of the patient. Age and nutritional status are particularly important. The earlier the age at which primary infection occurs the greater the risk of both clinical manifestations from the primary lesion itself and of the more serious complications of haematogenous spread, i.e. miliary tuberculosis and tuberculous meningitis. The greatest risk is in the first 5 years of life. From then until adolescence there is a period of relatively reduced risk followed by a second peak of incidence in adolescence and early adult life. As the disease becomes relatively uncommon, as it has in many parts of the United Kingdom, different patterns emerge. Nowadays, the disease frequently presents as a late breakdown of apparently stable disease in middle-aged or elderly individuals, often as a result of other disease which lowers resistance, for example, diabetes and alcoholism.

Trends in incidence and mortality

During this century there has been a steep decline in mortality from tuberculosis in most countries. In England and Wales this decline has been virtually continuous since death registration began in the 19th century (Fig. 2.1), except for some interruption in the trend associated with the two World Wars.

Most of the reduction in mortality occurred before the introduction of chemotherapy and the main reasons for it are thought to have been improvements in housing and nutrition. Mortality from the disease and its incidence decreased at a greater rate than previously after effective chemotherapy became available. This is apparent from examining the secular trend on a logarithmic scale (Fig. 2.2). However, at the end of the 1970s, even in England and Wales, there were still approximately 10 000 new reported cases each year (an incidence of 200 per million population) and in 1978, 900 deaths were attributed either to

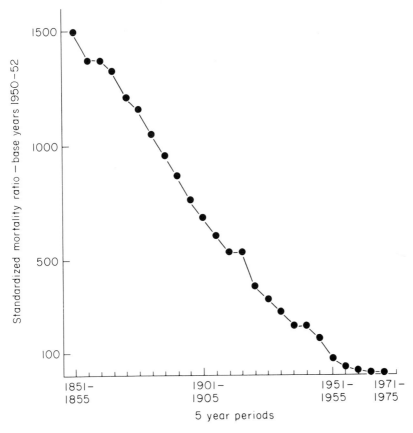

Fig. 2.1. Tuberculosis mortality in England and Wales in 5 year periods, 1851–1975.

tuberculosis or to its late sequelae. Although the accuracy of such figures is open to considerable dispute there is clearly a significant continuing mortality associated with this disease.

In the Third World the incidence of tuberculosis remains high (Table 2.1). Furthermore, the rate of decrease in incidence is modest in many of these countries. In the underdeveloped world overcrowding encourages the spread of infection, poor nutrition impairs resistance, and lack of resources prevents both the organization of care and the purchase of the now available but expensive drugs. In 1971 there were 315 million cases of this potentially curable and eradicable disease with a mortality of 585 682. The geographical variations in incidence are considered in detail by Bulla[1] and the most recent implications of epidemiological change are discussed in detail by Styblo[2].

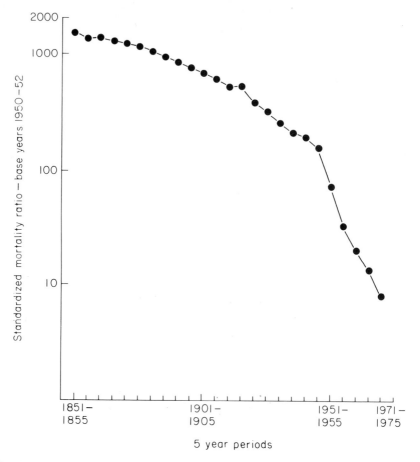

Fig. 2.2. Tuberculosis mortality in England and Wales in 5 year periods, 1851–1975 (log scale).

Table 2.1. Mortality from tuberculosis (death rate per 100 000 population).

Country		Year	Tuberculosis	
			Respiratory	Other
Argentina		1968	13.6	2.1
Sri Lanka		1968	12.9	1.6
South Africa Asiatic		1970	8.8	2.9
	Coloured	1970	49.2	6.9
	White	1970	2.4	0.3
USA		1971	1.6	0.5
Chile		1970	21.6	2.3
Belgium		1970	5.5	0.7
Denmark		1971	1.2	1.3
France		1970	7.1	1.1
Enland and Wales		1972	2.0	1.0

Indices of infection

Notifications

Diagnostic criteria and notification rates vary widely even within a single country. Even when an apparently firm criterion such as a direct positive sputum smear is used, assessment of incidence is very imprecise because many potentially positive patients do not come into contact with the diagnostic services and, of those who do, not all sputum-positive cases are notified. If less firm criteria are used notification rates become a much less secure index. Nevertheless a general indication of incidence is provided by notification rates and the figures internationally do give some indication of the extent of the problem.

Deaths

Data on mortality from tuberculosis also tend to be unreliable. In countries where the incidence of tuberculosis is high, the certification of causes of death is least accurate, and where the incidence is low, failure to make the diagnosis of tuberculosis is a frequent and increasing problem.

Tuberculin sensitivity

At the time of the primary infection, allergy to protein from the tubercle bacillus is acquired. This can be demonstrated by the intradermal injection of small quantities of protein derived from cultured tubercle bacilli. The allergic individual shows a positive reaction with induration around the site of the injection. Various methods of tuberculin testing are in common use – the Mantoux test (intradermal injection), the Heaf test (spring loaded 'gun' penetrating the epidermis) and the Tine test (pre-treated disposable prongs penetrating the epidermis). All these tests need care and experience in use and interpretation. The Mantoux test requires a skilled operator to make the injection. The Heaf test is simple but requires special equipment. The Mantoux and Heaf tests are relatively cheap to perform; the pre-treated Tine testing unit is relatively expensive. In the more advanced countries tuberculin testing by any of these methods can be readily carried out on large populations. The prevalence of positive reactions is a good index of the incidence of preceding primary infections. In the United Kingdom 5 year old children are routinely tested at school entry and the test is repeated at 13 years of age. The frequency of positive reaction at these times is a sensitive indicator of the extent of infection within the community and shows a steady decline. The value of these tests is less in communities with a high incidence of tuberculosis.

High risk groups

The groups which now have the highest incidence of tuberculosis are character-ized either by lack of resistance to infection due to poor nutrition or by environmental conditions which favour spread from infectious individuals, or by a combination of both these factors. The prevalence of the disease in migrant groups is affected by its incidence in their country of origin, though in time, as they are assimilated into the local community, they may assume the rate of the host population.

The problem is particularly severe in refugees and migrant workers who often originate in countries with high incidence and spend long periods in unsatis-factory living conditions, subsisting on poor diets. For example, migrant workers housed in camps have been a source of problems in some European countries.

In the United Kingdom, large scale immigration from East Africa and the Indian sub-continent has been associated with a rise in the incidence of tuberculosis. This has been largely confined to the immigrant populations themselves. There is now a disproportionately high incidence of tuberculosis in these communities. The cause of these problems is not clearly established. The incidence of disease in the Asian immigrant community may be no higher than it would have been had they not emigrated. However, they do present an addition to the potentially infective pool within the community.

The importance of occupation in tuberculosis is not great, except perhaps in the health care professions where a relatively high incidence of tuberculosis reflects excessive exposure to infectious patients or pathological specimens, whether or not tuberculosis has already been diagnosed. There seem currently to be few other significant factors of importance.

Therapeutic and preventive measures

Chemotherapy

With the drugs now available, particularly rifampicin and isoniazid, bacteriolog-ical cure is possible in over 90 % of cases. Sterilization of the lesions is the objective of the treatment which will break the chain of infectivity. In developed countries this is not particularly expensive, so that the control of tuberculosis now seems feasible and elimination of the disease is not an unrealistic possibility. The main problems are, firstly, patient compliance with the protracted period of treatment required to achieve sterilization of the lesion (9 months to 2 years), and, secondly, the need for good quality medical care with high standards of chemotherapy to prevent the emergence of drug resistance. Effective chemo-therapy has not only transformed the outlook for the individual patient for whom clinical cure is the normal expectation, but it has also had a major impact on the spread of disease.

In the Third World the contribution of chemotherapy is much more limited. The cost of drugs is an almost insuperable difficulty. Rifampicin, probably the single most effective drug, is very expensive and the cost of services required for the effective diagnosis and supervision of treatment is high. Chemotherapy, therefore, will make slow progress in the control of tuberculosis in this situation until cheaper regimes can be devised.

Bacille Calmette-Guérin (BCG) Vaccination

Intradermal injection of the attenuated strain of tubercle bacillus of Calmette and Guerin produces hypersensitivity to tuberculin and some immunity. It is cheap and can easily be given to large populations. Vaccination of tuberculin negative subjects, therefore, is an attractive potential control measure. It offers protection to the individual, particularly against the more serious complications of primary infection and, by improving community resistance, it should diminish the incidence of the disease. However, there is considerable disagreement about its overall efficacy. In the United Kingdom BCG vaccination at adolescence still results in approximately 75 % reduction of the incidence of tuberculosis over the succeeding 10 years. Results elsewhere are much less impressive, for example, in North America and in India, where a recent study failed to demonstrate any protective effect. The reasons for these differences are obscure. Although BCG vaccination has the disadvantage that the tuberculin test is sacrificed as a diagnostic procedure, it is probably unreasonable to abandon its use until firmer evidence of its lack of value is available. The present policy in the United Kingdom is to continue with BCG until the number of cases prevented makes the benefit unjustifiably small, a position which will probably be reached at about 1990. By then, even 75 % protection in vaccinated 13 year-olds will prevent fewer than 100 cases a year.

Control of the disease

The single most important measure in preventing the spread of tuberculosis, is treatment of sputum-positive individuals. Thus, case finding remains fundamental in any control policy. The most basic technique is the screening of the sputum of symptomatic individuals by direct microscopy of stained smears. This is a relatively easy and cheap procedure and will detect the most infectious individuals. The return from more sophisticated techniques is poor. Sputum culture is expensive, takes a long time and adds little to direct microscopy. It is not relevant as a control measure. Radiography of symptomatic subjects is probably the next most useful measure. The examination of close contacts of infectious cases is also rewarding. The return from mass screening procedures, including mass X-ray of 'normal populations' is poor. Case finding programmes must be backed up by effective therapeutic programmes which ensure that the drugs are taken for the full period of time required.

Segregation of infected individuals, hospital care and 'sanatorium' regimes have no place in control. They do not improve the efficacy of therapy nor do they diminish secondary cases. With modern chemotherapy infectivity can safely be assumed to cease at the time of diagnosis, and the resources used for institutional care would be much better spent on case finding, drugs or dispensary care.

Implications for health care planning

50 years ago there was no effective treatment for tuberculosis but the incidence and mortality were so high that governments in the United Kingdom and other countries set up committees to advise on the management of this health problem. As a result two special services were established, the Chest Clinic Service and the Sanatorium Service. Now that the disease has been largely controlled the sanatoria have been closed and the chest clinics are rapidly following suit.

These changes began before the introduction of chemotherapy but have been accelerating since. A similar situation now exists throughout the Western world. Over the next 10 years Western countries will face difficult decisions over the timing of any further run-down of the special tuberculosis services. Their premature abandonment could lead to recrudescence of the disease, though the continuation of a major service probably cannot be justified. The role of BCG in prevention will also have to be reconsidered within the next decade.

In underdeveloped countries the situation is different. Tuberculosis must have a high priority as a common preventable and treatable disease, which has a major impact on morbidity and mortality in relatively early life. It seems unlikely that control will be achieved until there has been significant improvement in the standards of living in the Third World. This is an economic rather than a medical problem. Until then the best use will have to be made of scarce resources. The emphasis will have to be on cheap, effective, case-finding programmes and cheap, effective, therapy. Short duration treatment will probably be useful if it can be shown to be effective, as it will reduce the problems of supervision. At the moment it seems reasonable to recommend continuation of BCG vaccination programmes, despite uncertainties about their efficacy.

References

1. Bulla A. Global review of tuberculosis morbidity and mortality in the world. *World Health Organization Statistics Report* 1977; **30**(1).
2. Styblo K. Recent advances in epidemiological research in tuberculosis. *Advances in Tuberculosis Research* 1980; **20**: 1.

Further reading

Epidemiology, indices of extent of disease, role of notification, etc.

Bulla A. Tuberculosis patients. *Bulletin of the International Union Against Tuberculosis* 1977; **52**: 35.

Medical Research Council Tuberculosis and Chest Disease Unit. National survey of tuberculosis notifications in England and Wales 1978–79. *British Medical Journal* 1981; **ii**: 895.

Styblo K, Meijer J. Recent advances in tuberculosis epidemiology with regard to formation and re-adjustment of control programmes. *Bulletin of the International Union Against Tuberculosis* 1978; **53**: 283.

Drug treatment

British Thoracic Association. Short course chemotherapy in pulmonary tuberculosis. *Lancet* 1975; **i**: 117, and 1976; **ii**: 1102.

Fox W, Mitchison DA. Short course chemotherapy for pulmonary tuberculosis. *American Review of Respiratory Diseases* 1975; **111**: 325.

Fox W. The current status of short course chemotherapy. *Bulletin of the International Union Against Tuberculosis* 1978; **53**: 268.

Infectivity of cases and contact policy

British Thoracic Association. A study of a standardized contact procedure in tuberculosis. *Tubercle* 1978; **59**: 245.

Leader article. Isolation of patients with pulmonary tuberculosis. *British Medical Journal* 1980; **ii**: 962.

BCG vaccination

Leader article. BCG: bad news from India. *Lancet* 1980; **i**: 73.

Problems in diagnosis

British Thoracic Association A survey of tuberculosis mortality in England and Wales in 1968. *Tubercle* 1971; **52**: 1.

McCulloch DK, Malone DMS. Presentation of tuberculosis in acute medical unit. *Lancet* 1980; **i**: 702.

Problems of immigrants

British Thoracic Association. Tuberculosis among immigrants related to length of residence in England and Wales. *British Medical Journal* 1975; **iii**: 698.

General

Keers RY. *Pulmonary tuberculosis. A journey down the centuries.* London: Balliere Tindall, 1978.

Pagel W, Simmonds FAH, *et al. Pulmonary tuberculosis* Oxford: Oxford University Press, 1964.

Chapter 3 · Infectious Diseases of the Nervous System

E M ROSS

Improvements in hygiene and the introduction of immunization have reduced the incidence of severe neurological diseases caused by infection in developed countries. In the developing world, they remain a major cause of death and suffering. The number of deaths from various infections of the nervous system are shown in Table 3.1. In all parts of the world the occurrence of these diseases continues to cause anxiety irrespective of their prevalence. Constant efforts are required to keep them at bay.

Table 3.1. Deaths due to infections of the nervous system (England and Wales, 1979).

	Male	Female
Tuberculosis of the meninges and CNS	8	10
Meningococcal meningitis	20	12
Poliomyelitis	0	0
Neurosyphilis	17	10
Bacterial meningitis	105	103
Unspecified meningitis	38	39
Encephalitis, myelitis & encephalomyselitis	36	21
Intracranial and intraspinal abscess	19	16
Acute infective polyneuritis	10	10
Slow virus infection	15	18
Non-arthropod-borne CNS virus	63	68

Many diseases of the nervous system of hitherto obscure aetiology are now being recognized as probably involving an infectious agent. These include a wide spectrum of diseases, for example, febrile convulsions, encephalopathy, Parkinson's disease and dementia. Different patterns of neurological disease occur at different ages. Neurological damage due to infection occurs most commonly in the young and the predominant infectious agents differ from those affecting older people. The passive immunity of the newborn protects him against viral exanthemata in the first 6 months, but his lack of large molecular immunoglobulins and little anatomical protection, facilitate Gram-negative bacterial septicaemia. Many viral infections cause less severe illness when acquired in early childhood. Their partial elimination by immunization can increase the hazard to older people when immunity wanes.

Sources of data

The World Health Organization (WHO) publishes regular bulletins of the world pattern of infectious diseases in their Weekly Epidemiological Record and Annual Statistics. These are supplemented by detailed national returns from the more organized countries. It is extremely difficult to draw meaningful international comparisons of the pattern of neuro-infective diseases because clinical diagnoses are rarely supported by adequate laboratory investigation, especially in the poorer countries.

At present, about two-thirds of cases of the recognised neuro-infectious diseases in the United Kingdom are due to viruses, the remainder are mainly bacterial with only occasional cases due to fungi or parasites such as toxoplasmosis, malaria or amoebae.

In England and Wales, 28 infectious diseases are notifiable by statute; these include meningitis. However, the neurological sequelae are not recorded, nor are the neurological sequelae of non-notifiable infectious diseases. Consequently, it is necessary to rely on local studies, aided by reports from microbiological laboratories to the Public Health Laboratory Service. These are collated and published in the Communicable Disease Report by the Communicable Disease Surveillance Centre (CDSC). Other sources of data include records of hospital admissions and General Practice registers; these are not satisfactory for epidemiological study.

Bacterial meningitis

Patterns of meningitis vary widely between countries; this variation reflects the prevalence of local bacterial types and the pathogenity of different strains. The resistance of the population to bacterial meningitis is influenced by climate, purity of food and water, the presence of vector insects and by local customs. Within Western Europe, bacterial meningitis tends to cluster in small scale local outbreaks, causing occasional tragic deaths. This contrasts with the experience in the savannah lands of North Africa where over 1 million cases are estimated to have occurred in the past 40 years during annual epidemics.

The newborn

Newborn babies have an immature immune system and have little anatomical protection against infection; they are particularly vulnerable to Gram-negative meningitis. It can be difficult to diagnose as it presents merely as irritability or poor feeding. About 1 in 10 000 newborn infants in England and Wales die from meningitis in the first 4 weeks of their life. Many of the survivors are left with permanent handicaps[1,2]. The disease occurs most often in prematurely born babies, in those with neural tube defects and those babies born more than 24 hours after the amniotic membranes had been ruptured. In a study from the North West Thames Region of England by Goldacre[3], it was found that 2.6 cases per 10 000 live-born occurred in the first 4 weeks. Goldacre estimated that that rate was one-tenth of the rate prevailing 50 years before.

A wide range of bacterial organisms have been demonstrated in sporadic cases. However, about 70 % are caused by either group B streptococci or coliforms. The group B β-haemolytic streptococcus has emerged as a major pathogen in recent years[4]. The spectrum of neonatal disease due to this organism ranges from asymptomatic colonization to serious and fatal illness with two main patterns of clinical disease. Early-onset infection presents with acute respiratory distress, septicaemia and meningitis. It is usually acquired from the mother's lower genital tract[5]. Symptoms are often present at birth, if not, they usually develop within 24 hours of delivery. The course of the illness is fulminating with a high case fatality rate. Late-onset disease usually presents after the tenth day of life as purulent meningitis. Infants may acquire this form of infection from their attendants, from other parts of their own body or from other colonized infants with whom they have contact. The lethality of the established late-onset disease has provoked studies into the immune status of the mothers of affected infants. The majority of normal babies appear to be protected by specific immunoglobulin IgG antibodies; it has been postulated that affected infants may be partially immuno-deficient.

Coliforms are the second commonest cause of neonatal meningitis. A study in Glasgow of 36 such cases[6] in the period 1960–74 showed that the disease often presents as a septicaemia with blood stained but sterile cerebro-spinal fluid in the early stage of the illness. Even early systemic administration of aminoglycoside antibiotics failed to prevent meningitis from developing. Of the 36 babies, 14 died and 13 survived with varying degrees of handicap, leaving only 9 who survived unscathed. Two-thirds of the cases were caused by *Escherichia coli*, the remainder involved a wide range of other coliforms. In these, increasing lethargy and failure to feed were common presenting features. Many survivors had gross neurological damage, the remainder were thought to be at risk of deafness and other handicaps.

The older child and adult

The clinical features and bacterial causes of meningitis in children and adults are different from those in the newborn. A North London study of children aged under 10 years[3] with bacterial meningitis identified the main organisms as: *Neissevia meningitis* 45 %, *Haemophilus influenzae* 33 % and *Streptococcus pneumonia* 11 %. The case fatality rates were 11 %, 6 % and 16 % respectively. All infections occurred more frequently in males than in females. Although meningitis due to these organisms can occur at any age, 80 % occur before the age of 15 years. Those children who live in institutions are particularly vulnerable.

The predominant organisms tend to vary in time and between epidemics. In the USA *H. influenza* is 3 times more commonly a cause of meningitis than it is in the United Kingdom. This may be because the greater frequency of commensal respiratory infection with *H. influenzae* in the UK gives children a greater chance of developing antibodies. A host of other organisms can be isolated from sporadic cases of meningitis but they are usually found under exceptional circumstances such as immune suppression, following brain surgery, through unhealed fractures of the cribriform plate, and by upward spread from dental abscesses. In theory, bacterial meningitis should respond to antibiotics and be curable if treated at an early enough stage with appropriate intensive antibiotics. In practice, the failure rate of treatment is considerable. There is continuing debate concerning the optimal selection of antibiotics, duration of treatment and whether intrathecal use is beneficial. Fatalities have occurred due to incorrect intrathecal use of penicillin. (It is vital to remember that special intrathecal preparations are required and must be given in doses not exceeding 10 000 iu to adults and correspondingly less to children).

Prevention of meningitis

Neonatal meningitis is a constant threat to the newborn but it is avoidable by cleanliness, light, space, breast feeding, by letting the mother care for her infant, and by watching very carefully for unexplained lethargy or respiratory problems. For the older child and adult, early detection and treatment remains the key to unscathed survival. Meningococcal infection is contagious and siblings of affected children need protection with antimicrobial drugs. Although vaccines to the main causal organisms have been prepared they have not been widely used in the United Kingdom. In the USA, army recruits are successfully immunized against meningococcal infection.

Virus infection of the central nervous system

Most viral illnesses have some effects on the central nervous system (CNS); these range from temporary depressive symptoms to permanent brain damage or death. In viral illnesses it is unusual for the brain and spinal cord to be the only affected system. However, its inability to self-repair and its unique response to infection means that it is more likely to suffer permanent damage than other parts of the body. Virus-associated illness may be due to direct viral invasion, as in herpes simplex and poliomyelitis, or indirect immune reactions where a virus cannot be recovered from the brain, for example, measles encephalitis, long-term sequelae to an infection by reactivation of dormant symbiotic virus in varicella-zoster, slow virus response in subacute sclerosing pan-encephalitis (SSPE), or kuru, and the wide variety of viruses isolated in 83 % of children with febrile convulsions.

Virus infections of the central nervous system in infants can have serious consequences. Among 49 British infants under 1 year with intra-cranial infections due to a wide variety of viruses, 1 died and 3 became severely retarded (2 with herpes encephalitis)[7]. 7 years later all of the apparently undamaged survivors were attending normal schools, but had lower intelligence quotients (IQ) and reduced academic achievements compared with their controls. The original illness occurred more frequently in babies with low birthweights and poor social backgrounds. When adjustments for these factors were made, it was found that the illness had not affected the verbal IQ, but was associated with a small but statistically significant deficit in the performance IQ.

It can be assumed that most non-bacterial diseases associated with acute alteration of consciousness and abnormalities, either in the cell count or distribution of immunoglobulins within the cerebro-spinal fluid, have a virus-associated aetiology. Failure to detect a virus does not prove that the disease is not of viral origin. Nor does the isolation of an unexpected virus mean that the true cause of the disease has been demonstrated. For purposes of simplification, virus-associated diseases can be separated into 2 groups.

1   Diseases predominantly associated with central changes, particularly fits and changing consciousness, are grouped together as 'encephalitides'.

2   Diseases causing peripheral damage, especially paralysis with poliomyelitis and Coxsackie B.

Encephalitis and encephalopathy

The terms 'encephalitis' and 'encephalopathy' both refer to the same group of brain symptoms. In the case of encephalitis an infectious cause has either been demonstrated or is strongly suspected. The commoner causes include parasites and fungi (especially in patients with impaired immunity), viral infections – particularly mumps, measles, herpes, echo and arbo viruses – and a few bacterial infections such as pertussis. Between 1969 and 1978 the annual number of cases of infectious and post-infectious encephalitis, notified in England and Wales, fluctuated between 102 and 256. Non-infectious encephalopathies can be caused by poisons such as lead, reactions to drugs – including phenytoin or pencillinamine – malignant diseases, and pathological states such as hypertension. Although immunization against pertussis and other organisms has been incriminated, this seems to be a rare cause of encephalopathy in the previously intact brain.

It is in the patient's interest that every effort be made to find a cause of encephalitic illnesses so that appropriate treatment, prognostic and genetic advice, can be given. In viral cases the judicious early use of anti-viral agents such as acycloviv or other deoxyribonucleic acid (DNA) chain inhibitors may improve the chance of survival[9]. Accurate diagnosis requires a high index of suspicion, expert laboratory facilities, and a preparedness to perform brain biopsy in appropriate cases in order to demonstrate virus. The epidemiology of these conditions is extremely difficult to explore. Diagnoses are not easy to make and depend both on the acumen and the facilities available to the examining physician. In the past, many cases were never diagnosed during life, making epidemiological trends impossible to decipher. Improvement in virology and ancillary means of investigation, including computer assisted tomography together with better electro-encephalography, make definite diagnosis possible in an increasing proportion of cases.

The herpes viruses

The herpes viruses are DNA viruses; they are members of a large group of viruses which affect a range of living organisms from fungi upwards. Human strains include herpes simplex, varicella-zoster (V-Z), Epstein-Barr (EB) and cytomegalovirus (CMV). All of these usually live in symbiosis with their human hosts.

The proportion of the population with antibodies to these viruses is highest in underdeveloped countries, but serious illnesses due to them occur most often in developed countries. This suggests that infection in adult life may be more harmful than when infection is acquired in infancy. The manifestation of an infection with one of these viruses varies. Frequently there are no symptoms. They may cause a minor illness in childhood. The most devastating effects are the rarest; these are intra-uterine spread to the fetus causing death or serious congenital malformation and encephalitis in children and adults.

Herpes simplex

An endemic pathogen: although cases cluster in families and in institutions, widespread epidemics are not seen. The virus has at least 2 different serotypes. Lesions on the skin, eye and buccal mucosa are usually caused by type 1 virus. It is spread by contact through broken skin and by kissing. Type 2 (see also Chapters 5 and 23) is usually confined to the genital tract of both sexes and is at least partially venerally spread, however, the virus can be transferred from the genital mucosa to mucosa elsewhere by oro–genital contact.

About 1 in 7500 newborn infants in the USA and 1 in 50 000 in the United Kingdom are infected with type 2 herpes simplex. This is more frequent to young primigravida. Prophylactic Caesarean section before rupture of the membranes has been advised in women with active lesions. Without this, there is a high perinatal mortality, 62 % in one series with 50 % survivors having central nervous system lesions[10].

In the older child and adult herpes 1 is the commonest known cause of encephalitis in the United Kingdom; currently it accounts for about 100 cases each year. It is more common in males than females, especially those under 10 years of age. Only a small proportion of the 80 % of adults who have antibodies to the virus ever get encephalitis. The reasons for this are not understood. The virus appears to migrate from the nose, via the olfactory nerves, to the brain. Since active herpetic skin lesions are rarely seen in people with encephalitis, it is presumed that the virus lies dormant within the brain until activated by an as yet unknown stimulus. Until the advent of viral chemotherapy, up to 70 % of people diagnosed died. Many survivors were left handicapped. The advent of viral chemotherapy is giving modest hope although early definite diagnosis is needed if it is to have any chance of success. The management and the place of brain biopsy are discussed by Longston and Bailey[9]. No protection against this disease is available yet. The introduction of a vaccine is hindered by anxieties relating to the involvement of herpes viruses in malignant and auto-immune diseases.

Varicella-zoster

This usually manifests itself as chickenpox or shingles. The virus can infect the fetus in the first trimester of pregnancy and in very rare instances, cause brain damage and poor intra-uterine growth. Christie[11] makes the point that chickenpox is often much less dangerous than the common cold, although on occasions it can be virulent, particularly in individuals whose immunity has been suppressed. In the rare case where encephalitis ensues, particularly in childhood, cerebellar signs and cranial nerve palsies tend to develop. These usually remit spontaneously and lasting brain damage is uncommon. The severity of the disease and likelihood of neurological complications varies markedly through-out the world, it is at its worst in the tropics. The lack of notification statistics in the United Kingdom means that it is not possible to work out the epidemiology of the disease in any detail.

Varicella-zoster, manifest as shingles, can occur at any age, although predominantly in the elderly. It is presumed that the virus dwells in symbiosis with its host in sensory root ganglia. It emerges to cause its characteristic signs when immunity wanes, thus permitting spread along the peripheral nerves. In Hope-Simpson's General Practice in Gloucestershire, England[12], V-Z occurred at a rate of 3.4 per 1000 persons per year.

Infectious mononucleosis

The Epstein-Barr virus, another member of the herpes group, was identified as the cause of infectious mononucleosis in 1968. It appears to be associated with a variety of reactions ranging from mild pharyngitis in childhood to Burkitt's lymphoma and carcinoma of the naso-pharynx.

The role of this virus is continuing to emerge; it appears to be a common factor in some cases of Hodgkin's disease, and acute lymphatic leukamia (where Epstein-Barr virus is commonly found in the mothers of affected children), but many unanswered questions remain, not the least the reason for its association with so many diseases.

Most prevalence studies have come from the USA. The disease seems to run a less virulent course in the United Kingdom. Neurological complications other than a non-specific depressive illness are rare but include encephalitis and polyneuritis. These generally resolve, though sequelae do occur and death can result from respiratory paralysis.

Chronic virus disease ('slow virus reactions')

The discovery that the cerebro-spinal fluid of some children with remorseless cerebral degeneration and fits, contained a high content of oligoclonal IgG measles antibody, has increased interest in the concept that some chronic neurological illness might be due to atypical virus behaviour within the brain[13,14]. Subacute sclerosing pan-encephalitis (SSPE) is a rare lethal disease affecting about 1 per million children with measles in the United Kingdom. It has a peak mortality at 4 years. In recent years, it has caused more deaths than measles encephalitis. The condition seems to be on the wane in the USA, possibly an extra benefit from their high rate of measles immunization.

Experience with subacute sclerosing pan-encephalitis and the observation that immune-deficient children are prone to chronic encephalopathic states, has stimulated interest in other diseases. From New Guinea the fact that fewer East Highlanders are getting kuru is probably due to more hygenic burial practices not, as previously supposed, to the abandonment of the practice of eating the brains of the deceased. The finding that inadequately sterilized neuro-surgical probes and corneal transplants can transmit Creutzfeldt-Jakob's type of spongiform degeneration of the brain, supports the hypothesis that some neuro-degenerative diseases may have a viral aetiology. The similarity of multiple sclerosis to animal neuro-degenerative diseases of viral cause, such as scrapie in sheep and mink encephalopathy, suggests that viral agents, possibly coupled with abnormal human leucocyte antigen (HLA) types*, may be involved.

---

* The HLA system consists of 4 series of inherited markers on leucocytes which may be identified using lymphocytotoxic antibodies (for the A, B and C series) or a mixed lymphocyte culture reaction (D series).

Main damage-causing viruses

Pico ribonucleic acid (RNA) Viruses.

This is a large group of viruses that affect man, animals, insects and plants. In man they can cause a wide spectrum of illness ranging from undifferentiated febrile illness to lethal paralysis. The enteroviruses are a major subgroup which includes 3 types of poliovirus, over 30 types of Coxsackie virus (A & B), 31 types of echoviruses and some unclassifiable enteroviruses.

Poliomyelitis

Although this disease has only been recognized as a clinical entity over the last 200 years, and been shown to behave as a virus by transmittion to monkeys since 1908, its effects were described in early antiquity. Most infected individuals are asymptomatic or have only mild respiratory symptoms. It has been estimated that as few as 1 per 1000 infected children develop paralysis, though the rate can be 12 times higher in adults. Infectivity through close human contact is very high. Before the advent of immunization, whole schools could be infected. Paralysis occurs more frequently in children taking strenuous exercise, or following recent tonsillectomy. Paralysis is most common around the site of intra-muscular immunizations, particularly where alum-containing adjuvants have been incorporated.

Millar[15] described the pattern of poliomyelitis in Great Britain and its control, firstly with killed vaccine in 1956, and subsequently with live vaccine in 1962. The national incidence had been rising rapidly since 1947, causing an average of 330 deaths each year between 1947–58. Most cases occurred between July and November. Large outbreaks were usually followed by lower attack rates in the following years. Most deaths occurred in young adults living in prosperous areas. The virus is spread through faecal contamination, ingested, then borne through the blood from intestinal or regional lymph nodes. It invades the peripheral nerves and ascends to the central nervous system.

Although immunization has virtually eliminated the disease in the United Kingdom and other developed countries, in underdeveloped countries cases still occur, mainly in very young children, amongst whom paralysis tends to be mild. Older people in these countries usually develop antibodies. There is particular danger to non-immunized Europeans visiting regions where the disease is endemic. They are at risk of developing severe paralysis and should be immunized before travel. The near eradication of polio in developed countries carries dangers of complacency and utmost efforts must be made to maintain immunization levels. National immunization practices differ. The Netherlands, which only uses killed vaccine, has had outbreaks among members of an unimmunized extreme religious group. Oral vaccine has a 1 in a million dose risk of precipitating vaccine-associated paralysis. Nathanson and Martin[16] have reviewed these issues and the enigmas posed by this disease.

Other enteroviruses

At present there are no immunizations available to protect against Pico RNA viruses other than polio. They remain rare but noxious causes of sporadic cases of acute paralysis and other devastating neurological disease, an example being the Coxsackie virus which was discovered in the small town of that name in New York State where a polio-like epidemic was raging. Other enterovirus infections are also associated with central nervous system disorders. As an example, among 24% of 335 Japanese children[17] with hand, foot and mouth disease associated with enterovirus, 71 developed a predominantly cerebellar form of temporary encephalitis with a very high incidence in those under 1 year. Echo viruses are potent causes of outbreaks of encephalitis in nurseries.

Paramyxoviruses

Measles (see also Chapter 1) is a member of the paramyxovirus group, there is no strain variation. The illness has a fascinating history. It is presumed to be an adaptation of rinder pest or canine distemper virus. It probably first appeared on the human scene about 2500 BC. Massive epidemics were known in ancient Rome and in China. The virus was isolated by Enders and Peebles in 1954 and led to the development of killed virus vaccines. These failed to give full protection and were replaced by a live-attenuated vaccine, which induces a greatly attenuated illness. It has not proved popular in the United Kingdom and currently large epidemics continue to occur every 4 years. In contrast, measles is a disappearing disease in the USA where immunization uptake is much higher[18]. Encephalitis[19] follows about 1 in 1000 cases of measles. It presents with drowsiness, fits and coma when the rash is fading. This encephalitis is probably not a separate disease entity but rather an immunological reaction to the virus, which cannot be identified in the cerebro-spinal fluid.

Many affected children are left with serious neurological sequelae. The extent of milder cases of persistent neurological deficit that follows measles, in the absence of clear-cut encephalitis, remains unknown. Many children with uncomplicated measles have transitory electroencephalogram (e.e.g.) changes.

Mumps

Mumps (see also Chapter 23) is caused by *Myxovirus parotidis*, a member of the influenza and parainfluenza group. This is a single strain of RNA virus spread by droplet infection. In the First World War it was the single most common disease causing loss of service among American soldiers in France. In some respects, mumps behaves as a neurotropic virus, and temporary neurological involvement can be detected in a high proportion of those affected. A Finnish survey shows 4 % subsequently had reduced hearing. In the USA, a live-attenuated mumps vaccine was introduced in 1967. Previously, up to 250 cases per 100 000 population had been recorded annually. The national rate fell to under 10 per 100 000 by 1979, and the disease was virtually eliminated in some states.

Mumps vaccine has not been widely advocated in the United Kingdom[20]. The population continue to be exposed to a condition with an associated meningo-encephalitis which affects about 2.5 per 1000 cases. In England and Wales there were 287 cases of mumps encephalitis in 1976 in people aged under 15 years. The majority seem to recover, but as mumps is not a notifiable disease, firm epidemiological data are lacking.

Pertussis and pertussis vaccine

Apart from meningitis, pertussis (see also Chapters 1 & 12) is the main bacterial cause of brain damage in the United Kingdom. This damage appears to be due to minute haemorrhages scattered through the cerebral substance. These changes are probably reversible in milder cases and are probably due to vascular stasis rather than an encephalopathy. Brief fits are seen in mild cases, though at the worst, blindness and the changes of severe cortical atrophy can be found. Only the most severe cases are recognized in clinical practice and early stages are rarely diagnosed. During the period July 1976–June 1979, 104 336 cases of pertussis were notified in England, Scotland and Wales, of whom 25 died. Preliminary findings of the first 1000 cases reported to the National Childhood Encephalopathy Study[8] which explored the natural history of severe brain illnesses in children in the same time period, revealed 19 cases of severe non-fatal brain illness (mainly encephalitis and prolonged fits) requiring hospital admission, that occurred within 2 months of the diagnosis of pertussis. One year later only 3 had persistent neurological sequelae.

There have been sporadic case reports of encephalitis and other neurological complications, particularly seizures, time-associated with pertussis vaccine. These formed the basis for a major British media campaign against the use of the vaccine which began in 1975. The immunization rates fell nationally from 80 % to 35 % though some areas reported rates as low as 9 %.

An analysis of the first 1000 of the 1182 children with encephalitis or other severe acute onset neurological illness reported to the National Childhood Encephalopathy Study, showed that 3.5 % had been immunized with diphtheria-tetanus-pertussis (DTP) vaccine within 7 days before onset of acute neurological illness. By comparison with controls, cases showed a significant, though slight, increase in risk of having received DTP immunization within 7 days before the onset of illness. The risk was greatest within 72 hours and in those with a history of convulsions or encephalopathy. The clinical findings did not reveal any characteristic illness unique to DTP vaccine.

Of the 35 DTP vaccine-associated cases, 32 were regarded as neurologically normal before their illness, 21 of these recovered completely. There were only 8 cases (3 with minor defects and 5 with major defects) in which no alternative explanation for their condition was found.

The estimated attributable risk was 1 per 110 000 immunizations for previously normal children, irrespective of eventual clinical outcome, and 1 per 270 000 for those with evidence of subsequent neurological damage (the confidence limits were very wide). The authors stressed that these figures must be interpreted with great caution and the nature of the assumptions on which the calculations were based appreciated.

These findings suggest that the problems associated with pertussis immunization are small in comparison with the natural toll of the illness. At the worst, the vaccine can only have a very marginal role in the overall picture of early childhood encephalopathy in Great Britain.

References

1. Davies PA. Neonatal bacterial meningitis. *British Journal of Hospital Medicine* 1977; **2**: 425–34.
2. McSwiggan DA. Neonatal and perinatal infection: routes of transmission and prevention. *Journal of Antimicrobial Chemotherapy* 1979; **5** (A): 1–12.
3. Goldacre MJ. Acute bacterial meningitis in childhood. *Lancet* 1976; **i**: 28–31.
4. Reid TMS. Emergence of group B streptococci in obstetrics and perinatal infections. *British Medical Journal* 1975; **ii**: 533–5.
5. Baker CJ, Barrett FF. Transmission of group B streptococci among women and their neonates. *Journal of Pediatrics* 1973; **83**: 919–25.
6. Heckmatt JZ. Coliform meningitis in the newborn. *Archives of Diseases in Childhood* **1976**: 569–75.
7. Chamberlain R, Christie P, *et al*. A study of school children who had identified virus infection of the CNS during infancy. 1982 In press.
8. Miller DL, Ross EM, *et al*. Pertussis immunization and serious acute neurological illness in children. *British Medical Journal* 1981; **282**: 1595–9.
9. Longston M, Bailey A. Early diagnosis and treatment of virus infections of the cerebral nervous system. *The Practitioner* 1978; **222**: 47–56.
10. Nahmias AJ, *et al*. Perinatal risk associated with maternal genital herpes simplex virus infections. *American Journal of Obstetrics and Gynecology* 1971; **110**: 825–37.
11. Christie AB. *Infectious diseases, epidemiology and clinical practice*. 3rd ed. London: Churchill-Livingstone, 1980.
12. Hope-Simpson RE. The nature of herpes zoster. A long term study and a new hypothesis. *Royal Society of Medicine. Proceedings* 1965; **58**: 9–20.
13. Bellman MH, Dick GWA. Surveillance of subacute sclerosing pan-encephalitis. *Royal College of Physicians of London. Journal* 1978; **12**: 256–61.
14. Mims CA. Slow virus infections. In Heath RB, ed. *Virus diseases* Tunbridge Wells: Pitman, 1979: 97–105.

15. Millar ELM. Poliomyelitis epidemiology and control. *Public Health* 1971; **85** 103–6.
16. Nathanson N, Martin JR. The epidemiology of poliomyelitis: enigmas surrounding its appearance, epidicity and disappearance. *American Journal of Epidemiology* **110** (6): 672–92.
17. Ishimaru Y, Nakano S, *et al. Archives of Diseases in Childhood* 1980; **55** 583–8.
18. Hinman AR, Brandling-Bennett AD, Nieburg PI. The opportunity and obligation to eliminate measles from the United States. *JAMA* 1979; **242**: 1157–62.
19. Miller DL. Frequency of complications of measles. *British Medical Journal* 1963; **ii**: 75–8.
20. Editorial. Prevention of mumps. *British Medical Journal* 1980; **ii**: 1231–2.

Further reading

Coid CR, ed. *Infections and pregnancy*. London: Academic Press, 1977.
Evans AS, ed. *Viral infections of humans. Epidemiology and control.* Chichester: John Wiley, 1978.
Legg N. How viruses affect the nervous system. In Williams D, ed. *Modern trends in neurology.* London: Butterworth, 1975.
Rose FC. *Clinical neuro-epidemiology.* Tunbridge Wells: Pitman, 1980.

Chapter 4 · Gastro-intestinal Infections and Food Poisoning

N S GALBRAITH

Enteric fever

Enteric fever is a septicaemic illness caused by *Salmonella typhi* and *Salmonella paratyphi* which are transmitted by food, water and occasionally directly from person to person. Other organisms of the salmonella group may also rarely cause a septicaemic illness (Table 4.1).

The disease

S. typhi, the commonest cause of enteric fever worldwide, is exclusively a human pathogen and the only source is an infected person, either a case or a carrier. The organism is conveyed to the mouth of another person and after an incubation period of 10–14 days a septicaemic illness begins, characterized by the gradual onset of continued fever with headache, severe malaise, sometimes a cough and usually constipation. As the disease progresses the organism localizes in three main sites: the spleen, clinically evident by splenic enlargement; the lymphoid tissue of the ileum, which may ulcerate causing diarrhoea and sometimes haemorrhage and perforation; and the gall bladder, where in the presence of gall-stones it may persist indefinitely giving rise to the chronic faecal carrier state. Organisms lodging in the skin sometimes produce the characteristic transient rash of rose spots on the abdomen at the end of the first week of the illness, but in other sites they may multiply and subsequently cause chronic abscess formation. This most often occurs in bone but occasionally it involves the urinary tract when there is pre-existing disease and may result in the chronic urinary carrier state.

S. typhi can be isolated on blood culture from over 90% of patients in the first week of the illness, from the urine in over 25% during the septicaemia, and from faeces of most patients from the second week of the illness. The discharge of organisms from the gut is particularly profuse during the second to fourth weeks and persists in over 50% of cases for 7 to 8 weeks. Most are clear by 4 months but in about 3% persistent gall bladder infection leads to chronic continuous or intermittent excretion. Chemotherapy cuts short the illness and reduces the fatality rate from about 10 to 1% but has a variable effect on the carrier state. Diagnosis of the clinical illness and the carrier state should be by culture of the causative organism because the agglutination reaction (Widal test) has many limitations and the isolation of the organism enables precise identification

Table 4.1. Salmonella infections in man: summary of main features.

Organism	Source	Usual methods of spread	Incubation period	Clinical illness
Salmonella typhi	Exclusively human	Water Food Rarely person-to-person	Usually 10–14 days limits 3–35 days	Enteric fever
S. paratyphi A	Exclusively human	Food Occasionally person-to-person Rarely water	As *S. typhi*	Enteric fever
S. paratyphi B	Human Rarely animal		Usually less than *S. typhi* 1–7 days	Enteric fever Sometimes acute gastroenteritis
S. cholerae suis	Animal (pig) Rarely human	Food	Similar to *S. paratyphi B*	Septicaemia with local abscess formation Sometimes acute gastroenteritis
S. typhimurium and other serotypes	Animal Rarely human	Food Person-to-person in institutions	Usually 12–72 hours	Acute gastroenteritis (food poisoning) Rarely septicaemic illness

by serotyping and bacteriophage typing which is of great epidemiological value in tracing the source of infection.[1]

S. paratyphi A, *S. paratyphi B* and *S. paratyphi C*, like *S. typhi*, are also essentially human pathogens, although *S. paratyphi B* infection occasionally occurs in cattle. They cause a similar but less severe illness of shorter duration, and symptomless infection – the so-called symptomless excreter – is more frequent with these organisms than with *S. typhi*. *S. paratyphi B* sometimes causes an acute gastroenteritis, with a short incubation period, resembling food poisoning (Table 4.1). There are over 1700 other salmonella serotypes only about 10% of which occur commonly. Some of these are primarily adapted to particular animals but most have no particular host preference; *S. typhimurium* is the commonest of these[2]. Infection in man usually gives rise to acute food poisoning, although on the one hand symptomless infection is frequent and on the other septicaemic invasion occasionally occurs. One serotype, *S. cholerae-suis*, a primary pathogen of the pig, often causes a septicaemic illness with subsequent focal abscess formation.

Mortality and morbidity data

Enteric fever became distinguished clinically and pathologically from other continued fevers from the middle of the 19th century onwards and mortality data are available since this time in many countries which had developed national systems of death registration and certification. Precise definition of the disease by microbiological techniques became available early in the 20th century which enabled the establishment of morbidity reporting systems. In England and Wales enteric fever became statutorily notifiable in 1911 and in 1938 typhoid and paratyphoid fevers were distinguished. Since the early 1970s data from statutory notification have been integrated with reports from microbiological laboratories to provide more complete information. Similar developments have taken place in other Western countries but in many underdeveloped countries accurate mortality and morbidity data are still lacking.

Incidence

There are wide geographical variations in the incidence of enteric fever associated with differences in the standard of hygiene and sanitation. The causative organisms and their bacteriophage types also vary geographically and these sometimes give a valuable clue to the area of origin of the infection[3]. Although indigenous enteric fever has almost disappeared in some Western countries, imported disease is increasing. The number of cases of typhoid fever reported each year in England and Wales has more than doubled to nearly 300 per year in the last 20 years, but in over 90% of these the infection was acquired abroad, usually in the Indian subcontinent (Fig. 4.1). Paratyphoid A fever has never been indigenous; about 50 cases per year are now reported, again most of them infected in the Indian subcontinent. Paratyphoid B fever has declined but the proportion of cases infected abroad, mainly in the Mediterranean and Middle East, has increased (Fig. 4.2).

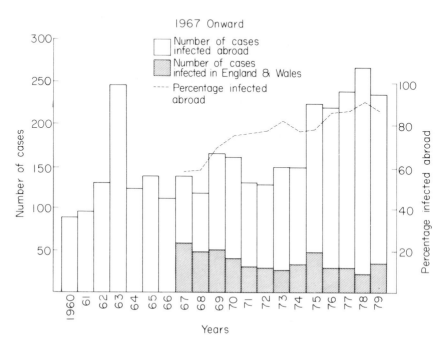

Fig. 4.1. Typhoid fever: notifications and laboratory reports, England and Wales, 1960–79. (From *British Medical Journal* 1980; **281**: 546.)

Special features

The special features which determine the incidence are the opportunities for the spread of the causative organisms by water or food. The dramatic decline in incidence in North-West Europe, North America and Australia over the past 100 years has been attributed to improvement in water supplies, the main mode of spread of typhoid fever, although occasional outbreaks still occur when purification breaks down[4]. Paratyphoid fever rarely spreads by water but like typhoid fever may be spread by faecal contamination of milk or food. At least 6 outbreaks of typhoid fever in the United Kingdom, the largest of over 500 cases in Aberdeen in 1964, were due to canned meat, which was contaminated by cooling the cans in sewage-polluted river water, the organisms

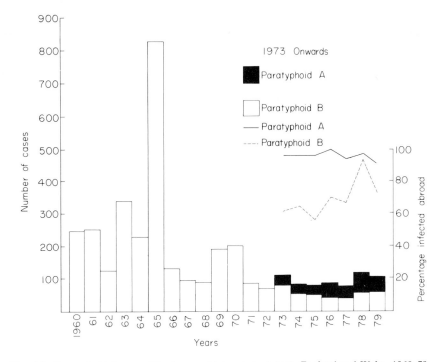

Fig. 4.2. Paratyphoid fever: notifications and laboratory reports, England and Wales, 1960–79. (From British Medical Journal 1980; **281**: 546.)

entering the cans through minute temporary leaks in the vulcanite seal[5]. Bakery products were implicated in the spread of many outbreaks of paratyphoid B fever in Britain in the 1950s and early 1960s and the source was eventually found to be bulk frozen egg products from China and desiccated coconut from Ceylon, presumably contaminated during unhygienic production. These materials are now heat-treated and this source of infection has been controlled.

Few outbreaks of enteric fever traced to food contaminated directly by carriers have been reported in recent years. In Britain occasional cases have occurred in hospital and laboratory workers due to direct transmission, but person-to-person spread of typhoid fever without the interposition of water or food is unusual and the communicability of the disease is often exaggerated. Hospital cross infection by endoscopes has been reported and an outbreak of 4 cases of typhoid fever in a gall-stone clinic in London, due to contaminated duodenal tubes, was described in 1977. Paratyphoid B fever is more likely to spread from person to person particularly in children but this mode of spread is much more common with the salmonellae causing acute gastroenteritis (Table 4.1).

Prevention

Prevention of enteric fever comprises controlling the source and methods of spread, and prophylactic immunization.

The source

Identification of cases, their early isolation or barrier nursing and treatment, and the detection and surveillance of carriers, are the main means of controlling the source of the disease. After recovery from illness persons should be kept under bacteriological surveillance for at least 12 months and a minimum of 3 specimens of faeces and urine examined at weekly intervals at the end of this period. More stringent clearance is necessary for food handlers. In countries with a low incidence of enteric fever screening of food handlers and water-works employees for the carrier state should be selective. Persons with a past history suggestive of enteric fever, a history of intestinal illness or fever contracted abroad, or recent residence in an area of high incidence of the disease, should have 3 faecal specimens examined but other employees need not be examined[4].

Method of spread

Control includes proper sewage disposal, the provision of a pure water supply, high standards of personal and food hygiene, the pasteurization of milk, cream and bulk egg products, the heat treatment of desiccated coconut and care to prevent post-processing contamination of tinned foods.

Prophylactic immunization

Moderately effective vaccines are available against *S. typhi* and are recommended for persons likely to be exposed to infection, such as laboratory workers and those visiting areas of high incidence, but immunization is no substitute for the hygienic control discussed above. Immunization is contra-indicated in the control of an outbreak, because if given during the incubation period it may increase the severity of the disease. Previous immunization invalidates the results of the agglutination reaction (Widal test) for diagnosis.

Food poisoning

Food poisoning can be defined as an acute gastroenteritis or other acute illness caused by the recent consumption of contaminated food.

The disease

Food poisoning may be caused by inherently poisonous foods, by chemical contamination of normally wholesome foods and by contamination of foods with certain pathogenic micro-organisms. Bacterial food poisoning is much the commonest form of food poisoning worldwide and the 6 main causative agents are listed in Table 4.2. These may cause symptoms by multiplication in the gastro-intestinal tract – infection type; by production of a toxin during multiplication in food – toxin type; or by releasing toxin on growth in the intestine – intermediate type. In general, toxin types of food poisoning have a short incubation period before the onset of vomiting, whereas infection types of food poisoning have a longer incubation period with diarrhoea predominating. Symptoms are usually confined to gastro-intestinal disturbance, except in botulism when muscular paresis occurs soon after the onset of the disease, characteristically ocular paresis, producing diplopia. Salmonella infections are often severe in the young, the elderly and those who have undergone gastric surgery, probably related to low gastric acidity, and occasionally produce a septicaemic illness (see enteric fever above).

The diagnosis of bacterial food poisoning is made by the isolation of the causative organism from the stools or vomit and confirmed by its subsequent isolation from suspect food. Serotyping and/or phage typing of the organism assists in the epidemiological identification of the source of infection.

In 1958 a widespread outbreak of 90 cases of *S. typhimurium* infection in South-East England was detected by phage-typing of the strains isolated from cases of human food poisoning, and an important clue to the source was obtained by the identification of the same organism from an outbreak of enteritis in calves. Without the aid of phage-typing it would not have been possible to link together the human cases, which comprised about 17 % of *S. typhimurium* infections reported at that time in a population of about 17 million. The calf outbreak focused attention on calf meat, which proved to be the vehicle of infection in most of the cases, and it was discovered that the sick calves had been obtained from the same dealer who supplied calves for veal. Although the origin of the calf infection was not found, cross infection in the dealer's premises was identified as an important factor in potentiating the outbreak[6].

The presence of food poisoning organisms in the stools of convalescent patients or symptomless persons does not have the same epidemiological significance as in typhoid fever, because the human faecal excreter or carrier of food poisoning bacteria does not constitute a source of secondary infection except in salmonellosis (Table 4.2). The most frequent types of non-bacterial food poisoning are listed in Table 4.3, but all of them are rare in most parts of the world.

Mortality and morbidity data

Mortality data are of limited value because deaths from food poisoning are uncommon. Morbidity data are available from many countries but it is recognized that there is considerable variation in reporting; for example, it has

Table 4.2. Bacterial food poisoning: summary of main features.

Organism	Type of food poisoning	Source	Usual circumstances of food poisoning	Incubation period	Clinical illness	Duration
Salmonella sp.	Infection	Intestinal contents of animals Rarely man	Cross contamination of cooked food by raw materials with subsequent inadequate refrigeration	6–48 hours	Diarrhoea, vomiting, fever	2–4 days but may extend to 2–3 weeks
Clostridium perfringens (type A)	Intermediate	Raw meats Environment	Cooked or reheated meats promoting anaerobic growth of organism for several hours	8–24 hours	Diarrhoea, abdominal pain	About 3 days
Staphylococcus aureus (enterotoxin producing)	Toxin	Staphylococcal lesions of man or of cattle	Hand contaminated cooked meats at room temperature for at least 6 hours Raw milk and dairy products inadequately	2–6 hours	Vomiting, diarrhoea, collapse	1–2 days

			food kept under...	limits.	...paresis	week of recovery
(types A, B and E)		(types A & B) Fish (type E)	anaerobic conditions and not subsequently cooked before eating	6 hours to 8 days	Extension of paresis to pharyngeal and respiratory muscles	over several months
Bacillus cereus	Toxin Possibly infection	Dried and powdered foods and ingredients Environment	Contaminated food kept moist and warm permitting profuse growth of organisms	1–6 hours 8–16 hours	Vomiting, diarrhoea Diarrhoea	12–24 hours
Vibrio parahaemolyticus	Infection	Fish and marine environment	Raw sea food or cross contamination of cooked sea food with subsequent inadequate refrigeration	2–48 hours	Diarrhoea, abdominal pain, vomiting	2–5 days

Table 4.3. Non-bacterial food poisoning: summary of main causes.

Type	Usual circumstances of food poisoning	Clinical illness All usually of rapid onset
Mushroom poisoning	Eating poisonous fungi of species *Amanita* containing muscarine or amantadine	Abdominal pain, vomiting, diarrhoea, convulsions and coma Poisoning with amantadine has high mortality
Potato (solanine) poisoning	Eating skin of sprouting potatoes or those exposed to light during growth, which often contain high levels of solanine	Headache, vomiting, diarrhoea and weakness Recovery in 3–4 days
Mussel poisoning	Eating mussels which have fed on toxin-producing dinoflagellates of genus Gonyaulax	Paraesthesiae, numbness, headache, weakness and paresis Recovery usual
Fish poisoning	Scombroid poisoning due to spoiled scombroid fish e.g. mackerel, tuna	Hot flushing, headache, diarrhoea Recovery in a few hours
	Ciguatera poisoning due to various poisonous fish of coral reefs	Paraesthesiae, numbness, vomiting, diarrhoea Recovery may take several weeks
	Tetraodon poisoning due to toxic puffer fishes	Numbness, weakness, vomiting, diarrhoea, paralysis, coma High mortality
Metallic poisoning	Consuming acid foods or drinks which have been prepared or stored in zinc or copper lined containers	Sudden vomiting Recovery within a few hours

been noted that the incidence is usually highest in areas with the best developed surveillance systems. There are variations also in the definition of food poisoning both within and between countries, which further complicates the interpretation of the available data. For example, in the United Kingdom it is not the usual practice to include foodborne dysentery, *Escherichia coli* or campylobacter infection, as food poisoning, even though they cause an acute gastroenteritis; cases where the causal agent is not identified are often not notified; and in salmonella infections symptomless excreters are included in some statistics and not in others, and cases arising from person-to-person spread of salmonellosis, for example in hospitals, are sometimes not differentiated from those due to food poisoning.

Most developed countries have statutory reporting systems. In England and Wales food poisoning has been statutorily notifiable since 1938, but there are in addition two other separate reporting systems, namely, a laboratory reporting system and reports by medical officers for environmental health to the Department of Health and Social Security. Since 1949 data from these three sources have been brought together centrally and published in a series of comprehensive reports describing annual trends.

Incidence

The wide variations in the reported incidence of food poisoning between countries are difficult to interpret, but there are also differences in the types of food poisoning experienced which reflect the geography of food habits. For example, in North-West Europe and North America species of salmonella are the commonest reported cause of food poisoning, a disease related to intensive rearing of animals[7], whereas in Japan food poisoning due to *Vibrio para-haemolyticus*, a marine organism often present in fish (the staple diet of many Japanese) is reported most frequently. Botulism is frequently reported in Poland due to home-preserved food and is also reported in the USA (usually type A), associated with home canning of vegetables; in northern Europe (usually type B), associated with sausages and meat products; and in Japan and Canada (usually type E), associated with fish and fish products. In non-bacterial food poisoning the most striking geographical differences occur in fish poisoning related to the local availability of the toxic fish involved[8].

In Britain the overall trends in the incidence of food poisoning in recent years are illustrated by notifications which have increased since 1972, mainly due to a rise in salmonella food poisoning caused by serotypes other than *S. typhimurium* (Fig. 4.3). This has been attributed to changes in animal husbandry, in particular the intensive production of poultry and to a rise in the consumption of poultry meat[9]. In contrast staphylococcal food poisoning and *Clostridium perfringens* food poisoning have declined, probably due to improvements in catering practice

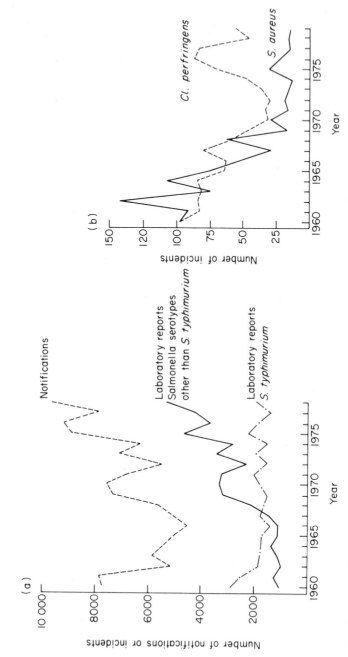

Fig. 4.3. Food poisoning, England and Wales, 1960–79. (a) Notifications of food poisoning and laboratory reports (incidents) of salmonella infections. (b) Laboratory reports (incidents) of *Staphylococcus aureus* and *Clostridium perfringens*. (From *British Medical Journal* 1980; **281**: 546.)

and personal hygiene but possibly also associated with changes in food habits. Bacterial food poisoning has a characteristic seasonal incidence reaching a peak in the summer months, most evident in staphylococcal food poisoning in Britain (Fig. 4.4) and in *V. parahaemolyticus* food poisoning in Japan[8].

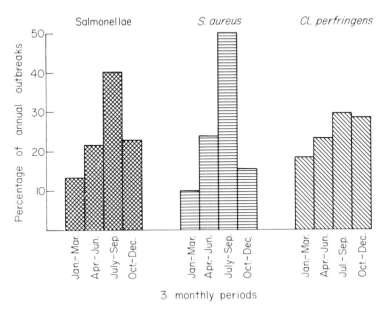

Fig. 4.4. Food poisoning outbreaks: seasonal distribution, England and Wales, 1954–68.

Special features

The incidence of food poisoning is determined by methods of food production and the food habits of populations, but cases of bacterial food poisoning only arise when the circumstances of time and temperature favour the growth in food of the pathogenic bacteria concerned (Table 4.2)[2]. In non-bacterial food poisoning, time and temperature errors in food hygiene are only important in scombrotoxic fish poisoning (Table 4.3)[10].

The main source of salmonellae is the gastro-intestinal tract of animals. Mass production of animal feeding stuffs and intensive farming increase the prevalence of salmonella infections in food animals[7]. The large scale processing of meat and meat products and other human foodstuffs and their wide geographical distribution tends to increase the incidence of salmonella food poisoning in the human population[9]. The organisms are heat-sensitive and although they often enter food factories and kitchens on raw meat or in other raw materials, can only give rise to human food poisoning if transferred to the finished cooked food product and given sufficient time at a suitably warm temperature to multiply to produce an infecting dose. The human faecal excreter is rarely the source of salmonella food poisoning, and when found in association with an outbreak is usually the result and not the cause of the incident. However, non-foodborne person-to-person spread is not uncommon, particularly in nurseries, institutions and hospitals, and outbreaks due to contaminated pharmaceutical preparations, such as pancreatin, have been reported.[2]

Antimicrobial drug-resistant strains of salmonellae have increased in recent years because of the widespread use of these drugs in veterinary and medical practice. These strains may arise after the treatment of salmonella infections, but they may also arise by transfer of resistance from non-pathogenic enterobacteria of animals or man produced by the use of antimicrobial drugs for prophylaxis, or in animals for growth promotion. Sometimes the acquisition of resistance may be accompanied by enhanced virulence and communicability.[2] Although anti-microbial drugs of value in human or veterinary medicine are no longer used as animal growth promoters, limitation of the therapeutic use of these drugs is necessary. Human salmonella food poisoning is usually a self-limiting disease for which symptomatic treatment is appropriate and for which antimicrobial drugs are contra-indicated because they do not affect the course of the illness and prolong the period of excretion. They are justified only in systemic infections[11].

Staphylococcal food poisoning is the only other type of bacterial food poisoning with clearly defined sources; these are staphylococcal lesions of man and cattle (Table 4.2). Certain strains of *Staphylococcus aureus* from such lesions produce a heat-resistant enterotoxin during growth but this can only occur under suitable conditions of temperature and time. This is usually at least 6 hours at room temperature.

The causative organisms of the other types of food poisoning are widespread in the environment and are frequently and often continuously present in certain foodstuffs in small numbers, but do not produce disease unless provided with suitable conditions of time, temperature, moisture and atmosphere to promote profuse growth (Table 4.2). *C. perfringens* food poisoning is usually due to meat dishes, cooled slowly and stored at room temperature or slowly reheated, in which the relatively heat-resistant organism has had time to multiply under partially anaerobic conditions. Such dishes include stews, pies, soups and sliced meat covered with gravy. Botulinum toxin is heat-sensitive and is produced during growth of *C. botulinum* under anaerobic conditions provided the pH is above 4.5. These conditions are usually found in smoked fish or sausage which have been allowed to remain at room temperature for some time and then eaten raw or inadequately cooked, or in canned or bottled foods inadequately heated during preparation and not subjected to further cooking. *Bacillus cereus* food poisoning follows the profuse multiplication of the organism in farinaceous food under warm and moist conditions. In Britain most outbreaks have been due to rice dishes maintained at room temperature overnight and then reheated. *V. parahaemolyticus* food poisoning follows the consumption of raw sea food which has been allowed to stand at room temperature or of cooked foods contaminated by raw sea food or sea water and then maintained at room temperature, conditions promoting the rapid growth of the organism during warm weather.

Prevention

The main aim is to prevent the multiplication of pathogenic bacteria in food by hygienic production and distribution methods, and by health education to achieve high standards of food preparation and of personal hygiene in kitchens and food factories, thus avoiding the circumstances which lead to bacterial food poisoning (Table 4.2). The prevention of salmonella and staphylococcal food poisoning depends also on the control of the source of the organism: in the former, improved animal husbandry to reduce the prevalence of infection in animals, in the latter exclusion from work of food handlers with septic lesions of the skin. The prevention of non-bacterial food poisoning is by education about the special circumstances in which it occurs (Table 4.3) so that these may be avoided.

Shigella infections

Bacillary dysentery is an acute intestinal infection caused by the shigella group of organisms and characterized by diarrhoea with blood and mucus in the stools.

The disease

Shigellae are primarily human pathogens which cause a localized disease of the large intestine. There are 4 subgroups of shigellae: group A – *Shigella dysenteriae*; group B – *S. flexneri*; group C – *S. boydii*; and group D – *S. sonnei*. The first 3 of these are divided into several serotypes. Infection has been demonstrated in monkeys, usually with *S. flexneri*, but this is of little epidemiological importance in man (Table 4.4)[12].

The organisms gain access to the body by the mouth and subsequently multiply in the wall of the colon, giving rise to diarrhoea and fever within 2–7 days. The severity of the disease is very variable. The diarrhoea may be profuse and watery with blood, pus and mucus in the stools; in the very young, the elderly and debilitated, high death-rates occur especially with *S. dysenteriae* infections. However, sometimes diarrhoea is slight or absent, symptomless excretion being particularly frequent in *S. sonnei* infections. A similar clinical picture of acute dysentery may also be caused by protozoal infections, the commonest being amoebic dysentery due to *Entamoeba histolytica*.

Table 4.4. Dysentery and other gastro-intestinal infections: summary of main features.

Organism	Type	Source	Usual methods of spread	Incubation period	Clinical illness
Shigellae	*Dysenteriae* *Flexneri* *Boydii* *Sonnei*	Human cases or carriers, *Flexneri* rarely from monkeys	Flies, food, water in areas with poor standards of hygiene and sanitation *Flexneri* faecal–oral route in adults in mental institutions *Sonnei* faecal–oral route in children	2–7 days	Diarrhoea with fever Blood, pus and mucus in the stools *Dysenteriae* severe illness with deaths in very young, old and debilitated *Sonnei* mild diarrhoea often symptomless
Escherichia coli	Enteropathogenic (EPEC) Enterotoxic (ETEC) Enteroinvasive (EIEC)	Human cases or excreters	Person-to-person, dust, Fomites. Rarely food Usually food, person-to-person. Rarely water Person-to-person, food Occasionally water	Short, usually less than 48 hours	Infantile gastroenteritis Travellers' diarrhoea Dysentery-like illness in older children and adults
Campylobacter	Thermophilic strains related to *Campylobacter fetus*	Cattle, poultry, dogs Human cases Other unknown	Unpasteurized milk Raw or uncooked poultry Rarely person-to-person Other unknown	2–5 days	Fever, malaise, abdominal pain, diarrhoea
Viruses	Rotavirus Parvovirus-like agents Others, including adenoviruses, astroviruses, coronaviruses and caliciviruses	Human cases	Person-to-person by faecal–oral route Person-to-person Shellfish	24–48 hours	Infant and childhood winter gastroenteritis Sudden vomiting, abdominal pain and diarrhoea Children and adults Winter vomitting disease or gastroenteritis

The diagnosis of bacillary dysentery is made by the isolation of the causative organism from the stools. Subsequent typing of the isolate is valuable for epidemiological purposes. Large numbers of organisms are present in the stools in the early stages of the disease when the patient is most infectious, only very small numbers of organisms providing an infective dose. Although excretion may continue during convalescence and become chronic, the number of organisms diminishes and persons with formed stools are not usually a source of infection.

Mortality and morbidity data

These data have been available in developed countries for many years but ascertainment is incomplete and dependent upon the availability of diagnostic laboratory services, because it is not possible to make the diagnosis of bacillary dysentery with certainty without the isolation of the causative organism. Dysentery was made statutorily notifiable in England and Wales in 1919, and since 1946 these data have been supplemented by laboratory reports of isolations of shigellae.

Incidence

In areas where sanitation is poor many shigella types exist in endemic form affecting all age groups with occasional outbreaks of foodborne or waterborne disease, the incidence reaching a peak in the summer months. In Western countries with improved sanitation person-to-person spread predominates and *S. sonnei* infection is endemic with the highest incidence in children in the winter months. In recent years in Britain *S. sonnei* infection has declined, probably due to improved hygiene in schools and nurseries and other shigella infections have increased due to infection acquired abroad (Fig. 4.5)[13]. There were under 4000 notifications of dysentery in 1978 and laboratory reports indicated that most of these were due to *S. sonnei* and about 15 % due to *S. flexneri*. There were less than 100 laboratory reports of the other 2 shigella types in the year.

Worldwide, *S. dysenteriae*, the most virulent organism for man, predominated in the early part of this century. This was replaced by *S. sonnei* and *S. flexneri* as the commonest types in the inter-war years but in the past decade *S. dysenteriae* has reappeared in Central America and India in epidemic form. The reasons for this change are obscure[12].

Special features and prevention

Bacillary dysentery can only occur as a result of the transfer of shigellae from human faeces from a case or a carrier to the mouth of another person. Because

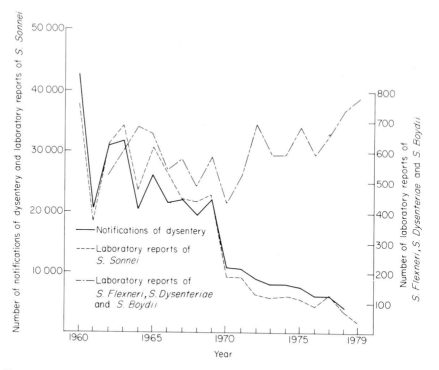

Fig. 4.5. Dysentery: notifications and laboratory reports, England and Wales 1960–79.
(From Galbraith NS. Epidemiology of Infection in Britain today. *Medicine International* 1981; **1**:
V10–V15.)

the infective dose is low, spreading by fomites or flies is very much more common
than in typhoid and paratyphoid fevers and salmonellosis.

Prevention depends on proper disposal of faeces, provision of pure water,
protection of food from contamination by flies and dust and high standards of
personal hygiene. In Britain the prevention of *S. sonnei* dysentery is particularly
related to toilet hygiene in infant schools and nurseries.

Acute enteritis and gastroenteritis

The food poisoning organisms are well established causes of gastroenteritis and
the shigellae of enteritis, but the causative organisms and epidemiology of other
acute gastro-intestinal infections are less well defined. Recently, however, the
roles of *E. coli, Campylobacter* sp. and viruses have been partially clarified and
these infections will be considered separately following a general introduction.

The disease

Acute diarrhoea and vomiting, which may be caused by a variety of infectious
agents, mainly affects children, especially infants living in poor hygienic

conditions who have been artificially fed. In severe cases dehydration rapidly occurs and death follows unless the fluid and electrolyte balance is restored promptly.

Morbidity and mortality data

Mortality data of diarrhoea and enteritis are available in most developed countries and morbidity data derived from statutory notification of infantile gastroenteritis are also available in some of them. Because the condition is ill-defined, morbidity data are unreliable and mortality data in infants under 1 year of age probably provide the best measure of trends in incidence.

Incidence

In Europe and North America deaths from diarrhoeal diseases in infants had a peak incidence in the summer in the early part of this century – 'summer diarrhoea' – but as the disease declined this peak disappeared. Subsequently institutional outbreaks of the disease, mainly in the winter months, were frequent during the 1940s and 1950s but in the last 2 decades the disease has become uncommon. However, in underdeveloped countries it remains a major cause of mortality, often affecting older infants at the time of their weaning. Acute gastroenteritis is not confined to infants although in older children and adults the mortality is negligible and assessment of the incidence of the condition has to rely on surveys. In Britain these indicate an incidence of about 5 % per annum at all ages.

Escherichia coli **gastroenteritis**

Certain serogroups of *E. coli* have for many years been associated with infantile gastroenteritis and are known as enteropathogenic *E. coli* (EPEC)[14]. More recently strains of different serogroups have been shown to produce enterotoxins, enterotoxic *E. coli* (ETEC), and others to be capable of invading the cells of the gut wall, entero-invasive *E. coli* (EIEC), (Table 4.4)[15].

The disease

EPEC are the causative organisms of infantile gastroenteritis and were probably the main cause of 'summer diarrhoea' of the 1920s and 1930s and the winter hospital outbreaks of gastroenteritis in the 1940s and 1950s in Europe and America. The last reported outbreaks in Britain were in hospitals in Manchester in 1969 and in Glasgow in 1970–71. Spread is by the hands of the infants' attendants, dust or fomites. EPEC are probably not important causes of diarrhoea in adults although waterborne and foodborne outbreaks affecting adults have been described.

ETEC are an important cause of travellers' diarrhoea in persons arriving in countries with poor standards of hygiene and sanitation, but do not appear to be an important cause of infantile gastroenteritis in developed countries. However, in areas where standards of hygiene are low, all age groups are affected. Spread is probably mainly by food in travellers' diarrhoea but person-to-person spread by the faecal–oral route may occur where hygiene is poor. A few common-source community outbreaks have been reported in Western countries due to water and to food.

EIEC are a cause of an illness resembling dysentery, with fever and diarrhoea with blood and mucus in the stools, and affecting mainly older children and adults. Spread is probably mainly person-to-person as in dysentery, although several foodborne outbreaks have been reported, the most notable of which was an outbreak of nearly 400 cases in the USA in 1971 due to imported French cheese.

Prevention

The principles of prevention of *E. coli* gastroenteritis in the general population are the same as mentioned for dysentery (see above). In addition, the prevention of infantile gastroenteritis requires the preparation of artificial feeds under aseptic precautions, or preferably the continuance of breast feeding, and if a case occurs in hospital, strict cubicle isolation and barrier nursing techniques to prevent cross-infection.

Campylobacter enteritis

In the early 1970s microbiological techniques were developed for the isolation of campylobacter from faeces, and since this time the organism has been isolated from between 2 and 7% of patients with acute enteritis in various parts of the world. In Britain it is now the most commonly isolated pathogen from sporadic cases of diarrhoea. It may be an important cause of diarrhoeal illness in children in underdeveloped countries and of travellers' diarrhoea[16].

The disease

After an incubation period of about 2–5 days, but sometimes as long as 10 days, fever develops with malaise and abdominal pain and, later, diarrhoea although in many cases this may be the presenting symptom, and in children may be accompanied by blood. The symptoms may sometimes suggest appendicitis or intussusception. The diagnosis is made by microscopy of fresh stools and by culture; stools are positive from early in the illness and the organism may persist for several weeks. The causal organism comprises strains related to *Campylobac-*

ter fetus but which are thermophilic, growing best at 42°C and sometimes known as 'related campylobacters'.

The disease is a zoonosis, the infection occurring in farm and domestic animals. Small outbreaks have been attributed to poultry meat, to handling contaminated poultry and to contact with infected dogs with diarrhoea. Several outbreaks have been due to unpasteurized milk but no large foodborne outbreaks have been described. Person-to-person spread appears to be uncommon even within families and institutions, probably because the organism survives for only a short while outside the body.

Prevention

Methods of prevention must await the development of techniques for subtyping the organism so that the epidemiology of the disease can be studied more precisely and the exact modes of spread determined. Already, however, the milkborne spread of campylobacter enteritis strengthens the case for pasteurization of milk.

Viral gastroenteritis

For many years it has been assumed that viruses caused gastroenteritis from which no bacterial pathogens could be isolated but it is only since 1973, by the use of electron microscopy and human volunteers, that these agents have begun to be identified. They fall into 2 main groups: reo-like viruses (known as rotaviruses because of their wheel-like appearance on electron microscopy) which are about 70 nm in diameter; and parvovirus-like agents, small round viruses 25–30 nm in diameter. The former cause acute gastroenteritis of infants and young babies and the latter, winter vomiting disease of older children and adults, although the 2 groups of diseases overlap[17].

Rotaviruses are a major cause of gastroenteritis in infants and young children in many parts of the world. The peak incidence of the clinical disease is between 6 and 24 months of age, breast milk apparently having a protective effect in young infants in whom the infection is mild or symptomless. In temperate climates the disease occurs almost exclusively in the winter and studies have shown that up to three-quarters of children admitted to hospital with gastroenteritis in the winter have rotavirus in their stools. Outbreaks in hospitals and nurseries have been reported and the mode of spread is considered to be from person to person by the faecal–oral route.

Parvovirus-like agents are causes of the syndrome of winter vomiting disease, a self-limiting disease with the sudden onset of vomiting, abdominal pain and fever, followed later by diarrhoea and sometimes accompanied by vertigo and muscle pains. In 1972 a virus was identified by electron microscopy in an outbreak in a primary school in Norwalk, Ohio, and subsequently similar agents have been identified in Britain and Australia. Spread appears to be by person to person transmission by the faecal–oral route, but recently foodborne spread by shellfish has been demonstrated. Widespread outbreaks took place in England in 1976 due to inadequately cooked cockles harvested from a sewage polluted estuary, and in Australia in 1978 due to oysters which had not been purified.

Other viruses have been detected in association with acute gastroenteritis but their importance has yet to be assessed. These include astroviruses, caliciviruses, coronaviruses and adenoviruses.

References

1. Boyd JSK. Bacteriophage-typing and epidemiological problems. *British Medical Journal* 1952; **ii**: 679–85.
2. Turnbull PCB. Food poisoning with special reference to salmonella – its epidemiology, pathogenesis and control. *Clinics in Gastroenterology* 1979; **8**: 663–714.
3. International Committee for Enteric Phage-typing. The geographical distribution of *Salmonella typhi* and *Salmonella paratyphi A* and *B* phage types, during the period 1 January 1966 to 31 December 1969. *Journal of Hygiene, Cambridge* 1973; **71**: 59–84.
4. The Public Health Laboratory Service Standing Sub-committee on the Bacteriological Examination of Water Supplies. Waterborne infectious disease in Britain. *Journal of Hygiene, Cambridge* 1978; **81**: 139–49.
5. Anderson ES, Hobbs BC. Studies of the strain of *Salmonella typhi* responsible for the Aberdeen typhoid outbreak. *Israel Journal of Medical Sciences* 1973; **9**: 162–74.
6. Anderson ES, Galbraith NS, Taylor CED. An outbreak of human infection due to *Salmonella typhimurium* phage-type 20a associated with infection in calves. *Lancet* 1961; **i**: 854–8.
7. Payne DJH. Salmonellosis and intensive farming. *Public Health, London* 1969; **84**: 5–16.
8. Todd ECD. Foodborne disease in six countries – a comparison. *Journal of Food Protection* 1978; **41**: 559–65.
9. McCoy JH. Trends in salmonella food poisoning in England and Wales 1941–72. *Journal of Hygiene, Cambridge* 1975; **74**: 271–82.
10. Hughes JM, Horwitz MA, *et al*. Foodborne disease outbreaks of chemical etiology in the United States, 1970–74. *American Journal of Epidemiology* 1977; **105**: 233–44.
11. Anon. Salmonellosis – an unhappy turn of events. *Lancet* 1979; **i**: 1009–10.
12. Keusch GT. Shigella infections. *Clinics in Gastroenterology* 1979; **8**: 645–62.
13. Gross RJ, Thomas LV. Rowe B. *Shigella dysenteriae, Sh. flexneri* and *Sh. boydii* infections in England and Wales: the importance of foreign travel. *British Medical Journal* 1979; **ii**: 744.
14. Taylor J. Host specificity and enteropathogenicity of *Escherichia coli*. *Journal of Applied Bacteriology* 1961; **24**: 316–25.
15. Rowe B. The role of *Escherichia coli* in gastroenteritis. *Clinics in Gastroenterology* 1979; **8**: 625–44.
16. Butzler JP. Skirrow MB. Campylobacter enteritis. *Clinics in Gastroenterology* 1979; **8**: 737–65.
17. Banatvala JE. The role of viruses in acute diarrhoeal disease. *Clinics in Gastroenterology* 1979; **8**: 569–98.

Further reading

Benenson AS, ed. *Control of communicable diseases in man*. 12th ed. Washington: American Public Health Association, 1975.
Christie AB. *Infectious diseases: epidemiology and clinical practice*. 2nd ed. London: Churchill Livingstone, 1974.

Hobbs BC, Gilbert RJ. *Food poisoning and food hygiene.* 4th ed. London: Edward Arnold, 1978.
Riemann H. Bryan FL, eds. *Food-borne infections and intoxications.* 2nd ed. London: Academic Press, 1979.
Taylor J, ed. *Bacterial food poisoning.* London: The Royal Society of Health, 1969.
Wilson GS, Miles AA. *Principles of bacteriology, virology and immunity.* Vol 2. 6th ed. London: Arnold, 1975.

Chapter 5 · Sexually Transmitted Diseases

M W ADLER

A formal service for the treatment and control of sexually transmitted diseases (STDs) was created in the United Kingdom in 1916 following publication of the Report of the Royal Commission on Venereal Diseases. The service was established to deal with three conditions: gonorrhoea, syphilis and chancroid. Today a wider range of genital infections, many of which are spread not only by sexual intercourse, are seen by clinicians in STD clinics (Table 5.1). The most important amongst them are gonorrhoea, herpes genitalis (see also Chapters 3 and 23) and warts, trichomoniasis, parasitic infections, syphilis, non-specific urethritis and chlamydial infections. The epidemiology of each of these is not considered separately here. However, some of the factors which affect their distribution are identified and the general features of their epidemiology are described below.

Clinical problems

Aetiology

The causative organisms of most of the sexually transmitted diseases are known and are simplified in their diagnostic labels. However, the cause (or causes) of the commonest clinical form of STD – non-specific urethritis (NSU) – remains uncertain. Traditionally this diagnosis was made in patients with evidence of urethral inflammation, shown by the presence of polymorphonuclear leucocytes on a Gram-stained smear, in whom no specific cause of urethritis could be found. In recent years it has been shown that *Chlamydia trachomatis* can be isolated in approximately 50 % of men with NSU and in 30 % of their female contacts (rates from different series vary from 23–57 % in men and 22–35 % in women)[1, 2]. Occasionally other organisms, such as *Ureaplasma urealyticum* can be isolated from patients with NSU.

Diagnosis

The usefulness of information on the epidemiology of STDs depends on the accuracy of diagnostic discrimination between the different causative agents. The problems that arise in this respect are illustrated by a recent study of STD clinics which demonstrated the variations in diagnostic and reporting criteria used by venereologists in England and Wales[3]. For example, as has already been stated, a diagnosis of NSU is usually made on the basis of the presence of poly-morphonuclear leucocytes on a Gram-stained smear and the absence of a causative organism. In the clinic study, the consultants were asked to indicate the microscopic criteria that they used to make a diagnosis of NSU in male patients. The most common criterion, the presence of between 1 and 5 leucocytes per high power field (HPF), was applied in 66% of the clinics surveyed. The next most frequently used criterion, 10 or more leucocytes per HPF, was used in 16% of clinics, followed by 5–10 leucocytes in 10% of clinics. In the remaining clinics other criteria were used that did not involve quantifying the number of

Table 5.1. Sexually transmitted diseases.

Infecting organism		Disease
Bacteria	*Neisseria gonorrhoeae*	Gonorrhoea
	Haemophilus ducreyi	Chancroid
	Calymmatobacterium granulomatis (Donovania)	Granuloma inguinale
	Chlamydia trachomatis	Urethritis/Cervicitis/ Salpingitis
		Ophthalmia neonatorum
		Lymphogranuloma venereum
	Corynebacterium vaginale	Vaginitis/Urethritis
	Group B haemolytic streptococcus	Neonatal sepsis
	Shigella sp.	Shigellosis
Viruses	Herpes virus hominis type 2	Herpes genitalis
	Wart virus	Condyloma acunimate
	Molluscum contagiosum virus	Molluscum contagiosum
	Hepatitis A + B virus	Hepatitis
	Cytomegalovirus	Congenital infection
	Ureaplasma urealyticum (T-mycoplasma)	Urethritis/Cervicitis
	Epstein Barr virus	Infectious mononucleosis
	Marburg virus	Marburg's disease
Protozoa	*Entamoeba histolytica*	Amoebiasis
	Giardia lambia	Giardiasis
	Trichomonas vaginalis	Trichomoniasis
Fungi	*Candida albicans*	Candidosis
Parasites	*Sarcoptes scabiei*	Scabies
	Phthirus pubis	Pediculosis pubis
Spirochaetes	*Treponema pallidum*	Syphilis
	Treponema pertenue	Yaws
	Treponema carateum	Pinta
Unknown		Non-specific urethritis

leucocytes. It is unsatisfactory that the notifications of NSU, the commonest STD, is based on no consistent diagnostic criteria.

A further example of the lack of uniform criteria concerns 'epidemiological' diagnosis and treatment. These terms are currently used by many venereologists where a diagnosis is made and treatment instituted in named sexual contacts or infected persons after a history of exposure but without, or in advance of, confirmatory pathological findings. For example, in the case of a female contact of a male with gonorrhoea the patient would be examined and smears and specimens for culture would be taken but even if microscopy was negative, she would be treated as if she were a confirmed case of gonorrhoea. In the clinic survey referred to above[3] 'epidemiological' diagnosis and treatment was widely used for gonorrhoea contacts, and applied more frequently to female than to male patients. This practice of giving treatment at the initial consultation on the basis of the patient's contact history despite negative microscopy, has important implications in relation to measurement of the incidence of STD, because in 19 % of clinics using 'epidemiological' treatment, these cases were counted by the consultants as if they were proven cases of gonorrhoea. Notification of 'epidemiologically' treated patients and classifying them as cases of gonorrhoea will inevitably lead to an overestimate of the number of 'true' cases of gonorrhoea treated.

The clinical criteria used to diagnose salpingitis also vary. However, attempts have been made to standardize these by asking clinicians to record the presence of the following features: lower abdominal pain, vaginal discharge, cervical motion tenderness, adnexal tenderness, pyrexia, raised erythrocyte sedimentation rate, and fever. The use of the laproscope allows much more accurate diagnosis than these clinical criteria alone. Attempts have also been made to standardize criteria for a diagnosis at laparoscopy. These criteria are erythema of the Fallopian tubes, oedema and swelling of the tubes, sero-purulent exudate from the fimbriated ends of tubes when patent and sero-purulent exudate on the surface of the tubes. Studies comparing use of clinical and laparoscopic criteria indicate that the use of the former gives a correct diagnosis in only 65 % of cases, with a false positive diagnosis rate of 23 %. In the remaining 12 % of cases other conditions such as ectopic pregnancy, appendicitis and endometriosis were found by laparoscopy[4].

Complications

One of the most serious complications of some of the STDs is pelvic inflammatory disease with the risk of subsequent permanent sterility. Gonococcal, chlamydial and non-specific infections are particularly hazardous in this respect. It is reported that between 10 and 20 % of women develop salpingitis after a gonococcal infection. However, the proportion who develop salpingitis arising from an STD will depend on how long they have had the infection before proper treatment is instituted, which in turn depends on the availability and standard of medical services. In most countries, patients with salpingitis are frequent users of health services. It has been calculated that in the USA 1 million women suffer from pelvic inflammatory disease[5]. In some developing countries, the proportion of all gynaecological admissions due to this condition is extremely high (Zimbabwe 44 % and Uganda 30 %).

The proportion of these patients who eventually develop occlusion of the Fallopian tubes has been difficult to determine. Westrom[6] has reported occlusion in 13 % of patients with one attack of salpingitis, rising to 75 % in women who have had 3 or more attacks. The commonest cause was non-gonococcal infection.

Transmission and infection

An essential feature of most of these diseases is that they are rarely transmitted other than by sexual intercourse. Therefore, their epidemiology is substantially determined by sexual behaviour in communities. However, the picture is often confused because some infections are asymptomatic and transmission is not an inevitable consequence of exposure. For example, 5–10 % of men and up to 50 % of women attending STD clinics who are eventually diagnosed as suffering from gonorrhoea, have no symptoms. It is much more important to know about the prevalence of asymptomatic and symptomatic sufferers in the community who are not seeking medical care.

The probability of acquiring a sexually transmitted infection following intercourse with an infected individual has been difficult to study. Most of the work has involved studying special populations, such as members of armed forces, in whom it has been easier to carry out follow-up tests after exposure and also to examine the index case. Such studies suggest that the risk of a man contracting gonococcal urethritis is between 22 and 35 % per sexual exposure[7]. Other workers have suggested that the risk of contracting gonorrhoea is between 5 and 40 % per sexual exposure. These figures need to be treated with caution because the risk of infection will depend upon a large number of other behavioural variables. The most important point is that the infectivity of gonorrhoea and other STDs is not 100 %.

Sources of data

Notification system

There are 230 STD clinics within the United Kingdom and 120 consultants working in them. Consultants in charge of clinics are required to make quarterly returns to the Chief Medical Officers of their respective countries (England, Northern Ireland, Scotland and Wales) of the number of cases seen in their clinics. The cases are notified under the following headings: syphilis, gonorrhoea, non-specific genital infection, trichomoniasis, candidiasis, scabies, pediculosis pubis, *Herpes simplex*, warts (*Condylomata acuminata*), molluscum contagiosum, chancroid, lympho-granuloma venereum and granuloma inguinale and other conditions requiring and not requiring treatment. Additional data are required for cases of gonorrhoea and syphilis: these are age, whether the infection was contracted within or outside the United Kingdom and the number of sexual contacts sought, how many attended and the number found to have a positive diagnosis. Because the STDs are not legally notifiable the reporting system depends upon voluntary co-operation with clinicians and always has done.

There are many drawbacks and omissions in the current information system for sexually transmitted diseases. The reported figures relate to the number of cases, not patients. This means that a patient can reappear several times in the published statistics and can do so for a number of different reasons. Firstly, they may have more than one disease diagnosed at the same point in time. Secondly, they may contract one or more diseases on several separate occasions during the year. Finally, in many instances there may be difficulty in differentiating a reinfection, which should be counted as a new episode, from a relapse, which should not be counted.

The effect of this is that the number of diagnoses made and thus the number of cases reported misrepresents the size of the problem and leads to an over-estimate of persons involved. This has practical implications for the organization of the service and health education for STDs, as it is not known whether STDs are as common as is supposed or whether they are limited to a much smaller and potentially well-defined or high risk group of the population.

Some surveys have attempted to differentiate patients from cases. A study of all new patients attending the clinic at the Royal Victoria Hospital, Belfast, during 1969, showed that there were 2093 diagnoses among 1753 patients, a patient/case ratio of 0:84[8]. In Aberdeen, the notes of all female attenders at the clinic over a 9 year period were examined and it was found that 1197 women contributed 1686 cases, a ratio of 0:7[9]. A similar study in England and Wales showed that 1071 patients contributed 1909 cases, a ratio of 0:6[10]. Of these patients, 55 % had one disease or diagnosis and thus constituted only a single case; 39 % had 2 to 3 diagnoses. 8 % of the patients had 4 diagnoses; these accounted for 22 % of the total cases. The second drawback with clinic statistics is the lack of uniform criteria for diagnosis and notification which has already been discussed.

There are 3 omissions from the routine statistics for STDs. Firstly, there is no notification of patients treated in General or Private Practice or in antenatal and gynaecological clinics. Secondly, there is no way of identifying people in the community who do not seek treatment either because they have no symptoms or because they choose to ignore them. These two groups will only come to notice through contact tracing. However, despite the drawbacks and omissions in the routine statistics in the United Kingdom, they are probably better than in most other countries in the world.

Incidence and prevalence

International trends

From returns made to the World Health Organization it is estimated that about 200 million new cases of gonorrhoea and 40 million new cases of syphilis occur in the world each year. These are probably underestimates because, firstly, some countries do not report to the World Health Organization and secondly, within some countries there are inadequacies in their reporting systems which lead to underestimation of the actual frequency of the diseases. Fig. 5.1 shows the recent trends in the reported rates for gonorrhoea in 8 countries between 1950 and 1977. Although the rates vary between countries the trend in most was for the rates to increase over most of the period with a recent flattening-out or decrease. The

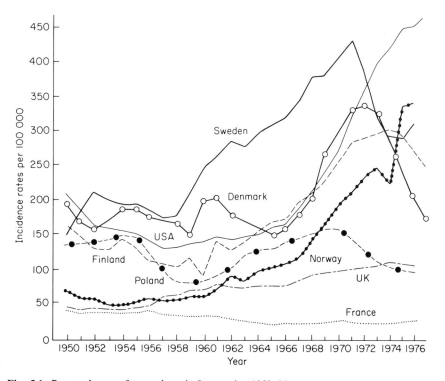

Fig. 5.1. Reported rates of gonorrhoea in 8 countries, 1950–76.

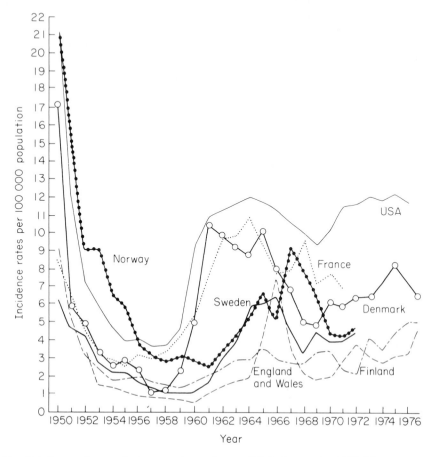

Fig. 5.2. Reported rates of primary and secondary syphilis in 8 countries, 1950–77.

trends in the reported rates for early syphilis (primary, secondary and latent infection in the first 2 years of the disease) in the same years for 7 countries are shown in Fig. 5.2.

There are explanations for some of the apparent international variation. For example, France has a particularly high reported rate for syphilis, but the rate for gonorrhoea is low. This may be because in France most patients with sexually transmitted diseases are seen by doctors who are paid a fee for notifying a case of syphilis but not for gonorrhoea. It is therefore likely that the incidence of gonorrhoea is much higher in France than is apparent. Likewise, until recently, Sweden had a particularly high reported rate for gonorrhoea, but the Swedish notification system and public clinical service is highly developed, resulting in the majority of cases being reported. The Americans developed an excellent venereal disease service after the First World War, but dismantled it after the discovery of penicillin and an initial drop in the incidence of both gonorrhoea and syphilis. The majority of patients are now seen by physicians who are not required to make returns. In 1977, the number of reported cases of gonorrhoea in the USA was 100 0177, but the reporting of primary and secondary syphilis and gonorrhoea in the USA is probably grossly underrepresented[11].

Trends in the United Kingdom

Table 5.2 shows the number of new cases of STDs reported for the years 1975–78. The total number of new cases seen in clinics each year is now about 340 000. Non-specific urethritis accounts for about one-third of these. A further 107 000 attendances are for conditions not requiring treatment (patients seeking reassurance, advice and check-ups). The workload in clinics is now generated mainly by diseases other than the original venereal diseases of syphilis, gonorrhoea and chancroid. Figs. 5.3 and 5.4 show the trends in the numbers of cases of syphilis and gonorrhoea notified each year since 1925. The number of cases of syphilis declined rapidly after a post-war peak. This is thought to be due largely to the discovery of penicillin as an effective treatment.

Table 5.2. Clinic returns for the United Kingdom of new cases of STD., by diagnosis, 1975–78.

Diagnosis	1975	1976	1977	1978*
Syphilis	3 964	4 306	4 780	4 802
Gonorrhoea	65 880	65 281	65 963	63 080
Chancroid	76	59	49	61
Lymphogranuloma venereum	40	39	43	34
Granuloma inguinale	14	36	56	14
Non-specific genital infections	94 483	101 651	105 210	107 788
Trichomoniasis	21 912	21 903	22 145	21 483
Candidiasis	37 740	39 414	41 144	42 220
Scabies	3 145	2 749	2 562	2 569
Pubic lice	5 838	6 168	6 769	7 443
Herpes simplex	6 762	7 547	8 399	8 957
Warts	23 126	25 035	26 063	27 133
Molluscum contagiosum	801	954	1 019	1 031
Other treponemal diseases	1 014	1 142	1 117	1 131
Other conditions requiring treatment	44 515	44 848	48 461	52 032
New cases of disease seen	309 310	321 132	333 780	339 778
Other conditions not requiring treatment	92 955	97 491	104 539	107 761
Total new cases	402 265	418 623	438 319	447 539

* Provisional.

Infectious Diseases

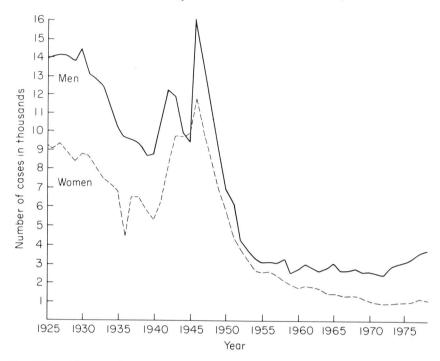

Fig. 5.3. Syphilis: annual cases (all stages) dealt with for the first time at any centre in the UK, 1925–78. Northern Ireland figures not included before 1958. (First produced for an article entitled: Sexually transmitted disease surveillance 1978. Report by Academic Department of Genito-Urinary Medicine, Middlesex Hospital Medical School, Communicable Surveillance Centre and Communicable Diseases (Scotland) Unit. *British Medical Journal* 1979; **ii**: 1375–6. I am grateful to Dr. N. S. Galbraith for allowing me to reproduce this figure.)

The widespread use of penicillin for other infections may also have contributed. However, in the last 10 years, the case notification rate of primary and secondary syphilis has risen again by 35 %. Gonorrhoea also showed a post-war peak, but has differed from syphilis in that this peak has been exceeded during the last 10 years, with a greater rise among women than men. In the last 10 years, the case notification rate has risen by 42 % for gonorrhoea. The notification rate of non-specific urethritis in males has more than doubled over the last decade.

Age-specific rates indicate the peak for primary and secondary syphilis in both sexes occuring in the age group 20–24 years (Table 5.3). The picture is similar for gonorrhoea.

Factors involved in increased incidence

The reasons for the increase incidence of sexually transmitted disease are not adequately understood and like many of the current health problems, the

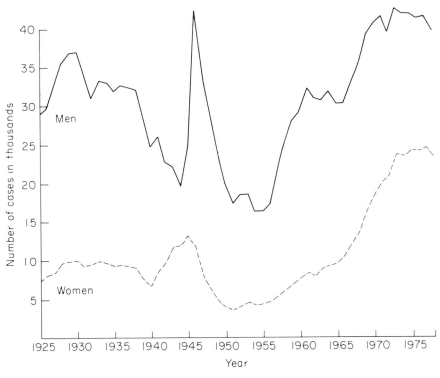

Fig. 5.4. Gonorrhoea: annual cases (all stages) dealt with for the first time at any centre in the UK, 1925–78. Northern Ireland figures not included before 1958. (First produced for an article entitled: Sexually transmitted disease surveillance 1978. Report by Academic Department of Genito-Urinary Medicine, Middlesex Hospital Medical School, Communicable Surveillance Centre and Communicable Diseases (Scotland) Unit. *British Medical Journal* 1979; **ii**: 1375–6. I am grateful to Dr. N. S. Galbraith for allowing me to reproduce this figure.)

Table 5.3. New cases of primary and secondary syphilis, and gonorrhoea, rate per 100 000 population, by age, 1978, United Kingdom clinic returns.

Diagnosis			Age group (years)		
			< 20	20–24	25 +
Primary and	Men	Number	95	349	1 233
secondary syphilis		Rate	4.2	17.0	17.0
	Women	Number	51	80	146
		Rate	2.4	4.1	2.1
Gonorrhoea	Men	Number	5 182	13 194	21 402
		Rate	228	643	295
	Women	Number	7 649	8 468	7 133
		Rate	354	436	101

explanation is probably multi-factorial. Demographic, social, organizational and medical factors have to be considered.

Demographic and social

The age of sexual maturity has decreased throughout this century. The figures given earlier suggest that the young are at particular risk from STDs. There are very little other routine data which help to identify high risk groups more specifically. Special studies have described particular risk groups, including homosexuals, prostitutes and itinerant sections of the community. The proportion of homosexually acquired cases of syphilis in the United Kingdom between 1971 and 1977 has risen from 42% to 54%[12]. Over the same period, the proportion of homosexually acquired cases of gonorrhoea had risen from 9.8% to 10.9%. These changes were particularly noticeable in London clinics. Prostitution is no longer considered to be a major factor in the spread of disease in Western countries and reports suggest that within the United Kingdom they rarely act as the source of infection[13].

Many studies have described the various demographic and socio-economic features of patients attending clinics. Most need to be treated with caution since they were all carried out on patients attending particular clinics and are not necessarily representative, either of all clinics or of all patients. Finally, studies examining demographic variables have been criticized since bland measurements of social standing indicate very little about sexual behaviour and treatment-seeking patients, both of which are important variables if adequate control strategies are to be developed.

An important social factor that has to be considered is the change that has occurred in sexual attitudes and behaviour over the last decade. The age of first sexual intercourse within the United Kingdom has decreased. In 1964, 16% of a sample of 15–19 years olds claimed to have experienced sexual intercourse[13]. In a different survey carried out in 1974 this had increased to 51%[14]. A higher proportion of women now have pre-marital sexual intercourse than previously. In the United Kingdom, 35% of women first married between 1956 and 1960 had had intercourse with their husbands before marriage. This had increased to 74% of women who married between 1971 and 1975[15]. Cohabitation before first marriage increased from 1% to 9%. The reduction in age of menarche, and an increase in people having intercourse earlier and before marriage, does not indicate promiscuity but, despite this and the lack of scientific data on sexual behaviour, promiscuity must be an explanatory factor in the changing pattern of incidence. Another important factor related to the incidence of STDs is the development of non-barrier contraceptives, such as the oral contraceptives and intra-uterine devices which have replaced the barrier techniques such as the sheath which afforded some protection against infection.

Other important social factors are the effects of war and an increase in the mobility of populations both nationally and internationally. It has been suggested that military personnel, seafarers, immigrants, tourists, professional travellers and similar groups who are separated from their families and normal social restraints, are more likely to have intercourse with unknown contacts outside a stable relationship.

Organizational and medical

The existence of a good clinical service and a contact tracing system which are free, help in the control of these diseases. However, their existence may result in people who previously would not have sought treatment seeking care or being brought into clinics by active contact tracing. Therefore, it is uncertain whether the increase in the number of recorded cases during the last 30 years reflects a real increase in the incidence of STDs.

Over the years the resistance of the gonococcus to penicillin has increased. This is not necessarily seen in all parts of the world. For example, it has not occurred in the Scandinavian countries, the United Kingdom and the USA. In 1963 the WHO Expert Committee on gonococcal infections recommended that international reference methods for the determination of sensitivities of current strains of gonococcus to various drugs should be established. Recently β-lactamase procuding gonococci have been found. A specific plasmid (R) carries the coding for β-lactamase and has probably transferred from other bacteria such as *Escherichia coli*. Once this transference has occurred the gonococcus involved becomes totally resistant to penicillins. This development has probably resulted from the widespread use of suboptimal dosages of antibiotics in the treatment of gonococcal infections.

Methods of control

The most important methods available for the control of the STDs are the provision of adequate diagnostic and treatment facilities and the training of health professionals. In the United Kingdom, it has always been considered that a hospital-based clinic service staffed by physicians specially trained in genito-urinary medicine, was the most effective approach. Special features of this system are that the service is free and that patients can walk into clinics without having to be referred by general practitioners. The existence of such a service does not mean that it will be used in an optimal fashion. This is partly because many of the diseases are asymptomatic and also because those with symptoms do not necessarily seek care. An understanding of why individuals ignore their symptoms and fail to consult deserves high priority in behavioural and epidemiological research.

One possible method of controlling the STDs is to screen all women attending antenatal and gynaecological clinics. Table 5.4 shows the results of a number of surveys carried out in the United Kingdom to determine the prevalence of gonorrhoea and trichomoniasis found in gynaecological and obstetric clinics[16-21]. These types of surveys are not representative of the general problem because they screen patients who have sought medical care and do not refer to a defined population at risk. What is required is a survey that measures both symptomatic and asymptomatic disease in a defined population of all those at risk. This type of total screening suggests that the proportion of women with a gonococcal infection is low (0.2%)[22]. In view of the low yield obtained by screening hospital or community populations, it is probably more cost effective to control STDs by providing good centralized facilities and health education programmes.

Table 5.4. United Kingdom patients with gonorrhoea and trichomoniasis, gynaecology (G) and antenatal (AN) clinic surveys.

Series	Type of clinic	Patients with disease (%)
Gonorrhoea		
Hughes (1971)	G	0.3
Silverstone (1974)	G	0.3
Driscoll (1970)	G	2.9
Cassie (1973)	AN	0.2
Rees (1972)	AN	0.6
Trichomoniasis		
Hughes (1971)	G	3.5
Driscoll (1970)	G	23.5
Rees (1972)	AN	4.0
Thin (1970)	AN	8.9

Reference has already been made to the importance of contact tracing in the control of disease and more widespread provision of this type of service will be of use in control. The final potential control measure will be through the development of a vaccine against gonorrhoea, syphilis and herpes genitalis.

References

1. Philip RN, Hill DA, *et al.* Study of chlamydiae in patients with lympho-granuloma venereum and urethritis attending a venereal disease clinic. *British Journal of Venereal Diseases* 1971; **47**: 114.
2. Schachter J, Hanna L, *et al.* Are chlamydial infections the most prevalent venereal disease? *JAMA* 1975; **231**: 1252.
3. Adler MW, Belsey EM, *et al.* Facilities and diagnostic criteria in sexually transmitted disease clinics in England and Wales. *British Journal of Venereal Diseases* 1978; **54**: 2.

4. Jacobson L, Westrom L. Objectivized diagnosis of acute pelvic inflammatory disease. *American Journal of Obstetrics & Gynaecology* 1969; **105**: 1088.

5. Curran JW. Economic consequences of pelvic inflammatory disease in the USA. *Journal of Obstetrics and Gynaecology* 1980; **138**: 848.

6. Westrom L. Effect of acute pelvic inflammatory disease on fertility. *American Journal of Obstetrics & Gynaecology* 1975; **121**: 707.

7. Homes KK, Johnson DW, Trostle HJ. An estimate of the risk of men acquiring gonorrhoea by sexual contact with infected females. *American Journal of Epidemiology* 1970; **91**: 170.

8. Pemberton J, McCann JS, *et al.* Socio-economic characteristics of patients attending a VD clinic and the circumstances of infection. *British Journal of Venereal Diseases* 1972; **48**: 391.

9. Thompson B, Rutherford HW. Aberdeen venereal disease clinic 1960–69: perspective on female attenders. *British Journal of Venereal Diseases* 1972; **48**: 209.

10. Woodcock K. How useful are our present statistics on sexually transmitted diseases? *British Journal of Venereal Diseases* 1975; **51**: 153.

11. McKenzie-Pollock JS. Physicians reporting of venereal disease in the USA. *British Journal of Venereal Diseases* 1970; **46**: 114.

12. British Co-operative Clinic Group. Homosexuality and venereal disease in the United Kingdom. *British Journal of Venereal Diseases* 1980; **56**: 6.

13. Schofield M. *The sexual behaviour of young people.* London: Longmans, 1965.

14. Farrell C. *My mother said.* London: Routledge and Kegan Paul, 1978.

15. Dunnell K. *Family formation 1976.* London: HMSO. Office of Population Censuses and Surveys, 1979.

16. Hughes WH, Davies JM. Better specimens from the female genital tract. Letter. *British Medical Journal* 1972; **iv**: 424.

17. Silverstone PI, Snodgrass CA, Wigfield AS. Value of screening for gonorrhoea in obstetrics and gynaecology. *British Journal of Venereal Diseases* 1974; **50**: 53.

18. Driscoll AM, McCoy DR, *et al.*, Sexually transmitted diseases in gynaecological out-patients with vaginal discharge. *British Journal of Venereal Diseases* 1970; **46**: 125.

19. Cassie R, Stevenson A. Screening for gonorrhoea, trichomoniasis, moniliasis and syphilis in pregnancy. *The Journal of Obstetrics and Gynaecology of the British Commonwealth* 1973; **80**: 48.

20. Rees DA, Hamlett JD. Screening for gonorrhoea in pregnancy. *The Journal of Obstetrics & Gynaecology of the British Commonwealth* 1972; **79**: 344.

21. Thin RNT, Michael AN. Sexually transmitted diseases in antenatal patients. *British Journal of Venereal Diseases* 1970; **46**: 126.

22. Adler MW, Belsey EM, Rogers JS, Sexually transmitted diseases in a defined population of women. *British Medical Journal* 1981; **i**: 29.

Chapter 6 · Viral Hepatitis

A J ZUCKERMAN

Viral hepatitis has emerged as a major public health problem occurring endemically in all parts of the world. The general term viral hepatitis refers to infections caused by at least 3 different viruses – hepatitis A (infectious or epidemic hepatitis), hepatitis B (serum hepatitis) and the more recently identified form of hepatitis, non-A/non-B hepatitis which is almost certainly caused by more than one virus.

Acute viral hepatitis is a generalized or systemic infection with particular emphasis on inflammation of the liver. The clinical picture of the infection ranges in its presentation from inapparent or subclinical infection, slight malaise, mild gastro-intestinal symptoms and the anicteric form of the disease, acute icteric illness, severe prolonged jaundice to acute fulminant hepatitis. The incidence of individual symptoms and signs varies, therefore, both in different outbreaks and in sporadic cases. In addition, hepatitis B and non-A/non-B hepatitis may progress to chronic liver disease, which may be severe, and there is substantial evidence of a close association between hepatitis B virus and primary liver cancer.

Hepatitis A and hepatitis B can now be differentiated by specific laboratory tests for antigens and antibodies associated with these infections. Laboratory tests for non-A/non-B hepatitis are under development.

Hepatitis A

Viral hepatitis type A occurs endemically in all parts of the world, with frequent reports of minor and major outbreaks. The exact incidence is difficult to estimate because of the high proportion of subclinical infections without jaundice, differences in surveillance and differing patterns of disease. The degree of underreporting is believed to be very high. The incubation period of hepatitis A is between 3 and 5 weeks with a mean of 28 days. Subclinical and anicteric cases are common and although the disease has, in general, a low mortality, patients may be incapacitated for many weeks. There is no evidence of progression to chronic liver damage.

Mode of spread

Hepatitis A virus is spread by the faecal–oral route, most commonly by person-to-person contact, and infection occurs readily in conditions of poor sanitation and overcrowding. Common source outbreaks are most frequently initiated by faecal contamination of water and food, but waterborne transmission is not a major factor in the maintenance of this infection in the industralized communities. On the other hand, many food-borne outbreaks have been reported. This can be attributed to the shedding of large quantities of virus in the faeces during the incubation period of the illness in infected food handlers, and the source of the outbreak can often be traced to uncooked food or food that has been handled after cooking. However, although hepatitis A remains common in the developed countries, the infection occurs mainly in small clusters, often with only few identified cases. The infection is highly endemic in many tropical and subtropical areas, with the occasional occurrence of large epidemics. Hepatitis A is not infrequently acquired by travellers to areas of high endemicity.

Age incidence

All age groups are suceptible to hepatitis A. Until recent years the highest incidence in the civilian population was observed in children of school age, but in a number of countries in Western Europe and in North America most cases occur in adults, a shifting age pattern reflecting improvement in socio-economic and hygienic conditions.

Seasonal pattern

In temperate zones the characteristic seasonal trend is for a marked rise in incidence in late autumn and early winter months falling progressively to a minimum during midsummer. In many tropical countries the peak of the infection tends to occur during the rainy season with low incidence during the dry periods.

Laboratory tests and the nature of hepatitis A virus

The identification in 1973 by immune electron microscopy of virus particles in extracts of faeces (Fig. 6.1) during the early acute phase of illness, provided the long-awaited lead to further studies of this infection. The availability of viral antigen permitted in turn the identification of specific antibody, the development of serological tests for hepatitis A and determination of susceptibility to infection in both human and non-human primates. Human hepatitis A has been transmitted to certain species of marmosets and to chimpanzees shown to be free of homologous antibody, thereby providing a model for experimental infection and also a source of reagents.

Large numbers of virus particles are detectable during the incubation period in experimental infection in chimpanzees, beginning as early as 9 days after

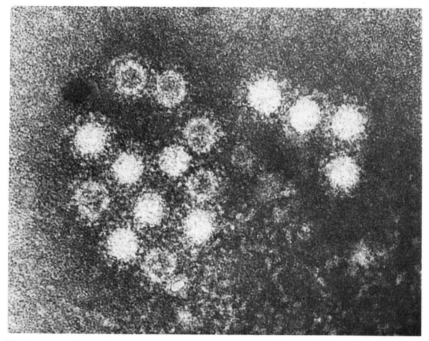

Fig. 6.1. Hepatitis A virus particles found in faecal extracts by immune electron microscopy. Both 'full' and 'empty' particles are present. The particles are surrounded by a halo of hepatitis A antibody. The virus measures 27–9 nm in diameter. × 252,000.

exposure and continuing, in general, until peak elevation of serum amino-transferases. Similar observations have been made in the course of natural infection in man; virus is also detected in faeces early during the acute phase of illness, but relatively infrequently after the onset of clinical jaundice. Interestingly, antibody is also detectable late in the incubation period coinciding approximately with the onset of biochemical evidence of liver damage, and the antibody persists.

A variety of serological tests are now available for hepatitis A antigen and antibodies, including immune electron microscopy, complement-fixation, immune adherence haemagglutination, radioimmunoassay and enzyme immunoassay. Immune adherence haemagglutination is specific and sensitive and has been widely used. Several methods of radioimmunoassay are now available and of these a solid-phase competitive type of assay is particularly convenient. Very sensitive enzyme immunoassay techniques have also been developed. Both radioimmunoassay and enzyme immunoassay for detection of hepatitis A antibodies of the immunoglobulin IgM and IgG classes are now available.

Only one serotype of hepatitis A virus has been identified in volunteers infected experimentally with the MS-1 strain of hepatitis A, in patients from different outbreaks of hepatitis in different geographical regions, in random cases of hepatitis A, and in naturally and experimentallly infected non-human primates. The possibility of some strain differences is under investigation. Because of the availability of specific serological tests for hepatitis A, it became possible to study the incidence and distribution of hepatitis A in various countries. These studies have shown that infections with hepatitis A virus are widespread and endemic in all parts of the world, that chronic excretion of hepatitis A virus does not occur, the infection is not transmitted by blood transfusion and evidence of progression to chronic liver disease has not been found.

Recent studies on the nature of hepatitis A virus have shown that this virus contains single-stranded ribonucleic acid (RNA) and polypeptides with similar molecular weights to the 4 major polypeptides of the Enterovirus genus within the picornaviridae. The virus is ether resistant, stable at pH 3.0 and relatively heat resistant. It is partially inactivated by heat at 60° C for 60 minutes, mostly inactivated at 60° C for 10 hours and inactivated at 100° C for 5 minutes. Hepatitis A virus is inactivated by 1:4000 formalin at 37° C for 72 hours, by ultraviolet irradiation and by chlorine 1mg/litre for 30 minutes. The successful propagation of hepatitis A virus in primary monolayer and explant cell cultures and in several continuous cell strains of human or simian origin opens the way to the detection and assay of the virus *in vitro* and eventually to the preparation of hepatitis A vaccines.

Control

Control of the infection is difficult. Spread of hepatitis A is reduced by simple hygienic measures and the sanitary disposal of excreta. Normal human immunoglobulin (a 16 % solution in a dose of 0.02–0.12 ml/kg body weight) before exposure to the virus or early during the incubation period, will prevent or attenuate a clinical illness, while not always preventing infection, and inapparent or subclinical hepatitis may develop.

Hepatitis B

Serological markers of infection

The discovery of Australia antigen in the circulation in 1965 and subsequently its association with hepatitis type B resulted in rapid advances in this field. Infection with hepatitis B virus (serum hepatitis) results in the appearance in serum of at least 3 serological markers; firstly hepatitis B surface antigen (originally referred to as Australia antigen) and later the homoligous antibody, the surface antibody. The second antigen, located in the core of the 42 nm hepatitis B particle (Fig. 6.2)

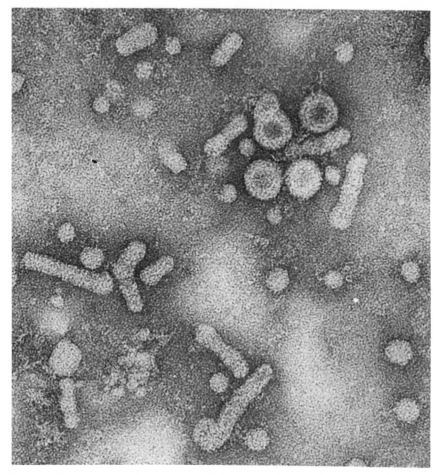

Fig. 6.2. Electron micrograph of serum containing hepatitis B virus after negative staining. The 3 morphological forms of the antigen are shown:
(1) small pleomorphic spherical particles 20–2 nm in diameter.
(2) tubular forms
(3) the 42 nm double-shelled virus.
× 239 400.
(Reproduced with permission from Zuckerman AJ, *Human viral hepatitis*. Amsterdam: North Holland/Elsevier, 1975.)

gives rise to the core antibody. The third marker of hepatitis B virus infection, which correlates closely with the number of virus particles and the relative infectivity of serum containing hepatitis B surface antigen, is the *e* antigen. This is a distinct soluble antigen which is specifically associated with hepatitis B and is located within the core of the virus particle. There is evidence that serum antibody to *e* indicates, in general terms, relative low infectivity of serum.

All these serological markers, which can now be detected by sensitive techniques such as radioimmunoassay and enzyme immunoassay, have proved extremely useful for unravelling the epidemiology of hepatitis B, established the global dissemination and public health importance of this infection, led to the routine screening of blood donors for the surface antigen and resulted in remarkable advances in the knowledge of the virology and pathogenesis of hepatitis B and its associated chronic liver disorders.

Hepatitis B virus

There is substantial evidence that the 42 nm particle is the hepatitis B virus. Double-stranded deoxyribonucleic acid (DNA) has been isolated from circulating virus particles and also from cores extracted from the nuclei of infected hepatocytes.

Hepatitis B surface antigen carries a common group determinant, termed *a*, and a number of major subdeterminants, *d*, *y*, *w* and *r* in various combinations, which are coded by the virus genome. The major subtypes have differing geographical distribution. For example, in northern Europe, the Americas and Australia subtype *adw* predominates. Subtype *ady* occurs in a broad zone which includes North and West Africa, the eastern Mediterranean, Eastern Europe, Northern and Central Asia and the Indian subcontinent. Both *adw* and *ady* are found in Malaysia, Thailand, Indonesia and Papua New Guinea, while the *ady* subtype predominates in other parts of South-East Asia including China, Japan and the Pacific.

Carrier state and epidemiology

Infection with hepatitis B virus may be followed by the persistent carrier state. Such a carrier state may be associated with liver damage. Survival of hepatitis B virus is ensured by the reservoir of carriers, estimated to number about 176 million. It appears that the prevalence of carriers, particularly among blood donors, in North America, northern Europe and Australia is 0.1 % or less; in Central and Eastern Europe up to 5 %, a higher frequency in Southern Europe, the countries bordering the Mediterranean and parts of Central and South America; and in some parts of Africa, Asia and the Pacific region as many as 20 % of the apparently healthy population may be carriers.

The importance of the parenteral route of transmission of hepatitis B is now well established and infectivity appears to be especially related to blood. However a number of factors have altered the epidemiological dogma that hepatitis B was spread exclusively by blood and blood products by the parenteral route. These include the findings that under certain circumstances the virus is infective by mouth, that it is endemic in closed institutions and is more prevalent in adults in urban communities and in poor socio-economic conditions, and that the carrier rate and age-distribution of the surface antigen varies in different regions.

Considerable circumstantial evidence is available for the transmission of hepatitis B by intimate personal contact and by the sexual route. Various body fluids such as saliva, menstrual and vaginal discharges, seminal fluid, breast milk and serous exudates have been implicated in the spread of infection, although in low prevalence areas the inoculation of blood and some blood products continues to be a major factor. Transmission may result from transfusion or accidental inoculation of minute amounts of blood such as may occur during medical, surgical and dental procedures, intravenous and precutaneous drug abuse, immunization with inadequately sterilized syringes and needles, tattooing, ear piercing, acupuncture, laboratory accidents, and accidental inoculation with objects such as razors that have been contaminated with blood.

Although the modes of transmission of hepatitis B in the tropics are similar to those in other parts of the world, additional factors may be of importance, including traditional tattooing and scarification, ritual circumcision and re-peated biting by blood-sucking arthropod vectors. Preliminary results of investig-ations into the role which biting insects may play in the spread of hepatitis B are conflicting. Hepatitis B surface antigen has been detected in several species of mosquitoes which have either been trapped in the wild or experimentally fed on infected blood, and in bed bugs, but no convincing evidence has been obtained either of replication of the virus or of persistence of the antigen after digestion of the blood meal. Mechanical transmission of infection may occur, however, particularly as a result of interrupted feeding in high prevalence areas.

Transmission of hepatitis B infection from carrier mothers to their babies can occur during the perinatal period. The risk of infection may reach 40 %, although it varies from country to country and appears to be related to ethnic groups. The risk is greatest if the mother has a history of transmission to previous children, a high titre of surface antigen and/or hepatitis B *e* antigen. There is also a substantial risk of perinatal infection if the mother has an acute infection in the second or third trimester of pregnancy or within 2 months after delivery. Most children infected during the perinatal period become persistent carriers.

Links with chronic liver disease and hepatocellular carcinoma

The role of viral hepatitis in the pathogenesis of chronic liver has been debated for many years. The outcome of acute hepatitis may be either complete resolution, massive necrosis, chronic hepatitis or resolution with scarring and cirrhosis. So chronic liver disease following hepatitis may be the result of necrosis, collapse of the reticulin framework, the formation of scars or nodular hyperplasia. Other factors include immunological processes, persistence of the virus in the liver and various host factors. There is a firm association between hepatitis B and chronic active hepatitis. Chronic active hepatitis patients with persistent hepatitis B antigens are usually male, and older than patients without the antigen(s). Auto-antibodies are usually absent from the serum, and multisystem involvement is not present. A proportion of patients with cryptogenic cirrhosis have evidence of persistent infection with hepatitis B virus.

Although primary hepatocellular carcinoma is rare in Europe, the USSR, North America and Australia, and it appears to be relatively infrequent in Central and South America, it is common in many communities in Africa and South-East Asia and probably less so in Japan. In some parts of Africa, this carcinoma is the commonest type of cancer in adult males. Hepatocellular carcinoma may therefore be among the most common human cancers.

Many studies show a highly significant occurrence of markers of hepatitis B infection in patients with primary hepatocellular carcinoma. Indeed, hepatitis B is ubiquitous in areas of the world where macronodular cirrhosis and primary liver cancer are common. Important factors in this possible aetiological association may be the early age of exposure to infection and the high prevalence of carriers. More recent laboratory studies have shown the presence of virus DNA base sequences in host cells derived from patients with persistent hepatitis B infection and chronic active hepatitis, and also in patients with hepatocellular carcinoma. These findings are consistent with hepatitis B viral DNA being integrated into host chromosomal DNA molecules. However, the actual mechanisms involved in the pathogenesis of hepatocellular carcinoma remain unknown. It is possible that liver cancer is the cumulative result of several cofactors including genetic, nutritional and hormonal factors, mycotoxins, chemical carcinogens and other environmental factors, and that hepatitis B virus acts either as a carcinogen or as a co-carcinogen in persistently infected hepatocytes.

Prevention

Passive immunization

The availability of laboratory tests for hepatitis B surface antibody has allowed the selection of plasma for the preparation of hepatitis B immunoglobulin, which may confer temporary passive immunity.

The major indication for the administration of hepatitis B immunoglobulin is a single acute exposure, such as when blood or other material containing hepatitis B surface antigen is accidentally inoculated, ingested orally or splashed on the conjunctiva. The optimal dose of hepatitis B immunoglobulin is not known but doses in the range of 0.04–0.07 ml/kg have been used with success. Based on available data, 2 doses administered 30 days apart are required for efficacy. The timing of the first dose appears to be important and the immunoglobulin should be administered as early as possible and prefer-ably within 48 hours. It should not be administered after 7 days following exposure.

Hepatitis B immunoglobulin administered within 2–6 days of birth to babies born to surface antigen-positive mothers yielded encouraging results if the baby was treated within 48 hours of birth. More recently, interruption of maternal–infant transmission of hepatitis B virus was achieved, and the carrier state prevented by the administration of hepatitis B immunoglobulin within 48 hours of birth, with further doses of immunoglobulin monthly for 6 months, reinforcing the impression that the timing of immunoglobulin was critical in determining its efficacy.

Pre-exposure prophylaxis with immunoglobulin has also been recommended in endemic settings such as haemodialysis units, where transmission of hepatitis B virus is known to occur and where preventive hygienic measures cannot be implemented.

Active immunization

The high rate of infection with hepatitis B virus in certain defined populations in the developed countries and among the general population in many developing countries points to the urgent need for a hepatitis B vaccine. Among the groups which might benefit from such a vaccine are health care and laboratory personnel, patients and staff of haemodialysis units, residents and staff of institutions for the mentally handicapped, persons requiring multiple transfu-sions of blood or plasma or injection of plasma derivatives, and individuals living in regions where hepatitis B infection is prevalent and especially where hepatocellular carcinoma is common.

The repeated failure to grow and passage hepatitis B virus serially in tissue culture has hampered progress toward the development of a conventional vaccine. Attention has therefore been directed toward the use of other preparations for active immunization. The foundations for such hepatitis B immunogens were laid by the demonstration of the relative efficacy of diluted serum containing hepatitis B virus heated to 98° C for 1 minute in preventing or modifying the infection in susceptible persons. Since the separated viral coat material, in this instance, hepatitis B surface antigen, leads to the production of protective antibody as shown in serological surveys and experimental studies, the possibility of using purified 22 nm spherical hepatitis B surface antigen particles appeared feasible. Such experimental vaccines have been prepared from the plasma of apparently healthy carriers of this antigen. Human hepatitis B infection has been successfully transmitted to chimpanzees, and although the infection is mild, the biochemical, histological and serological responses in these primates is very similar to that in man. A number of susceptible chimpanzees have now been shown to be protected by the 22 nm particle immunogens that had been treated with formalin. Trials in volunteers of such subunit vaccines are now in progress. Although it is generally accepted that the viral subunit preparations, when pure, are free of nucleic acid and therefore noninfectious, the fact that the starting material for their preparation is human plasma obtained from persons infected with hepatitis B virus, means that extreme caution must be exercised to ensure their freedom from all harmful contaminating material. Indeed, the plasma is collected from individuals who are persistent carriers of hepatitis B surface antigen, which is a marker of hepatitis B virus. Some concern has also been expressed on the possible induction of harmful immunological reactions to host components, including pre-existing structures of the liver cells, which may be present in such vaccine preparations, but reactions of this type have not been observed in the chimpanzees and individuals immunized so far.

In addition to the development of experimental hepatitis B vaccines composed of intact 22nm spherical forms of the surface antigen, vaccines are being prepared from the constituent polypeptides. Vaccines prepared from such polypeptides would have an added margin of safety since they would be even less likely than the 22 nm particle subunit vaccines to contain infectious viruses, or contaminating host proteins, which might lead to untoward reactions in some individuals.

An alternative source of hepatitis B surface antigen is the use of antigen produced by cell lines derived from antigen-producing hepatocellular carcinoma. Here both the production and quality of the antigen may be more precisely controlled. Obviously rigorous purification of the antigen is essential to eliminate any contaminants, but the relatively simple biochemical composition of the cell line antigen and its ready availability make this an attractive source of material either for a highly purified intact 22nm particle vaccine or polypeptide vaccines.

The rapidly advancing field of recombinant DNA technology provides the possibility of producing large quantities of immunizing antigens in a prokaryotic system.

The third form of hepatitis

The specific laboratory diagnosis of hepatitis A and hepatitis B has revealed a previously unrecognized form of hepatitis which is clearly unrelated to either type, and it is referred to as non-A/non-B hepatitis. It is now the most common form of hepatitis occurring after blood transfusion and the administration of certain plasma derivatives in some areas of the world. The infection has also been transmitted experimentally to chimpanzees. Although specific laboratory tests for identifying this new type of hepatitis are not yet available and the diagnosis can only be made by exclusion, there is considerable information about the epidemiology of this infection. Non-A/non-B hepatitis has been found in every country in which it has been sought and it has a number of features in common with hepatitis B.

This form of hepatitis has been most commonly recognized as a complication of blood transfusion, and in countries where all blood donations are screened for hepatitis B surface antigen by very sensitive techniques, non-A/non-B hepatitis may account for up to 90 % of all cases of post-transfusion hepatitis. Outbreaks of non-A/non-B hepatitis have also been reported after the administration of blood clotting factors VIII and IX. Non-A/non-B hepatitis has occurred in haemodialysis and renal transplantation units and among drug addicts. In several countries a significant number of cases are not associated with transfusion and such sporadic cases of non-A/non-B hepatitis have been found to account for 15–20 % of all adult patients with viral hepatitis. In general, the illness is mild and often subclinical or anicteric. However, there is evidence that the infection may be followed by prolonged viraemia and the development of a persistent carrier state. Several recent studies of the histopathological sequelae of acute non-A/non-B infection indicate that chronic hepatitis may occur in as many as 40–50 % of the patients.

Clinical, epidemiological and experimental studies in a number of laboratories suggest that non-A/non-B hepatitis may be caused by 2 or more infectious agents. Clinical evidence is based on the observation of multiple attacks of hepatitis in individual patients. Epidemiologically, short-incubation and long-incubation forms of non-A/non-B hepatitis have been described, although it is possible that differences in the incubation period represent differences in the infective dose. Experimental evidence for the existence of at least 2 distinct non-A/non-B hepatitis viruses has been obtained from recent cross-challenge transmission studies in chimpanzees and the finding of 2 different types of ultrastructural cytoplasmic and nuclear changes in the hepatocytes of infected chimpanzees.

Serological procedures for antigens and antibodies specifically associated with this recently recognized form of viral hepatitis are under development.

General References

Dienstag JL, Purcell RH. Recent advances in the identification of hepatitis viruses. *Postgraduate Medical Journal* 1977; **53**: 364–73.

McColloum RW, Zuckerman AJ. *Viral hepatitis.* Report on a WHO internal consultation. *Journal of Medical Virology* 1981; **8**: 1–29.

World Health Organization. *Viral hepatitis.* Technical report series. No 570. Geneva: WHO, 1975.

World Health Organization. *Advances in viral hepatitis.* Technical report series. No 602. Geneva: WHO, 1977.

Zuckerman AJ. *Human viral hepatitis.* 2nd ed. Amsterdam: North Holland/Elsevier, 1975.

Zuckerman AJ. The three types of human viral hepatitis. *Bulletin of the World Health Organization* 1978; **56**: 1–20.

Zuckerman AJ. Specific serological diagnosis of viral hepatitis. *British Medical Journal* 1979; ii: 84–6.

Zuckerman AJ, Howard CR. *Hepatitis viruses of man.* London: Academic Press, 1979.

SECTION 2 · DISEASES OF THE HEART, BLOOD VESSELS AND BLOOD

Chapter 7 · Coronary Heart Disease

H TUNSTALL PEDOE

Definition and clinical problems

Coronary heart disease is the leading cause of death in economically advanced countries and the subject therefore of many epidemiological studies. The term is synonymous with ischaemic heart disease defined by the World Health Organization as 'the cardiac disability, acute or chronic, arising from reduction or arrest of blood supply to the myocardium in association with disease processes in the coronary arterial system.' As neither the blood supply to the myocardium, nor the coronary arteries, can be inspected in life without sophisticated investigations, the disease is usually recognized through its common syndromes. Non-atheromatous coronary disease is comparatively rare so that coronary heart disease usually implies atheroma. This consists of fatty deposits in the arterial wall which increase slowly in size, narrowing the arterial lumen. They may calcify or ulcerate providing a raw surface for thrombi to form, which can embolize or occlude the lumen. Critical narrowing of the lumen by atheroma, thrombus and/or spasm, (a recently rediscovered factor), cause regional myocardial ischaemia and infarction which predispose to fatal cardiac arrhythmias. The clinical syndromes of coronary heart disease are as follows.

1 *Angina pectoris* of effort. Usually a chronic and sometimes intermittent symptom detectable in prevalence surveys by symptom questionnaires[1].

2 *Cardiac (myocardial) infarction.* The clinical evidence of the pathological process is an acute episode characterized by central chest pain, serial electrocardiographic changes and raised serum levels of cardiac muscle enzymes[2]. Chest pain may be atypical or absent so that a proportion of attacks are misdiagnosed or are silent at the time. These may be detected later by looking for electrocardiographic evidence of old infarction. The electrocardiogram can be used in populations to measure the prevalence of old infarctions or, by repeated re-examination, the incidence of infarction.

3 *Sudden death* from coronary heart disease. Death from ventrical fibrillation or asystole may occur in subjects with severe coronary artery stenoses, with or without evidence at necropsy of recent cardiac infarction or coronary thrombosis. Most such deaths are instantaneous, but different studies have defined sudden death as death within 1 hour, 3 hours, 12 or 24 hours of the onset of acute symptoms.

Other manifestations of coronary heart disease include cardiac failure and non-fatal arrhythmias. Cardiac infarction is virtually specific to coronary heart disease; angina pectoris and sudden death are not, but in Western countries other causes are now comparatively rare. In other countries rheumatic heart disease and cardiomyopathy are potential sources of diagnostic confusion.

Sources and quality of data

Mortality rates are generally used to compare incidence of coronary heart disease where no specially mounted epidemiological study exists. The World Health Organization's International Classification of Diseases coding group for coronary heart disease (410–414) has remained unchanged since 1968 although specific items within the group were changed with the substitution of the Ninth for the Eighth Revision in 1979 (Table 7.1). In 1968 there was a break in disease coding since, prior to that date, the terms 'arteriosclerotic' and 'degenerative' heart disease were used. The discontinuity in terminology and coding is a source of difficulty in plotting long term mortality trends. The changes in classification reflect the progression of medical beliefs. Sudden cardiac deaths used to be ascribed to myocardial degeneration, angina, fatty heart, hypertension or arteriosclerosis. Nowadays myocardial infarction is frequently certified by doctors without pathological evidence of actual infarction. A more recent trend is to diagnose cardiac arrest and to record it on death certificates as the immediate cause of death.

Because most coronary deaths are sudden, 70–80 % occur outside hospital without diagnostic tests in life. In some Western countries they are usually the subject of medico-legal necropsy; in others this is exceptional. Necropsy criteria are not standardized and case series vary greatly in the reported proportion of coronary deaths showing infarction or thrombosis. In the absence of these, a diagnosis of death from coronary heart disease is based partly on the presence of coronary artery stenoses and partly on the exclusion of other causes of death such as drug overdose. Without a necropsy there is a tendency to over-diagnose coronary heart disease, to explain the sudden deterioration and death of subjects suffering from another longstanding illness or who have just had a major surgical operation.

Despite its importance coronary heart disease is not a notifiable disease and morbidity data are not routinely collected. Hospital discharge statistics depend on admission policies; many cases of infarction are looked after at home. The European Office of the World Health Organization coordinated the setting up of community myocardial infarction registers[2] in the early 1970s. These collate all cases of definite and possible myocardial infarction and sudden death coming to medical or medico-legal attention within defined communities and apply previously missing, uniform diagnostic criteria. (The attack rate and case fatality rate are very sensitive to differences in diagnostic criteria[3]). The results showed a

Table 7.1. International Classification of Diseases –changes in coding.

7th Edition (before 1968)		8th Edition (1968–78)		9th Edition (1979–)	
420–422	Arteriosclerotic & degenerative heart disease	410–414	Ischaemic heart disease (IHD)	410–414	Ischaemic heart disease (IHD)
420	Arteriosclerotic heart disease	410	Acute myocardial infarction	410	Acute myocardial infarction
421	Chronic non rheumatic carditis	411	Other acute and subacute IHD	411	Other acute and subacute IHD
422	Other myocardial degeneration	412	Chronic IHD	412	Old myocardial infarction
		413	Angina pectoris	413	Angina pectoris
440	Essential benign hypertensive heart disease (any condition in 422 with hypertension)	414	Asymptomatic IHD	414	Other forms of chronic IHD
		402	Hypertensive heart disease	402	Hypertensive heart disease
795	Sudden death (cause unknown)	795	Sudden death (cause unknown)	798	Sudden death (cause unknown)

good correlation between locally measured attack or incidence rates and nationally published mortality rates, validating the use of the latter for comparative purposes.

Strict comparison of morbidity rates, including angina pectoris, is possible only in special epidemiological studies. The Minnesota code for the electrocardiogram[1], developed specifically for epidemiological studies, enables bias-free estimates to be made of the prevalence rates of previous non-fatal cardiac infarction (using the Q and QS codes) and of myocardial ischaemia (ST and T wave codes). The London School of Hygiene[1] (Rose) questionnaire for chest pain on effort has proved to be a useful investigative tool for measuring the comparative prevalence of angina, although it is not entirely free of cultural bias because of subtleties in the meaning of words in different languages.

Mortality

In most Western countries deaths attributed to cardiovascular disease account for 50% of the total, and coronary heart disease for one-half to two-thirds of this proportion. It is thus the leading cause of death. Differences in coronary mortality rates between these countries account for much of the overall differences in mortality between nations, regions, social classes and ethnic groups, and by age and sex.

Mortality rates for coronary heart disease for England and Wales in 1977 are displayed in Fig. 7.1. Coronary heart disease in middle age is predominantly a male problem. The cumulative risk of death from coronary heart disease in men is 9% by the age of 65 and 19% by the age of 75 years. In women, breast cancer is of greater importance below the age of 65 years. The cumulative risk is 2.4% by the age of 65 and 8% by the age of 75 years.

International differences

Despite its predominance as a cause of death there are large international differences in mortality rates. These might be even greater if national statistics were available for the bulk of Afro-Asian countries, as coronary heart disease tends to be associated with affluence and routine vital statistics tend to be more complete in wealthy countries. National figures for 1977, (or the nearest available year), for certain countries for the age groups 35–74, age standardized to the population of England and Wales for 1977 are shown in Fig. 7.2[4]. In general, male and female rates are very different but highly correlated. The highest coronary mortality occurs in Northern Europe and in English-speaking countries, while Southern European rates are much lower, and those in Japan, albeit a rich industrialized country, are extremely low.

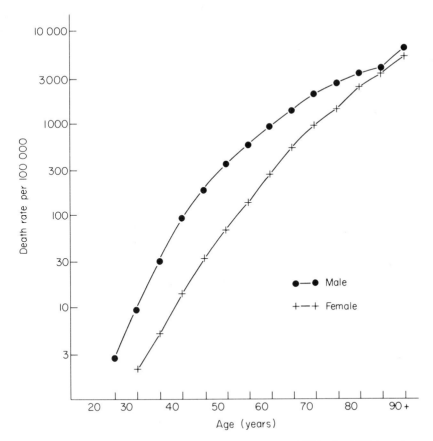

Fig. 7.1. Death rates from coronary heart disease in England and Wales for 1977 (note log scale)

Regional differences

National differences in mortality can be ascribed to cultural differences both in life-style and medical diagnosis; regional differences within one country are less easily dismissed. In Britain there is a large South-East to North-West gradient with low rates in the southern counties and very high rates in South Wales, around Glasgow and in Northern Ireland[5]. Many other countries report similar unexplained differences. In Finland there is a west to east gradient with the highest regional rates in the world in Karelia, against the Russian border.

Time differences

Coronary deaths occur throughout the 24 hours of the day but more occur between 8 and 10 in the morning and less in the very early morning. Slightly more

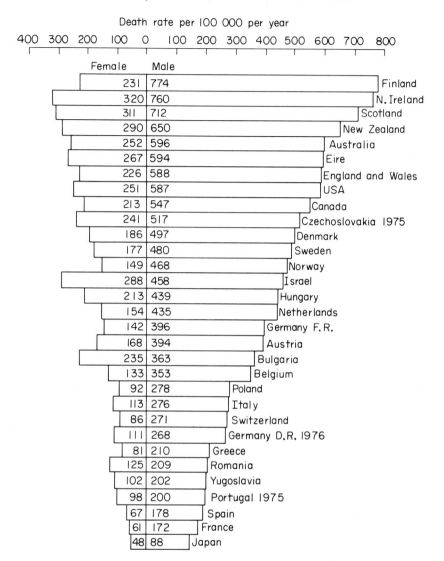

Fig. 7.2. Death rates from coronary heart disease in different countries. Rates for age 35–74 are standardized to the population of England and Wales in 1977. 1977 rates unless indicated.

occur on Mondays relative to other days[2]. In temperate countries coronary deaths increase in the winter months, and fluctuations can be attributed to periods of extreme cold but also, less often, to heat waves.

Long term trends in mortality are less easy to follow because of changes in certification and coding practice. Myocardial infarction was first described frequently from the USA between 1910 and 1920; case reports from elsewhere tended to come later. American coronary mortality was very high in the 1940s and 1950s, while those in European countries were climbing very rapidly. American male rates have been falling since the 1960s, so that they are now similar to those in England and Wales which have remained stable[6] (Fig. 7.3). Less marked declines have occurred in Canada, Australia, Finland and Belgium, while rates in Central and Eastern Europe and in many Afro-Asian countries are still rising. Male and female trends are not always parallel. In England and Wales, female rates apparently declined during the 1940s and 1950s, but there has been an increase in the last decade[7].

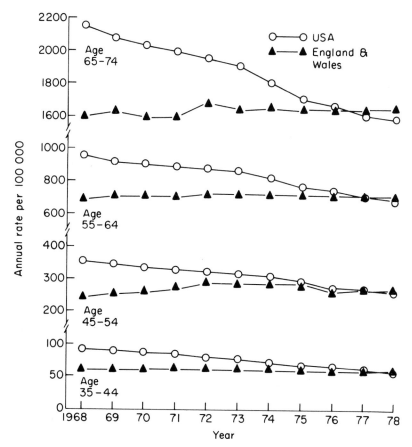

Fig. 7.3. Male death rates from coronary heart disease in the USA, and England and Wales, 1968–77.

Occupation, social class and ethnic group

Within coronary-prone cultures all sections of the community are susceptible, but several inequalities have been discovered. Many of the early case reports of coronary disease were described from Private Practice, and during the 1950s and 1960s it was considered to be a disease related to 'executive' life-style with manual labour acting as a protective factor. There is now evidence from several sources[8, 9] that professional and administrative workers are less susceptible than blue-collar workers so that coronary heart disease, like the bulk of other diseases has a positive social class gradient.

Cultural and genetic differences usually go together so that ethnic differences in susceptibility could be from either cause (hence the importance of migrant studies discussed later). Black Americans have less coronary disease when Whites although the gap is closing. In Britain the Tower Hamlets study in London[10] showed that West Indians had a very low coronary heart attack rate but in Bangladeshis it was high compared with native Londoners. Ethnic differences in susceptibility are difficult to demonstrate unless the size of different ethnic groups is recorded at census, as both numerator and denominator data are needed to calculate rates.

Incidence prevalence and natural history

Because of its different manifestations there are a number of different potential ways of reporting incidence rates for coronary heart disease within one population. If minor manifestations such as angina pectoris are included in the definition, repeated rescreening of the population is needed. In the Framingham study, with biennial examination, an annual incidence rate of 100 per 10 000 (1 %) was found in men aged 45–54 and 200 per 10 000 aged 55–64 and 65–74. In women rates were 30 per 10 000 at 45–54, 100 per 10 000 at 55–64, and 140 per 10 000 at 65–74[11]. However, repeated use of the Rose angina pectoris questionnaire has shown that many subjects are positive on one occasion and subsequently deny symptoms, so that the apparent incidence and period prevalence rates are linked to the frequency of examinations. Only a minority of questionnaire-positive angina sufferers consult doctors with their symptoms, so that the medically recorded incidence is only part of the total. This is also true of cardiac infarction which may be misdiagnosed or 'silent' in a proportion (estimated at 20–50 % of cases in different studies).

In the myocardial infarction community registers[2], all episodes of definite or possible infarction and sudden death that came to medical or medico-legal attention were included. In the London centre, Tower Hamlets[10], the attack rate was 100 per 10 000 per year in men aged 54–64 and 30 per 10 000 per year in women. Half of the attacks apparently occurred in the absence of a previous history of angina pectoris or infarction and were therefore presumed to be incidence cases; however, others were of equal interest and importance to the medical services, despite having had a previous history of coronary heart disease. The overall attack rate was, therefore, a more useful concept than incidence for some purposes.

The prevalence of coronary heart disease can be estimated from cross-sectional surveys. For example, in the United Kingdom Heart Disease Prevention Project[12] the prevalence of electrocardiographic evidence of old infarction (Q/QS items) was 0.9% in male industrial workers aged 40–59, while the proportion with a history of prolonged chest pain or possible infarction was 6.6%. Some 6.9% had other electrocardiographic signs of suspected ischaemic heart disease and 3.6% were positive to the angina questionnaire. The overlap between a positive history and electrocardiographic evidence of infarction was not very great. Only 23% of those who were positive for angina and 5% of those with a history of prolonged chest pain had ischaemic type electrocardiograms. Data from other European centres were comparable[12].

The natural history of coronary heart disease is highly variable as it is compatible with remission of symptoms and prolonged survival or with sudden death. The results from the heart attack registers[2] suggested that half of the clinical episodes of infarction or sudden death were preceded by angina pectoris or previous infarction, but repeated use of an angina questionnaire would raise the proportion with previous mild angina. The case fatality of a recognized attack was 35–40% at 28 days from onset (including all ages below 65) but would be lowered by inclusion of silent and misdiagnosed cases. Of the fatalities occurring within 28 days the majority were very rapid and in 69% death occurred at the place of onset (most frequently in the home) and often in the absence of an eye witness[3]. The survivors at 28 days ran an increased risk of further events amounting to 1% per month for the first year. By the end of the first year about 45% of attack victims had died. At 1 year over half of the survivors had angina pectoris, but most survivors had successfully returned to work. Those invalided out of work were a high risk group for subsequent fatal attacks. Coronary heart disease presents at a late stage in its natural history in many cases and there has therefore been intense epidemiological interest in its antecedents.

Aetiology and risk factors

Evidence that coronary heart disease has environmental determinants has come from observations of the wide differences in mortality between different countries, the large changes in mortality rates that have occurred over time and the fate of migrants. Of particular interest has been work on Japanese who have little coronary disease in Japan but acquire it after living in California. Other immigrant groups have also been studied with similar results.

Major risk factors

The characteristics identifying subjects at increased risk of coronary disease, or risk factors (Table 7.2), have been studied prospectively within high incidence

Table 7.2. Risk factors for coronary heart disease.

Major established factors*	Less established factors†
Individual	
Sex	High density lipoprotein cholesterol
Age	Other lipids
Blood pressure	Glucose intolerance, insulin levels
Serum (plasma) cholesterol	Obesity
Cigarette smoking	Physical activity
	Psycho-social factors
	Social class
	Social mobility
	Ethnic group
	Personality type
	Familial factors
	Contraceptive pill
	Clotting factors and fibrinolysis
	Diet
Group	
Diet	Water hardness

* Consistently shown to be powerful factors in many different studies over many years.
† Inconsistent, less powerful, less commonly or more recently investigated, or factors in which epidemiological techniques are poorly developed.

populations. A number of American studies have pooled their results[13] and these suggest that in middle-aged men 3 major factors predominate and these are of equal and independent predictive power; blood pressure (systolic or diastolic), cigarette consumption and serum or plasma cholesterol (Fig. 7.4). In each case the gradient of risk between those in the top and bottom fifths (or quintiles) of the population distribution is 2.5:1. Assessment of individual risk must be based on consideration of all 3 factors. A large British study showed similar results[14].

The determinants of risk within populations may not be the same as those between populations. In the Seven Countries Study an attempt was made to explain international differences in coronary incidence in terms of known coronary risk factors[15]. The results showed that hypertension, obesity, physical inactivity and cigarette smoking were prevalent in all the cohorts studied, but that serum cholesterol distributions varied so much that there was little overlap between that recorded in southern Japan, with the least coronary disease, and in East Finland with the most. There was a good correlation between mean serum cholesterol and coronary incidence. Mean serum cholesterol correlated with the percentage of food energy from saturated fat. Thus, international differences in coronary mortality may be explained by the dietary-fat theory.

Dietary-fat theory

Central to this theory is the serum cholesterol which is thought to contribute to the development and growth of atheromatous plaques. The serum cholesterol level of individuals and groups can be modified through dietary change. Saturated fats tend to increase it (as does dietary cholesterol) while poly-unsaturated (unmodified vegetable or fish oils) will lower it[16]. The logical conclusion of this theory is that coronary-prone societies should adopt cholesterol lowering diets, by reducing their intake of animal fats and dairy products and substituting vegetables, cereals and oils. The strength of the theory is that observations in the Seven Countries Study (among others) fitted it well: the Japanese had low fat diets, low serum cholesterols and low incidence while the

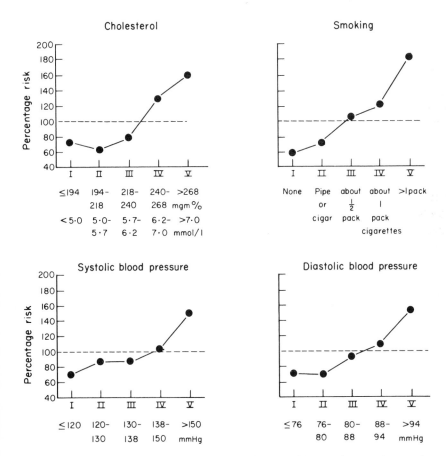

Fig. 7.4. Risk of major coronary event by initial risk factor level. Data refers to 658 events in 8381 men aged 40–64 followed on average 8½ years. Each data point concerns one-fifth (quintile) of the population except in smoking where groups are unequal. (Pooling project research group).

East Finns were at the other extreme. Also metabolic experiments confirm that levels of serum cholesterol can be modified by diets consistent with the international data. The weaknesses of the theory are that quite major differences in coronary mortality apparently occur in populations with similar fat intakes and cholesterol levels, that serum cholesterol can be changed only by a moderate percentage even with large changes in diet, and that no study has shown that, within groups, individual fat intake accounts either for individual cholesterol level, or for future susceptibility to coronary disease, although this may be related to problems of measurement of individual diet.

The dietary fat theory has major implications for the agricultural and food processing industries who have made much of its apparent weaknesses. However, there does not at present appear to be an alternative theory which is as comprehensive in its explanation of the aetiology of coronary heart disease.

High density lipoprotein cholesterol

Different lipid fractions in the blood are now known to behave differently so that the serum cholesterol, a robust standardized measurement that can be made in the non-fasting state, now appears rather crude. The high density lipoprotein cholesterol (HDL) correlates inversely with coronary risk and all the experiments on modifying total cholesterol are now being repeated whilst measuring HDL. Alcohol, exercise, weight loss and stopping smoking have all been claimed to raise HDL and it is higher in women, but HDL levels in different populations do not correlate perfectly with coronary risk and are less variable than low density lipoprotein cholesterol. In the past the *triglycerides* were claimed to be an independent risk factor; these are inversely related to HDL in some studies and so their effect is difficult to distinguish from it.

Polyunsaturated fats

These have functions other than their weak one in lowering serum cholesterol and there has been recent renewed interest in clotting factors and fibrinolysis in relation to diet and as coronary risk factors[17]. The distinction between saturated and polyunsaturated fats in their effects on cholesterol levels is a simplification as different specific fatty acids have different effects. There may be other dietary factors with effects on circulating lipids, for example, in milk and in fermented milk. The way food is prepared and eaten may be important.

Obesity

Obesity did not appear important in some prospective studies once cholesterol and blood pressure had been taken into account but other studies suggest that it is[18].

Glucose intolerance

This is unimportant in population terms except for a small percentage of people at the high end of the distribution. The suggestion that coronary disease is caused by consumption of refined sugar has little epidemiological evidence to support it compared with that for saturated fat.

Family

There is undoubtedly a strong familial element in susceptibility to coronary heart disease but evidence as to how much of this is mediated by the major recognized risk factors and how much by other means is conflicting. A familial tendency to coronary disease could be mediated by a genetic element, as probably occurs in blood pressure, or by shared environmental factors and habits such as cigarette smoking or diet. The genetic contribution to cholesterol level does not appear great since those of identical twins are not particularly similar. Inherited hyperlipidaemias are comparatively rare.

Physical activity

This may have a protective role. The effect of physical activity at work now appears to be small as manual workers have more coronary disease than non-manual workers. Leisure time activity both in British civil servants[19] and Harvard graduates appears to be protective but the effect is not so strong as to cancel out other risk factors.

Psycho-social factors

Psychosocial factors are difficult to measure. An American study has found that individuals with aggressive, competitive personalities who are always setting themselves deadlines have a high risk of coronary heart disease independent of other factors[20]. The study is being repeated elsewhere with varying results. It has also been shown from California that those Japanese who have similar risk factor levels to Americans but have retained traditional Japanese attitudes and life-styles have less coronary disease[21]. The importance of social class in Britain has already been mentioned. Americans have less data and find the subject embarassing, but they claim that social mobility increases coronary risk.

Oral contraceptives

The risk of myocardial infarction in women seems to be increased by oral contraceptives and the effect is additional to that of smoking[22]. There is some argument about whether the oestrogen or progesterone component is of greater importance; the role of both male and female sex hormones in relation to coronary risk is under investigation.

Regional factors

The large regional differences in coronary mortality have been related in several countries to water hardness, the higher mortality occurring in soft water areas. However, in Britain water hardness also correlates with rainfall, latitude and various socio-economic factors. The Regional Heart Study of the Medical Research Council is attempting to unravel this important problem and results from it are beginning to appear[23].

Treatment, prevention and control

The workload

A large proportion of angina pectoris and cardiac infarction is not recognized clinically but nonetheless coronary heart disease accounts for a significant proportion of the caseload of both general practitioners and acute hospitals. In 1971 coronary heart disease accounted for 1.6 % of consultations in General Practice; angina pectoris made up a quarter of this[24]. Now that angina pectoris is more intensively treated with beta-blockers it probably involves a higher proportion of consultations.

In 1975 in England and Wales an estimated 90 480 hospital discharges and deaths were attributed to myocardial infarction, 1.9 % of the total discharges from acute non-psychiatric hospitals. The average length of stay was 18 days with a median of 13 and on an average day 4400 hospital beds were so occupied, 2.4 % of the total. Other ischaemic heart disease, much of it probably admitted as possible myocardial infarction, led to another 47 000 discharges and deaths and because of a longer length of stay (averaging 24 days) needed 3200 beds, so that 4 % of acute hospital beds were occupied with coronary patients[25]. However, the proportion of patients with non-fatal myocardial infarction admitted to hospital varies as the different British community studies have shown[10, 26, 27, 28]. Over the decade 1965–75 discharge rates increased rapidly but by 1975 they were stabilizing. Length of stay fell steadily while hospital fatality rates fell contemporaneously with the rise in discharges. The number of deaths in hospital increased slightly.

Treatment objectives

Angina pectoris and cardiac infarction are both painful conditions and relief of pain is a major objective of treatment. However, the association of both conditions with a high mortality has led to the introduction of different treatments aimed at reducing the risk of death.

In cardiac infarction, bed rest, anti-coagulant therapy and anti-arrhythmic treatment in a coronary care unit have all been introduced as major life-saving procedures but in each case the original claims have not been substantiated, so that the life-saving element of hospital treatment remains in doubt[29]. Coronary care units were introduced to detect warning arrhythmias which presaged ventricular fibrillation. It is now known that these are often benign, are often missed by the nurse observers, and that ventricular fibrillation often occurs without any warning. Because 50 % or more of fatalities occur within 1 hour of the fatal attack and the median patient may take 4 hours to reach hospital[10], the great majority of coronary deaths occur outside hospital and many are not witnessed. Mobile coronary care units may be cost-effective compared with other emergency services, but their successes constitute a small percentage of the potentially fatal attacks even in the best centres[30], while results in some centres have led to their disbandment. Therefore, these units cannot be any more than a very partial answer to the problem of sudden death.

Patients are also admitted to hospital for coronary artery bypass surgery. This is a major activity in richer countries, so far practised less, but on an increasing scale in Britain. The objective is pain relief for angina but with the hope that the angina related mortality is also reduced. A number of studies suggest that the operation does reduce subsequent mortality in certain subgroups with serious anatomical lesions. However, a proportion of patients with poorly functioning heart muscle are unsuitable for surgery.

Primary and secondary prevention

With the disillusionment following the early promise of coronary care units, and the limitations posed by cost on coronary artery bypass surgery, there is increasing interest in intervention in the presymtomatic and early stages of coronary artery disease, in contrast to end-stage resuscitation and salvage.

Early trials of coronary disease prevention concentrated on one factor at a time. Two early trials of primary prevention employed dietary methods to lower cholesterol levels and resulted in a reduction of coronary events, but both were open to criticism[31, 32]. Dietary trials in secondary prevention have yielded mixed results[33, 34, 35]. Lowering of cholesterol levels by drugs has also been attempted. These have been unsuccessful in secondary prevention[36, 37] but in a recent large trial of the drug 'clofibrate' there was a significant reduction in non-fatal cardiac infarction. Unfortunately, an almost equal excess of gastro-intestinal deaths occurred in the treated group[38].

Those who stop smoking after cardiac infarction have a lower subsequent risk than those who continue to smoke. The risk appears to be halved. A large reduction in subsequent coronary risk also appears to occur in young and early middle-aged men who stop smoking before developing coronary disease. Unfortunately, these are observational findings rather than trials. The only large randomized controlled trial in smoking cessation is concerned with primary prevention of coronary disease and final results are not yet known[39].

Early trials of blood pressure reduction showed minor non-significant reductions in coronary events while stroke rates were grossly reduced[40]. However, the recent American Hypertension Detection and Follow-up Trial[41] (discussed further in Chapter 8) has shown substantial reductions in coronary mortality through a programme of stepped care for hypertension.

Other drug trials both of lipid-lowering drugs and hypotensive medication are in progress. In addition to these there is considerable interest in drugs which interfere with platelet function such as aspirin and sulphinpyrazone; some successes are claimed for both in secondary prevention. Beta-blocking drugs are also being evaluated as hypotensive agents and in the prevention of fatal arrhythmias. The results of secondary prevention with beta-blockers have been inconsistent from drug to drug, large apparent benefits occur with some and insignificant or no benefits with others. Further trial results are being reported every few months.

Recently, emphasis has swung away from the unifactorial to the multi-factorial approach[42] as being more consistent with the known aetiology of coronary heart disease, and from hospital clinic-based to community-based interventions. A large scale collaborative European trial of risk factor screening and intervention in industry is in progress[12]. Results available from the first individual centre to report, the United Kingdom Heart Disease Prevention Project, suggest that risk factor changes are poorly sustained without continued strong intervention[43]. In the USA a more intensive trial, confined to individuals identified as at high risk, the Multiple Risk Factor Intervention Trial (MRFIT),[44] is in progress. A third multifactorial trial is being run in Gothenberg, in Sweden, using randomly allocated members of a defined community[45].

At the same time that randomized trials of individuals or factory groups have been in progress, investigators in Stanford California and in Finnish Karelia have been attempting coronary prevention programme in whole communities. The first Stanford project suggested that widespread use of the media for health propaganda, with some personal challenge, could cause significant changes in risk factor levels in the test towns, compared with control communities, but the towns used were too small to study the effects on incidence[46]. A larger trial is now in progress. In the North Karelia project, intervention was attempted in the Finnish county with the highest coronary mortality in the world, at the request of the local population. Over 5 years significant falls in the prevalence of the 3 major risk factors occurred, compatible with a net reduction in risk of 17 % in men and

12 % in women. The incidence of myocardial infarction fell by 16 % in men and by 5 % in women while that of stroke fell 38 % in men and 50 % in women. North Karelia had been compared with a neighbouring county where, paradoxically, although the health education campaign had not taken place, similar reductions in coronary event rates also occurred; it is probable that this county was contaminated by the local and national interest in the project, but it does make interpretation difficult. However, the North Karelia project did demonstrate that coronary prevention campaigns are feasible, given a receptive population, and that they are compatible with a decline in coronary events[47, 48].

For a number of technical reasons the perfect coronary prevention trial may never be done. It is not surprising that the multi-factorial prevention message for coronary disease is meeting slow acceptance when the simpler and more powerful connection between cigarette smoking and major diseases has taken decades to seriously influence public behaviour and attitudes. Meanwhile a debate is in progress between the doubters and academics who feel that information is inadequate for widescale application of epidemiological knowledge[49] and the men of action who feel that to prevaricate in the face of a major epidemic and ignore the implications of aetiological research is foolhardy and negligent[50].

References

1. Rose GA, Blackburn H. *Cardiovascular survey methods.* Geneva: World Health Organization, 1968.
2. World Health Organization. Regional Office for Europe. *Myocardial infarction community registers.* Public health in Europe 5. Copenhagen: WHO, 1976.
3. Tunstall Pedoe H. Uses of coronary heart attack registers. *British Heart Journal* 1978; **40**: 510–15.
4. World Health Organization. *World Health Statistics Annual.* Geneva: WHO, 1979, 1980, 1981.
5. Fulton M, Adams W, *et al.* Regional variations in mortality from ischaemic heart and cerebrovascular disease in Britain. *British Heart Journal* 1978; **40**: 563–8.
6. Havlik RJ, Feinleib M, eds. *Proceedings of the Conference on the Decline in Coronary Heart Disease Mortality.* DHEW No (NIH) 79–1610. Washington: US Government Printing Office, 1979.
7. Clayton DG, Taylor D, Shaper AG. Trends in heart disease in England and Wales 1950–73. *Health Trends* 1977; **9**: 1–6.
8. Marmot MG, Adelstein AM, *et al.* Changing social class distributions of heart disease. *British Medical Journal* 1978; **ii**: 1109–12.
9. Marmot MG, Rose G, *et al.* Employment grade and coronary heart disease in British civil servants. *Journal of Epidemiology and Community Health* 1978; **32**: 244–9.
10. Tunstall Pedoe H, Clayton D, *et al.* Coronary heart attacks in East London. *Lancet* 1975; **ii**: 833–8.
11. Shurtleff D. *Framingham Study. Section 30. Some characteristics related to the incidence of cardiovascular disease and death: Framingham Study 18-year follow-up.* DHEW No (NIH) 74–599. Washington: US Government Printing Office, 1974.
12. World Health Organization European Collaborative Group. Multifactorial trial in the prevention of coronary heart disease: 1. Recruitment and initial findings. *European Heart Journal* 1970; **1**: 73–9.

13. Pooling Project Research Group. Relationship of blood pressure, serum cholesterol, smoking habit, relative weight and e.c.g. abnormalities to incidence of major coronary events: final report of the pooling project. *Journal of Chronic Diseases* 1978; **31**: 201–306.
14. Reid DD, Hamilton PJS, *et al.* Smoking and other risk factors for coronary heart disease in British civil servants. *Lancet* 1974; **ii**: 979–84.
15. Keys A, ed. Coronary heart disease in seven countries. *Circulation* 1970; **41** (Suppl. 1).
16. Tunstall Pedoe H, Rose G. Atherosclerosis as related to diet. In Neuberger A, Jukes TH, eds. Biochemistry of nutrition II. *International review of biochemistry*. Baltimore: University Park Press, 1979.
17. Meade TW. Diet and ischaemic heart disease. In Bennett AE, ed. *Recent advances in community medicine*. London: Churchill Livingstone, 1978: 20–36.
18. Garrow JS. Weight penalties. *British Medical Journal* 1979; **ii**: 1171–2.
19. Morris JN. Physical exercise. In Tybjaerg Hansen A, Schnohr P, Rose G, eds. *Ischaemic heart disease: the strategy of postponement*. Copenhagen: FADL Forlag, 1977.
20. Rosenman R, Friedman M, *et al.* Coronary heart disease in the Western Collaboration Group Study. *JAMA* 1966; **195**: 86–92.
21. Marmot MG, Syme SL. Acculturation and coronary heart disease in Japanese-Americans. *American Journal of Epidemiology* 1976; **104**: 225–47.
22. Mann JI, Inman WHW, Thorogood M. Oral contraceptive use in older women and fatal myocardial infarction. *British Medical Journal* 1976; **ii**: 445–7.
23. Pocock SJ, Shaper AG, *et al.* British Regional Heart Study: geographic variations in cardiovascular mortality and the role of water quality. *British Medical Journal* 1980; **ii**: 1243–8.
24. Office of Population Censuses and Surveys. *Morbidity statistics from General Practice 1970–71*. London: HMSO, 1974.
25. Office of Population Censuses and Surveys. *Hospital Inpatient Enquiry Main Tables 1975*. Department of Health and Social Security. London: HMSO, 1978.
26. Kinlen LJ. Incidence and presentation of myocardial infarction in an English community. *British Heart Journal* 1973; **35**: 616–22.
27. Armstrong A, Duncan B, *et al.* Natural history of acute coronary heart attacks – a community study. *British Heart Journal* 1972; **34**: 67–80.
28. Colling A, Dellipiani AW, *et al.* Teeside Coronary Survey: an epidemiological study of acute attacks of myocardial infarction. *British Medical Journal* 1976; **ii**: 1169–72.
29. Rose G. Contribution of intensive coronary care. *British Journal of Preventive Social Medicine* 1975; **29**: 147–50.
30. Briggs RS, Brown PM, *et al.* The Brighton resuscitation ambulances: a continuing experiment in pre-hospital care by ambulance staff. *British Medical Journal* 1976; **ii**: 1161–5.
31. Dayton S, Pearce ML, *et al.* A controlled clinical trial of a diet high in unsaturated fat in preventing complications of atherosclerosis. *Circulation* 1969; **40** (2): (I–II) 63.
32. Turpeinen O, Karvonen MJ, *et al.* Dietary prevention of coronary heart disease: The Finnish Mental Hospital study. *International Journal of Epidemiology* 1979; **8**, 99–118.
33. Research Committee. Low fat diet in myocardial infarction. *Lancet* 1965; **ii**: 501–4.
34. Research Committee to the Medical Research Council. Controlled trial of soya-bean oil in myocardial infarction. *Lancet* 1968; **ii**: 693–700.
35. Leren P. Effect of plasma cholesterol lowering diet in male survivors of myocardial infarction – a controlled clinical trial. *Acta Medica Scandinavica* 1966; **466** (Suppl.): 1–92.
36. Dewar HA, Oliver MF. Secondary prevention trials using clofibrate: a joint commentary on the Newcastle and Scottish trials. *British Medical Journal* 1971; **iv**: 784–6.
37. Coronary Drug Project Research Group. Clofibrate and niacin in coronary heart disease. *JAMA* 1975; **231**: 360–81.
38. Committee of Principal Investigators. A cooperative trial in the primary prevention of ischaemic heart disease using clofibrate. *British Heart Journal* 1978; **40**: 1069–118.
39. Rose G, Hamilton PJS. A randomized controlled trial of the effect on middle-aged men of advice to stop smoking. *Journal of Epidemiology and Community Health* 1978; **32**: 275–81.

40. Veterans Admin. Cooperative Study Group. Effects of treatment on morbidity in hypertension. *JAMA* 1970; **213**: 1143–52.

41. Hypertension Detection and Follow-up Program Cooperative Group. Five year findings of the Hypertension Detection and Follow-up Program. 1. Reduction in Mortality of persons with high blood pressure including mild hypertension. *JAMA* 1979; **242**: 2562–76.

42. Joint Working Party of the Royal College of Physicians of London and the British Cardiac Society. Prevention of coronary heart disease. *Journal of the Royal College of Physicians* 1976; **10**: 213–75.

43. Rose G, Heller RF, *et al.* Heart disease prevention project: a randomized controlled trial in industry. *British Medical Journal* 1980; **ii**: 747–51.

44. MRFIT collaborating investigators. The Multiple Risk Factor Intervention Trial (MRFIT). *JAMA* 1976; **235**: 825–7.

45. Wilhelmsen L, Tibblin G, Werko L. A primary prevention study in Gothenburg, Sweden. *Preventive Medicine* 1972; **1**: 153–60.

46. Farquhar JW, Maccoby N, *et al.* Community education for cardiovascular health. *Lancet* 1977; **i**: 1192–5.

47. Puska P, Tuomilehto J, *et al.* Changes in coronary risk factors during comprehensive five-year community programme to control cardiovascular disease (North Karelia project). *British Medical Journal* 1979; **ii**: 1173–7.

48. Salonen JT, Puska P, Mustaniemi H. Changes in morbidity and mortality during comprehensive community programme to control cardiovascular diseases during 1972–7 in North Karelia. *British Medical Journal* 1979; **ii**: 1178–83.

49. Mann GV. Diet heart: end of an era. *New England Journal of Medicine* 1977; **297**: 644–50.

50. Blackburn H. Diet and mass hyperlipidemia: a public health view. In Levy R, Rifkind BM, *et al.* eds. *Nutrition, lipids and coronary heart disease.* New York: Raven Press, 1979.

Chapter 8 · Hypertension

H TUNSTALL PEDOE

The association of left ventricular hypertrophy with contracted kidneys in man was recognized in the early 19th century. Stephen Hales had measured the blood pressure of a horse by arterial cannulation 100 years earlier. However, it was not until Riva Rocci invented his indirect mercury sphygmomanometer and then Korotkov described the sounds heard over the brachial artery during sphygmomanometry in 1905 that blood pressure measurements became well established.

The initial preoccupation was with hypertension as a disease, a condition with characteristic symptoms and signs and a distinct natural history. For patients with severe and malignant hypertension this was a valid concept. They presented with heart failure or organ damage, with retinal signs, renal impairment and albuminuria, and the prognosis was as devastating as that of an inoperable cancer. Because of this blood pressure measurement became an established part of medical and life insurance examinations.

With information from life insurance examination and with the development of effective and tolerable drugs for controlling blood pressure, has come progressive interest in lesser degrees of hypertension and in its natural history, and in whether it is changed by medication. The distinction between the hypertensive and normotensive state is now disputed for a number of reasons. The distribution of blood pressure in the population follows a normal curve skewed to the right. Risk appears to rise smoothly with each increment of pressure across the whole range. The point at which normal blood pressure becomes abnormal or raised is simply that at which either risk becomes unacceptable or treatment desirable. Criteria for these levels may be different for different age and sex groups and may change with time.

The popular presumed symptoms of hypertension are feelings of tension, anxiety and headache. Because both undiagnosed mild and moderate hypertension and such symptoms are highly prevalent in the population, they frequently occur together and the popular impression is reinforced. (By contrast in central Europe the disease of hypotension is widely diagnosed and associated with symptoms of fatigue and lassitude). However, population studies suggest that there are no symptoms indicative of the level of blood pressure, unless it is severely raised, nor are there very specific personality types or emotional states associated with it. Finally, the bulk of cardiovascular morbidity and mortality associated with hypertension is not usually attributed to it.

For all these reasons hypertension should be considered more as a risk factor for cardiovascular disease than a disease entity in itself. It is easier to define in statistical and epidemiological terms than as a diagnosis. The difficulty is further illustrated by the problem of variability and measurement of blood pressure.

Variability and measurement

Continuous recording of blood pressure in individuals using in-dwelling arterial catheters and portable tape-recorders has shown wide diurnal and minute-to-minute fluctuations with peaks during arousal, pain and isometric exercise, and troughs during relaxation, rest and sleep.[1] Blood pressure is also affected by posture, the ambient temperature and other circumstances at the time of measurement. The initial reading in an individual tends to be higher than subsequent ones, hospital clinic readings are greater than those recorded outside, and those recorded by an unfamiliar observer of a different sex or race to the patient also tend to be raised. There is considerable variability between different observers, some of which is systematic and can be minimized by standardizing the circumstances and technique of measurement and by training of staff.

For epidemiological studies it is recommended that blood pressure is recorded in standard circumstances. These usually are after 5 minutes rest in one specified posture and with no food, smoking, pain or exercise within the previous half hour.[2] The arm should be supported. Although several automatic electronic blood pressure measurement devices are available and may one day supersede it, the standard technique is still indirect sphygmomanometry using the mercury column sphygmomanometer and a stethoscope to listen for Korotkov sounds.

Two modified instruments are available for epidemiological research. The London School of Hygiene sphygmomanometer[3] is designed to obviate several sources of inaccuracy. It is equipped with a levelling device; inflation and deflation are automatic, the latter at a controlled rate of descent of 2mm per second, and readings of systolic and diastolic points are made blindly by freezing the descent of the mercury columns, their heights being measured subsequently using a mirror to minimize parallax error. Although the most sophisticated of its type this machine is less portable than the 'Random Zero Machine'[4] which is more widely used. A zero error is introduced to prevent the observer interpreting and censoring outlying readings before they are recorded; the zero error is then subtracted. Mercury sphygmomanometers, although simple in design, need to be regularly serviced and checked, like all blood pressure devices, as they are subject to sticking valves and blocked air filters which cause spurious readings. An appropriate sized inflatable cuff should be used, 12–14 cm wide for the average adult and long enough to go most of the way round the arm. Criteria must be established for the systolic and diastolic (phase 4 muffling of sounds or phase 5 disappearance of sounds). Observers should be trained and tested, and retested during the survey. Tape recordings are available for this purpose.[5]

If attempts have been made to minimize systematic observer error and bias, the blood pressure distribution of a population can be characterized accurately by single readings taken from an appropriately sized random sample of subjects. It is less easy to characterize the blood pressure of individuals as the standard deviation of measurements within subjects can be more than half as great as that between subjects.[6] A single reading is a sample of the personal range and may lead to a wrong estimate of that person's place in the population distribution. The more readings that are averaged the greater the precision of the estimate.

Within-person variability is responsible for the phenomenon of regression to the mean. A proportion of subjects classified on a single reading as being above a certain cut-off point will have been misclassified, and on repeating the reading in those subjects, the mean value will tend to be nearer to the mean of the original group; it will appear to have fallen. This phenomenon must be allowed for in any trial of treatment.

Clinical observation of the variability of blood pressure in some subjects has given rise to the idea that labile hypertension is a distinct condition. All blood pressure fluctuates and the higher it is, the more variable in absolute units for the same proportionate change. Some subjects may react more than others to having their pressure measured, but they are not physiologically or prognostically distinct from other subjects.

The inaccuracy of single base-line readings in characterizing individuals means that the importance of blood pressure as a risk factor may be underestimated; a better estimate of an individual's long term pressure than a single reading should be more discriminatory.[7]

Incidence, prevalence and mortality

The concept of incidence has limited value in hypertension because of the variability of consecutive readings in individuals. If repeated measurements are made, some normal subjects will cross an arbitrary threshold value to become cases, but a number of cases will now cease to be so by having lower readings. Instead, population distributions have been plotted for different age groups in cross-sectional studies, and prospective studies have been done to follow the phenomenon of 'tracking', that is, how consistently an individual's blood pressure remains in the same percentile of the distribution, over a period of years.

In Western populations mean blood pressure and the dispersion of readings rise with age. There is a tendency for individuals to retain the same place in the overall distribution but the pressure in those with initially high readings tends to rise faster than in those at the low end of the range. The prevalence of hypertension therefore rises with age. The prevalence of severe hypertension is low, but that for moderate hypertension is high, and for mild hypertension it is very high. However, any specific figure is meaningful only if the circumstances of

measurement and the diagnostic criteria have been specified. A cumulative
frequency distribution graph shows how the prevalence rises as the threshold
criterion is lowered. (Fig. 8.1). Either systolic or diastolic criteria can be used, or
both, in which case a multi-dimensional graph would be needed.

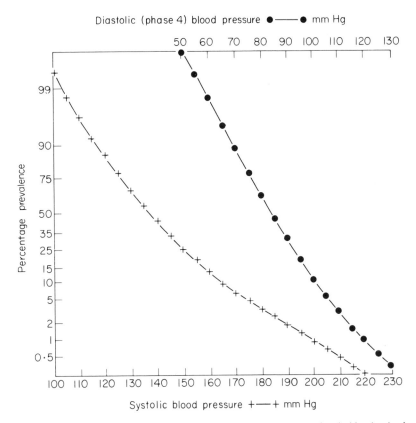

Fig. 8.1. Percentage prevalence of hypertension by systolic or diastolic threshold value in the
UK. (Data from men aged 40–59 in UK Heart Disease Prevention Project.)

Mortality rates from hypertension are misleading as it is a condition so
frequently not recognized in life, or recognized but left off the death certificate.
Out of 575 928 deaths in England and Wales in 1977, only 7225 (1.3%) were
coded to hypertensive disease (World Health Organization International
Classification of Diseases (ICD) codes 400–404) of which 200 were coded as
malignant hypertension[8]. However, hypertension was mentioned on the death
certificates of 13 432 deaths attributed to ischaemic heart disease and 10 110
stroke deaths. By contrast there were 292 596 deaths from all cardiovascular
causes. It is epidemiological research rather than routinely collected data that has

demonstrated that hypertension is a major and grossly underreported factor in cardiovascular mortality.

Risk

The excess risk of death in severe hypertension was readily recognizable from clinical case series, but the extent of disease associated with all levels of hypertension was only demonstrated through large scale follow-up studies such as pooled life insurance data in the Build and Blood Pressure Study, and prospective epidemiological studies of which the Framingham Study is the most extensively reported. Fig. 8.2 shows smoothed curves for mortality rates from all

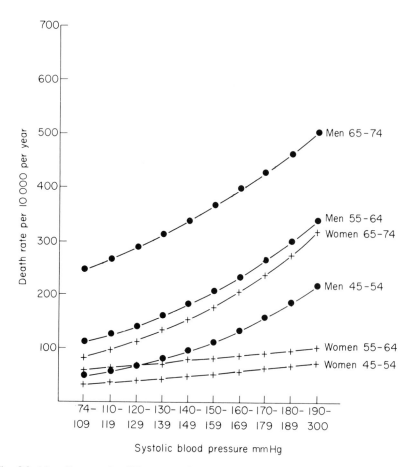

Fig. 8.2. Mortality rates for different systolic blood pressure levels. Framingham data[9]. Age-standardized smoothed rates for men and women aged 45–74.

causes for men and women in the 10 year age groups from 45–74 in the Framingham Study[9] in relation to systolic blood pressure.

All age-groups and both sexes show a gradient of risk with increasing blood pressure. Men aged 55 –64 years can be used as an example. Risk of death from any cause rises smoothly with no clear threshold; that in the highest class, above 190 mm of mercury is 340 per 10 000 per year, while those below 110 mm of mercury had a death rate of 111 per 10 000 per year. The relative risk of death is 3 times greater in the highest pressure group while the excess, or attributable risk, is 230 per 10 000 per year (over 2% per year). However, a graph such as this does not reveal the numbers of subjects in each class. Because of the skewed normal distribution curve the bulk of the population is concentrated in the intermediate blood pressure classes, and the majority of deaths attributable to blood pressure do not therefore occur at the extreme but at, and just above, average pressures where large numbers of subjects are exposed to a modest increase in risk. By subtraction of the risk in the lowermost class from that for all classes combined (181 per 10 000 per year) it is possible to calculate the population attributable risk as 70 per 10 000 per year (over a third of total mortality) and therefore the amount by which mortality might be diminished if the observed effects were completely reversible.

Fig. 8.2 illustrates some other important findings. For the same blood pressure and age men have a worse prognosis. Although the relative risk, the ratio between the right and left hand ends of each graph, diminishes with age, the attributable risk increases. As the mean blood pressure rises with age the population attributable risk rises even faster. These figures give some idea of mortality in the community attributable to hypertension, but the estimates are inevitably imprecise. Mortality rates at the extremes of blood pressure are based on small numbers and deviate from the ideal model curve. The raw results for men aged 65–74 are drawn in over the smoothed curve as an example; the first point is based-on 8 deaths and the second on 5. However, all prospective studies in Western populations have shown that death rates rise with blood pressure. The calculated risks are dependent on the age and sex of the subjects and the proportion of the population placed in the different classes at the extremes.

The variable used in Fig. 8.2 is the systolic blood pressure which has been found, despite past clinical teaching to the contrary, to be as good a predictor of prognosis as the diastolic pressure. The systolic blood pressure, diastolic phase IV (muffling) and diastolic phase V (disappearance of sounds) all produce a similar picture, which is not surprising as they are highly correlated.

The nature of the excess mortality associated with hypertension varies, but the bulk of it appears to be cardiovascular. In Western countries it is mainly coronary heart disease with stroke, heart failure, and aortic aneurysms also prominent. In Japan the main risk is stroke. Not only does blood pressure correlate with excess cardiovascular mortality, it also correlates with many causes of morbidity such as myocardial infarction, angina pectoris, intermittent

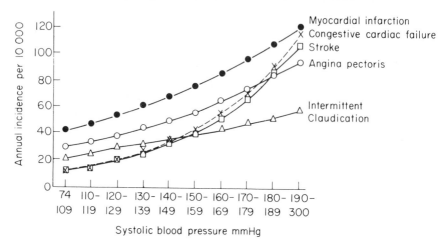

Fig. 8.3. Incidence rates for myocardial infarction, angina pectoris, stroke, intermittent claudication and congestive cardiac failure at different systolic blood pressure levels. Framingham data[9]. Age standardized smoothed rates for men aged 45–74.

claudication, stroke and congestive heart failure. The last two have particularly steep gradients of risk[9] (Fig. 8.3).

Aetiology

The younger the subject and the more severe the hypertension, the higher the probability that it is secondary to some identifiable and possibly even reversible cause such as renal abnormality, coarctation of the aorta or adrenal tumour. The great bulk of the symptomless mild and moderate hypertension of middle-aged Western man is primary or essential hypertension.[10] This would not be true in populations with a high prevalence of renal disease. Essential hypertension is unexplained but there are a number of clues. It could be multifactorial in causation or represent a common end-point for several mechanisms.

Genetics

Studies on inheritance of blood pressure show that it is familial and behaves more like a polygenic than a simple Mendelian factor. Blood pressure follows a unimodal distribution and over a long period of follow-up there is no tendency for a separate group of hypertensives to emerge[11]. Blood pressure is lower at birth, and between 6 weeks and 6 years, than it is subsequently but there is a definite tendency for individuals to 'track' along the same percentile line. This tendency is not strong enough to identify future hypertensives with any degree of certainty in infancy, but it does suggest that a large part of the future blood pressure tendency is determined near to or before birth.

The correlation of blood pressure between family members has been studied.

In monozygotic twins it is almost as good as that for repeated measurements in one individual. For dizygotic twins the correlation coefficient is less than half as good but better than for siblings and for parent and child. Different studies report a zero, or very poor correlation increasing with time, between parent and step- or adopted child; between spouses it is weak and does not (in Framingham data) increase with length of marriage, suggesting that a shared environment has less effect than choice of spouse. Attempts to find genetic markers that are associated with hypertension have been largely unsuccessful.

Environmental factors

Within cultural groups sharing similar environments and life-styles the genetic contribution to the between subject variance in blood pressure appears dominant; a high estimate of 80%[11] and a low one of 30% for systolic blood pressure have been made[12]. However, the same might be said of the determinants of lung cancer in a culture where everybody smoked 40 cigarettes daily. The determinants of differences in blood pressure distribution between groups could be largely environmental. However, within cultures blood pressure has been correlated with weight gain and loss, with consumption of alcohol and with oral contraceptive use. The small differences between monozygotic twins correlate with weight, triglycerides and high density lipoprotein but not consistently with levels of exercise or salt intake[11]. Blood pressure levels appear to show a social class gradient, being highest among manual workers and their families (who also tend to obesity). Further evidence for environmental effects on blood pressure is the impression that manifestations of severe hypertension are declining in Western countries. Malignant hypertension, hypertensive retinopathy, hypertensive heart failure and stroke are in decline. This decline apparently preceded the widespread use of hypotensive agents.

Despite the difficulties of standardization of measurement, it has proved possible to identify ethnic groups and subgroups with greater or lesser degrees of hypertension. In the USA Blacks have higher pressures than Whites, although it is not possible to differentiate genetic from socio-economic factors. A large study in Detroit[13] led to the suggestion that urban stress correlated with higher blood pressure levels, but blood pressure is not invariably higher in urban than in rural communities. Severe hypertensive disease is common in West Africans. Regional differences in blood pressure have been demonstrated in several countries, most notably Japan, where it correlates to some extent with stroke and gastric cancer mortality.

Of great interest are a small number of ethnic groups who have low blood pressure levels and no increase with age. These are found in the Pacific Islands, Asia, Africa and South America. In general these communities are small and isolated and the people are interdependent; they are physically active, thin, and subsist on a diet low in calories with a high fruit and vegetable content and low salt intake (below 40–50 mEq/day). They sometimes experience periods of starvation[14]. As they become less isolated and primitive, or their people migrate, they tend to put on weight, increase their salt intake and put up their blood pressure, a finding confirmed in a study in Kenya of Africans from traditional life-styles joining the army.

Theories of causation

Linked to these findings in low blood pressure communities theories of causation include exercise and chronic infection (allegedly protective), obesity, salt, other dietary factors and stress (allegedly causative). Obesity and exercise are not adequate explanations alone as hypertension can occur at all grades of both. The methodology of investigating stress is poorly developed[15]. It has been suggested that in societies where the group takes responsibility rather than the individual the population is less prone to hypertension. Other dietary factors tend to correlate positively or negatively with salt.

The salt story is the most popular hypothesis at present and has evidence from different sources for it. There is a danger, however, of a naïve version of the story becoming popularized as if hypertension were unifactorial.

Prevention and control

The different problems posed by attempting to control severe and mild hypertension are implicit in Figs. 8.1 and 8.2. The proportion of the population with severe hypertension is very small and the risk they run is great. Many cases are symptomatic so that traditional methods of consultation and management have been able to cope. In addition unpleasant and even hazardous treatments have been justified because of the poor prognosis. However, treatment of severe hypertension alone can have only a minimal effect on incidence of hypertension-related disease, although it is fully justified, even mandatory in the individuals concerned.

In attempting to control a risk factor two alternative strategies can be used. One is to identify individuals at the high end of the distribution curve, so called high risk individuals, and intervene in them alone. The second is to attempt to move the whole population distribution to the left which includes interference with low risk individuals but avoids the necessity for discrimination by screening. In hypertension the first strategy, which is an extension of clinical practice, has been adopted. The second would depend on the development of methods of mass control, probably by prevention rather than medication. However, calculations based on the assumption that hypertension-related risk is reversible by risk free interventions, suggest that a 10 mm of mercury fall in the mean population pressure caused by a shift in the whole distribution, would cause a bigger reduction in morbidity and mortality than the treatment of all subjects at present considered to be mildly or moderately hypertensive. Only by control of pressure in the range of 85–95 diastolic and 140–60 systolic could similar reductions be made. Reference to Fig. 8.1 shows that this would involve some 40 % or more of the population.

The history of hypertension control, therefore, has been that of a cautious extension downwards, building on previous experience of treatment of higher levels of pressure and using newer and, it is hoped, more tolerable and safer drugs. The problem at each level has been to demonstrate that the hypertension-related risk is reversible by treatment and that the treatment itself is acceptably safe and free from side effects. For this reason there has always been a gap between the level of blood pressure which is thought to denote increased risk and that which is conventionally treated. If treatment were completely effective, free of risk and cost nothing, this gap would disappear.

Trials of blood pressure treatment

As each level of pressure is investigated and it becomes ethically desirable to treat new cases above a certain threshold, the size, cost and duration of trials needed to investigate effect of treatment of lower levels increase enormously. Early blood pressure trials involved a few score of patients for a few months only; current trials involve tens of thousands of patients for several years. This is because the number of end-point events in the treated group must be shown to be significantly reduced compared with controls. As the level of individual hypertension-related risk is low for mild and moderate hypertension, the number of man- or woman-years of observation has to be large. For this reason trials can only be done in middle-aged subjects and have tended to be concentrated on men, who have greater hypertension-related risk.

The early controlled trials of which the American Veterans Administration Study[16] was the largest, showed that hypertensive medication could effect major reductions in the morbid events showing the steepest gradients in Fig. 8.3 (i.e. strokes and congestive cardiac failure). However, coronary events did not show a statistically significant decline in any one study, although pooling of results from the larger trials suggested that a useful and significant, but by no means dramatic, reduction might be occurring. Other problems with the Veterans' Study were the atypical nature of American veterans and the diagnostic criteria, which were based on blood pressure measurements after rest in hospital. The morbidity and mortality in the control group were appropriate to that of higher levels of outpatient blood pressure. In addition, the diastolic criteria (phase IV or V) were not explicitly stated, but it is known that this and other American studies used phase V which would be equivalent to a phase IV reading some 5 mm of mercury higher.

The Veterans Administration trial suggested that moderate hypertension should be treated to reduce the risk of stroke and cardiac failure. A later generation of trials was mounted to overcome some of its deficiencies. The British Medical Research Council Mild Hypertension Trial [17] has some years to run but Australian and American studies are reporting their results from 1979.

The initial results of the Australian Therapeutic Trial in mild hypertension [18] show a major reduction in mortality from all causes, but although entry criteria ranged from diastolic (phase V) 95 to 109 mm of mercury, this and other benefits seemed to be confined to those with entry diastolic pressure over 100 mm of mercury. The proportionate reduction in non-fatal strokes was, as in the American Veterans, much greater than the reduction of coronary heart disease but as the latter was more common the absolute reduction was similar. The trend of benefit seemed to occur both in men and women above and below the age of 50. The authors suggested that subjects with diastolic phase V pressure below 100 mm of mercury should be observed but not treated by drugs.

The American Hypertension Detection and Follow-Up Program (HDFP)[19] compared the outcome in subjects picked up in mass screening campaigns who were randomly allocated, either to a programme of stepped care with target blood pressure levels, or to a group who were referred to their ordinary medical attendants. The results showed a major advantage to stepped care with a 17 % lower all-causes mortality. This was accounted for by not only a 19 % lower mortality from cardiovascular disease, but a 14 % lower mortality from non-cardiovascular diseases including 18 % fewer cancers. Stroke deaths were 44 % lower and coronary deaths 26 % lower under stepped care. The largest benefits appeared to be occurring in the blood pressure stratum 90–104 mm of mercury diastolic phase V at entry, in contrast to the Australian findings. In the USA these findings have been widely accepted as the starting signal for mass medication for mild hypertension in middle-age because the benefits of treatment appear considerable and there is little evidence of drug toxicity.

There are, however, grounds for caution. The stepped care programme may have induced changes of behaviour other than taking tablets. The non-specific nature of the improvement in mortality is puzzling. The study included a large proportion of Black subjects who obtained the greatest benefit. It also included a proportion of subjects already on treatment for hypertension whose pre-treatment pressures would have been higher. Only one treatment regime was followed so the optimum medication is not known. White women failed to benefit. For these and other reasons this outstanding contribution to the problem cannot be considered entirely alone and needs to be corroborated and supplemented with data from other trials.

Community control of hypertension

The accumulating evidence of risk of hypertension from prospective studies and the success of trials demonstrating its reversibility by medication, have stimulated interest in methods of ensuring that it is detected and treated. 10 years ago a number of studies, particularly in the USA, produced evidence for the rule of halves. Half the hypertensives were undetected, half of those detected were untreated and half of those treated were inadequately treated, leaving 1 in 8 adequately treated. Major campaigns have altered this situation in America. In Britain there is also an increasing awareness of and interest in hypertension. However, a controlled trial of screening in General Practice suggested that 10 years ago[20] identification of hypertensives by general practitioners had little effect on subsequent blood pressure. Another London study in the middle 1970s showed that most hypertensives had had their blood pressure measured within the last 5 years.[21] The problem in both instances was not identification of cases but their follow-through.

With such a widespread problem the traditional clinical approach of individualized treatment and use of clinical judgement may prove inappropriate. The use of a standard protocol with target blood pressures, as in the HDFP, simple regimes employing paramedical help, and even self-recording of blood pressure by patients may all be of help. In countries such as the USA where General Practice is rare, hypertension detection and control clinics have to be specially organized. In Britain hypertension should be detected and controlled mainly in General Practice where 70% of the population makes contact every year and perhaps 90% within 5 years. In 1971 control of blood pressure accounted for 2.6%[22] of general practitioners' consultations; by 1977 it was estimated to be 3.7%

Compliance

Detection of hypertension and prescription of drugs is not enough, the patient has to take them and for this reason the results of special trials cannot necessarily be extrapolated to the general population, in whom compliance in drug taking may be different. Symptomless hypertensives have to be persuaded to take regular medication that may cause symptoms. Methods of securing improved compliance are under investigation[23] including the simplification of treatment schedules. Research has also been mounted into the psychosocial effect of being identified as hypertensive and its effects on sickness absence from work; there is some conflict in the findings.

Non-pharmacological approaches

Although based on good epidemiological evidence and trials, the prospect of mass medication of the middle-aged population for decades of their lives is unattractive. Two non-pharmacological approaches, loss of weight and salt restriction, lead to a significant fall in blood pressure and are also being investigated as methods for the prevention of subsequent hypertension in children. Yoga, biofeedback, transcendental meditation and psychotherapy are also under investigation though without large scale trials of their effect on morbidity and mortality. All of these behavioural approaches demand a higher degree of compliance than simple medication.

For diseases in which hypertension is one factor among several in the aetiology, such as coronary heart disease, lowering the pressure is only one of several alternative strategies for reducing overall risk. It is as important for mild hypertensives to run low cholesterol levels and not to smoke cigarettes as to have their blood pressure lowered (see sections on coronary heart disease and stroke). On the other hand mass control of hypertension appears to offer the best strategy for prevention of stroke.

References

1. Millar Craig MW, Bishop CN, Raftery EB. Circadian variation of blood pressure. *Lancet* 1978; i: 795–7.
2. Rose GA, Blackburn H. *Cardiovascular survey methods.* Geneva: World Health Organization, 1968.
3. Rose GA, Holland WW. Crowley EA. A sphygmomanometer for epidemiologists. *Lancet* 1964; i: 296–300.
4. Wright BM, Dore CF. A random-zero sphygmomanometer. *Lancet* 1970; i: 337–8.
5. Prineas RJ. *Blood pressure sounds: their measurement and meaning. A training manual.* Gamma Medical Products, 1978.
6. Armitage P, Rose GA. The variability of measurements of casual blood pressure. 1. A laboratory study. *Clinical Science* 1966; **30**: 325–35.
7. Gardner MJ, Heady JA. Some effects of within person variability in epidemiological studies. *Journal of Chronic Disease* 1973; **26**: 781–95.
8. Office of Population Censuses and Surveys. *Mortality Statistics. Review of the Registrar General on deaths in England and Wales, 1977.* London: HMSO, 1979.
9. Shurtleff D. *Framingham Study Section 30. Some characteristics related to the incidence of cardiovascular disease and death: Framingham Study, 18-year follow-up.* DHEW No (NIH) 74–599. Washington: US Government Printing Office, 1974.
10. Berglund G, Anderson O, Wilhelmsen L. Prevalence of primary and secondary hypertension: studies in a random population sample. *British Medical Journal* 1976; **ii**: 554–6.
11. Feinleib M. Genetics and familial aggregation of blood pressure. In Onesti G, Klimt C, eds. *Hypertension determinants, complications and interventions.* New York: Grune & Stratton, 1979: 36–48.
12. Miall WE. Genetic considerations concerning hypertension. *Annals of the New York Academy of Sciences* 1978; **304**: 18–25.
13. Syme SL. Psychosocial determinants of blood pressure. In Onesti G, Klimt C, eds. *Hypertension, determinants, complications and interventions.* New York: Grune & Stratton, 1979: 88–98.
14. Prior IAM. Hypertension risk factors; a preventive point of view. In Gross F, Strasser T, eds. *Mild hypertension: natural history and management.* Tunbridge Wells: Pitman Medical, 1979.
15. Page LB, Tobian L. Salt and hypertension: epidemiology and mechanisms. Interrelationships of sodium and hypertension. In Onesti G, Klimt C, eds, *Hypertension, determinants, complications and interventions.* New York: Grune & Stratton. 1979: 3–32.

16. Veterans Administration Cooperative Study Group on Anti-hypertensive Agents. Effects of treatment on morbidity in hypertension. II. Results in patients with diastolic blood pressure averaging 90 through 114 mmHg. *JAMA* 1970; **213**: 1143–52.
17. Medical Research Council Working Party on Mild to Moderate Hypertension. Randomized controlled trial of treatment for mild hypertension: design and pilot trial. *British Medical Journal* 1977; **i**: 1437–40.
18. Management Committee. Initial results of the Australian Therapeutic Trial in mild hypertension. *Clinical Science* 1979; **57**: 449S–452S.
19. Hypertension Detection and Follow-up Program Cooperative Group. Five year findings of the Hypertension Detection and Follow-up Program. 1. Reduction in mortality of persons with high blood pressure including mild hypertension. *JAMA* 1979; **242**: 2562–70.
20. D'Souza MF, Swan AV, Shannon DJ. A long-term controlled trial of screening for hypertension in General Practice. *Lancet* 1976; **i**: 1228–32.
21. Heller RF. Detection and treatment of hypertension in an inner London community. *British Journal of Preventive and Social Medicine* 1976; **30**: 268–72.
22. Office of Population Censuses and Surveys. *Morbidity statistics from General Practice. Second National Study 1970–71*. London: HMSO, 1974.
23. Taylor DW, Sackett DL, *et al.* Compliance with anti-hypertensive drug therapy. In Perry HM Jr, Smith WMcF, eds. Mild hypertension: to treat or not to treat. *Annals of the New York Academy of Sciences* 1978; **304**: 390–411.

Further reading

Gross F, Strasser T, eds. *Mild hypertension: natural history and management*. Tunbridge Wells: Pitman Medical, 1979.

Heller RF, Rose G. Blood pressure measurement in the United Kingdom Heart Disease Prevention Project. *Journal of Epidemiology and Community Health* 1978; **32**: 235–8.

Onesti G, Klimt CR, eds. *Hypertension determinants, complications and intervention*. New York: Grune and Stratton, 1979.

Paul O, ed. *Epidemiology and control of hypertension*. New York: Stratton Intercontinental Medical Book Corporation, 1975.

Perry HM Jr, Smith WMcF, eds. Mild hypertension: to treat or not to treat. *Annals of the New York Academy of Sciences* 1978; **304**.

Chapter 9 · Stroke

H TUNSTALL PEDOE

The clinical and diagnostic problem

The term 'stroke' and its older synonym 'apoplexy' are derived from the clinical appearance of the victim rather than the underlying pathology. A stroke patient is stricken, or to quote a World Health Organization (WHO) definition, has 'rapidly developed clinical signs of focal (or global) disturbance of cerebral function; lasting more than 24 hours or leading to death, with no apparent cause other than a vascular origin[1].' This definition excludes non-vascular causes, although clinically this is not always possible. Usually stroke is taken to mean the acute severe manifestations of cerebrovascular disease. (The term cerebrovascular accident is unfortunate as accident implies trauma). The 24 hour threshold in the definition is to exclude transient ischaemic attacks in which, however acute the onset, signs or symptoms do not persist beyond that time.

While the clinical diagnosis of stroke may be easy, that of the underlying pathology may not be and the World Health Organization's International Classification of Diseases (ICD)[2] covers a variety both of specific and non-specific diagnoses (Table 9.1). The problem for stroke epidemiology is that the aetiology, natural history, treatment and prevention of different stroke species is not necessarily the same. Subarachnoid haemorrhage (ICD 430) usually results from congenital berry aneurysms or vascular abnormalities. Cerebral or intraventricular haemorrhage (ICD 431) results from acquired microaneurysms. Cerebral infarction (ICD 432–434) results from thrombosis or embolism from atheromatous plaques in large and middle-sized arteries. Population studies

Table 9.1. Classification of stroke in ICD.

8th & 9th Edition of ICD	7th Edition
430 Subarachnoid haemorrhage	330
431 Cerebral haemorrhage	331
432 Occlusion of pre-cerebral arteries ⎫	
433 Cerebral thrombosis ⎬	332
434 Cerebral embolism ⎭	
435 Transient cerebral ischaemia	333
436 Acute but ill-defined cerebrovascular disease ⎫	
437 Generalized ischaemic cerebrovascular disease ⎬	334
438 Other and ill-defined cerebrovascular disease ⎭	

must either aggregate all strokes and conceal the different characteristics of the family members, or attempt to describe them individually, when the results may be affected by diagnostic habits and errors. The result is that definitions and classifications vary between stroke studies and this leads to bias in any comparisons of their findings. Some include presumed cerebral infarction alone, others include cerebral haemorrhage but not subarachnoid haemorrhage; some include strokes secondary to extra-cerebral disease and others do not. Persistent hemiparesis in survivors may or may not be a required criterion.

Accuracy and repeatability of diagnosis

A number of studies have been mounted in which death certificates or hospital discharge diagnoses for stroke have been reviewed, using the case notes and a strict protocol to validate the original diagnosis. Not surprisingly for a disease that predominantly affects elderly subjects, these have tended to show a large proportion of events where the diagnostic evidence was inadequate, or misinterpreted, or where there were multiple diagnoses, each of which might have been coded as the underlying cause of death. Although it was carried out in 1959 a large study in England and Wales is typical in illustrating these problems.

Heasman and Lipworth[3] asked clinicians in 75 hospitals to record mock medical certificates of cause of death before elective hospital necropsy; these were matched with those completed by the pathologists afterwards. The study was, therefore, relevant only to fatalities occurring among hospital in-patients in larger hospitals and it reflected only on the accuracy of clinical diagnosis, not necessarily on routine death certification, in which evidence from elective necropsies may contribute. Deaths at home, deaths not followed by necropsy, coroners' cases and, of course, non-fatal cases were not included.

Out of 9501 deaths cerebrovascular stroke was diagnosed 1096 times (11.5%) by clinicians and 886 times (9.3%) at necropsy, with agreement in 740 cases. The sensitivity of the clinical diagnosis was therefore 84% and the specificity 96% (see Table 9.2). The validity of different stroke diagnoses varied. Of 171 necropsied cases of subarachnoid haemorrhage only 65% were diagnosed clinically, but false positives and false negatives were almost equally common so that the clinical diagnosis was made 165 times. Cerebral haemorrhage was over-diagnosed. Of 377 necropsy cases 68% were diagnosed clinically, but the clinical diagnosis was made 539 times so that it was correct in only 48%. Cerebral embolism and thrombosis (classified together) were found at necropsy in 310 cases and, correctly diagnosed in 51%, but the clinical diagnosis was made 351 times so that it was correct on only 45% of occasions.

The major findings of this study, that stroke is a more valid diagnosis than its subgroups, that subarachnoid haemorrhage is the most valid of these, and that cerebral haemorrhage is overdiagnosed, are typical of findings in other studies.

Table 9.2. Accuracy of diagnosis of stroke as cause of death[3].

| | | Necropsy diagnosis | | |
		Stroke	Not	Total
Clinical	Stroke	740	356	1096
diagnosis	Not-stroke	146	8259	8405
	Total	886	8615	9501

In the last 20 years many new techniques have become available in specialized units for the diagnosis of non-fatal stroke – arteriography, ultrasound, radio-isotope scanning and computerized axial tomography; their impact on the overall level of accuracy of diagnosis must depend on the proportion of stroke victims admitted to and investigated in these units. Over the same time the proportion of deaths in hospital leading to elective necropsy has declined. Although stroke is a cause of medically unattended sudden death, the majority of patients with fatal strokes survive long enough for the victim to come under medical care. Forensic or coroners' post mortems therefore make a smaller contribution to the total diagnosed cases than they do in coronary heart attacks.

Mortality

Geographical variation

The stroke mortality-rate for men aged 35–74 for England and Wales in 1977 was 136 per 100 000 and for women 121 per 100 000 (8 % of male and 12 % of female deaths in these age groups). Using 1977 rates, the cumulative risk of a stroke death to the age of 75 from birth would be 4.4 % for men and 4.1 % for women. Stroke rates in Scotland are higher; within Britain there is considerable regional variation with a south-east to north-west gradient[4]. Stroke is a major cause of death in all countries publishing mortality returns. The most recently available international data are published by the World Health Organization[5] under the rubric A85, cerebrovascular disease. The 1979 report contains returns mainly for 1977 or 1976 but in a few countries, for earlier years.

Stroke mortality in the USA is lower than in England and Wales. If the 1976 returns are standardized to the England and Wales population, the male rate aged 35–74 was 101 per 100 000 and female rate 85. The south-east states of the USA have high stroke mortality while the rates in the mountain and south western states are low. The highest stroke mortality figures in the world used to come from Japan where rates are still very high and it is the leading cause of death. Recent returns suggest higher rates occur in Portugal (355 per 100 000 for males and 277 per 100 000 for females) and in Bulgaria, whilst very low rates are reported from the German Democratic Republic (65 per 100 000 for males and 58 per 100 000 for females – half those in England and Wales) and Switzerland. The most recent mortality rates available are shown in Fig. 9.1 (standarized for age). Countries with large proportions of vague diagnoses are excluded but diagnostic criteria standards do vary.

Time trends

Stroke mortality shows a seasonal variation which is more marked in some countries than in others. Cold countries show a winter peak while in hot countries the peak may occur at the hottest time of the year. The January peak in England and Wales is 44 % greater than the September trough.

Many countries have experienced a decline in stroke mortality over the last 30 years although this is difficult to estimate exactly because of changes in disease coding. In the USA, the decline was apparent in the 1920s except in non-White males, although the newly fashionable diagnosis of coronary heart disease might have attracted sudden deaths previously called stroke before the Second World War. However, the decline in stroke mortality continued into the 1960s when coronary rates had stabilized, and since 1968 has steepened to 5 % per annum, in all sex and colour groups, while coronary rates and overall mortality rates have been falling. Regional stroke mortality rates have tended to converge[6]. While cerebral haemorrhage accounted for the great majority of stroke death diagnoses in the 1920s, it currently accounts for the minority.

In England and Wales there has been a steady but slow decline in overall stroke mortality. Since 1950 death rates for subarachnoid haemorrhage have increased while rates for cerebral haemorrhage have declined; those for cerebral thrombosis rose during the 1950s and then declined[7]. The change in the ratio of cerebral thrombosis to cerebral haemorrhage was independently reported from a necropsy study[8]. The proportion of stroke deaths attributed to acute but ill-defined cerebrovascular disease has been increasing, reflecting either lack of care with the diagnosis or greater diagnostic humility.

Age, sex, race and occupation

Stroke mortality rises exponentially with age. Mortality for all stroke diagnoses, and for subarachnoid haemorrhage, cerebral haemorrhage and cerebral thrombosis in England and Wales in 1977 are shown in Fig. 9.2[9]. Out of 73 000 stroke deaths in that year, 88 % occurred in people aged 65 years and over and 62 % in people aged 75 years and over. Stroke mortality in males is higher than in females but the difference is small and varies between stroke subgroups and age groups; it also varies between countries and over time. Subarachnoid haemorrhage is more common in females and it is the most important stroke category in the younger age groups. All stroke categories have a positive social class gradient for

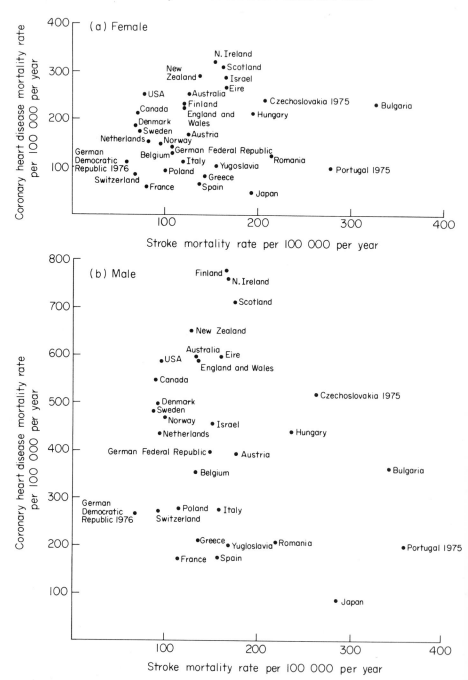

Fig. 9.1. Scatter diagram of male and female stroke and coronary heart disease mortality, ages 35–74, in 1977 unless otherwise stated, standardized to population structure of England and Wales.

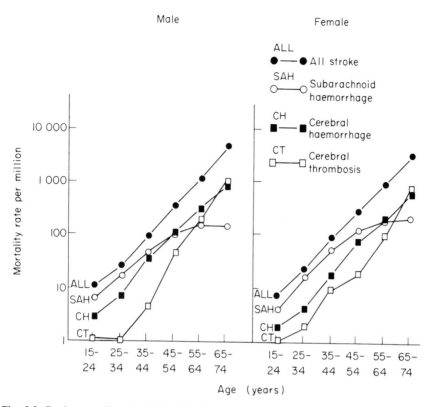

Fig. 9.2. Stroke mortality rates, England and Wales, 1977.

mortality, unskilled labourers suffering the highest rates and professional men the lowest. USA data show more stroke deaths in non-Whites, though Americans of Japanese stock who have adopted Western life styles are said to have similar stroke rates to Whites.

Incidence, prevalence and outcome

Numerous incidence studies have been undertaken but often using different diagnostic criteria and age groupings. A nationwide study of hospitalized cases in the USA has suggested that regional mortality differences correlated better with incidence than with case fatality[10]. A long term study in Rochester Minnesota[11] has shown a mean incidence rate (first attacks) of 164 per 100 000 total population per year, with cerebral infarction from all causes accounting for 79% of cases, intracerebral haemorrhage 10% and subarachnoid haemorrhage 6%. The 30 day survival rate was 82% for cerebral thrombosis, 16% for intracerebral haemorrhage and 48% for subarachnoid haemorrhage. Of the survivors 10% had a recurrent stroke within 1 year and 20% within 5 years, the stroke category sometimes changing. 38 % of stroke victims who died did so of the initial stroke, 10 % of a recurrence and 18 % of heart disease. However, of the survivors after 6 months only 4 % required total care, 30 % functioned normally, 54 % had some neurological deficit and 10 % some aphasia. The prevalence rate of stroke victims was about 700 per 100 000 population. Incidence, case fatality, prevalence and mortality all appeared to be declining. In contrast a stroke register[12] in southern England in the 1970s recorded an attack rate (including recurrences) of 209 per 100 000 with a 3 week overall survival of 50 % and an estimated prevalence rate of 549 per 100 000. These rates represent a higher incidence with lower survival and lower prevalence estimates than from America, however, the results are not age-standardized and the diagnostic criteria were different. 12 % had a recurrence within 4 years.

The British study used WHO definitions. A joint report from 17 WHO stroke registers has now been published[13] covering 4 Scandinavian, 3 other European, 5 Japanese, 4 other Asian and 1 African centre. Comparability between centres appeared good for the diagnosis of stroke but not for individual stroke species. The range of attack rates between most centres was smaller than for, say, coronary heart disease. Age-standardized rates for men were 2 per 1000 in Colombo, 4–8 in most European centres but 15 per 1000 in Akita in Japan. Female rates were on average 30 % lower. Cerebral haemorrhage did appear to be more common in centres with a high prevalence of hypertension such as Japan; coma, death or severe disability was more common in these patients. Overall, 23 % of subjects died within 1 week, 31 % within 3 weeks and 48 % within 1 year. Patterns of care varied enormously between cultures. In some, relatives undertook all the care at home but in others, as many as 25 % of survivors were in hospital 1 year later.

Hospital statistics

In 1975 there were 105 000 admissions to acute, non-psychiatric hospitals in England and Wales for stroke, 2.2 % of the total. However, on average 17 500 beds were needed, 9.6 % of total bed use[14]. The reason for this discrepancy is the long length of stay. While the median duration of stay was 15 days, the distribution was skewed with a mean of 61 days, and 6 % of cases were in hospital for more than 6 months. The hospital fatality rate was 42 % (26 % in the age group 45–64 and 54 % over 75 years). From this and national deaths it can be estimated that 57 % of stroke deaths occurred in those admitted to hospital for stroke during that year. 69 % of discharge diagnoses were for the ill-defined categories 436–438, in comparison with 46 % of deaths. Both cerebral haemorrhage and cerebral thrombosis were less than half as common as discharge diagnoses as they were on death certificates. Subarachnoid haemorrhage was $2\frac{1}{2}$ times more common as a cause of admission than as a cause of death.

Aetiology and risk factors

Except in Japan stroke is too rare a disease in middle age to be the subject of specific prospective studies, so that most research on risk factors comes from case–control studies or as a by-product of cohort (a segment of the population born around the same time period) studies on coronary heart disease where the number of events studied tends to be small. The identification of specific risk factors for specific stroke species is dependent on local diagnostic criteria.

Clinical antecedents of stroke appear to be heart disease, hypertension, transient ischaemic attacks and carotid bruits. The relative risk associated with these findings is age-dependent. While transient ischaemic attacks predict premature stroke (some 30% of subjects have 1 within 5 years) and the effect is independent of hypertension, only a minority of stroke victims have had preceding transient ischaemic attacks and these may be unreported at the time.

The largest and longest prospective study of cardiovascular disease is the Framingham study[15]. Table 9.3 shows the regression coefficients after 18 years for possible risk factors (measured biennially) against the frequency of cerebral infarction (haemorrhage of any kind is excluded).

Table 9.3. Regression coefficients for possible risk factors for stroke, Framingham data[15].

Factor	Regression coefficient	
	Men	Women
Systolic blood pressure	0.69	0.69
e.c.g. LVH	0.51	0.48
Serum cholesterol	0.27	0.13*
Cigarettes	0.31	−0.02*
Blood sugar	0.20	0.22
Relative weight	0.16*	0.44

* Not significant. LVH Left ventricular hypertrophy.

These results demonstrate the pre-eminence of hypertension as a risk factor (see also Chapter 8). Other risk factors are weaker and are also inconsistent between age groups and sexes. Of the different components of blood pressure, the systolic appeared to be as good a measure as any. A high haemoglobin level is a risk factor but not independently of blood pressure and smoking, as smokers have above average haemoglobins. Other studies have also shown the importance of blood pressure and heart disease and a varying importance for lipids, diabetes, smoking, alcohol consumption, use of the contraceptive pill, body weight, blood viscosity and clotting and fibrinolytic factors. Although these studies suggest that the risk factors for stroke are similar to those for coronary disease, their relative importance differs. International mortality rates show no good correlation between stroke and coronary disease rates (Fig. 9.1): men showing a weak positive, and women a weak negative, correlation. This suggests that the aetiological factors for the two diseases are unlikely to be similar.

Because subarachnoid haemorrhage and cerebral haemorrhage are less common they are more difficult to investigate. Hypertension appears to be the only consistently established risk factor for cerebral haemorrhage. Subarachnoid haemorrhage has been related to hypertension, cigarette smoking and the contraceptive pill.

Risk factors between cultures vary. Although hypertension appears to be a risk factor everywhere, Japanese workers have found higher stroke rates in communities with low cholesterol levels; however, the low cholesterol may not in itself be a factor so much as inadequate protein intake or a high salt diet. Regional differences in stroke rates are largely unexplained although a high salt intake, a soft water supply, other dietary constituents and low socio-economic status have all been correlated with high rates.

Treatment and prevention

The large differences in stroke mortality between different countries and regions, coupled with the decline in many countries, suggest that stroke is not an inevitable consequence of age and might be controllable. The most important known risk factor – blood pressure – is reversible with treatment. Trials discussed in Chapter 8 have shown stroke risk is one of the sequelae to high blood pressure most susceptible to drug therapy. It is likely that the decline in stroke has followed a decline in prevalence of hypertension in some countries, possibly related to the widespread consumption of canned and refrigerated foods in place of those preserved in salt. The stroke decline preceded widespread hypotensive medication and occurred in older age groups who are not often treated. Community control of hypertension should lead to a major decline in stroke.

Trials of blood pressure control in stroke survivors have produced contradictory results but the majority suggest benefit. Other attempts at secondary prevention have followed the same path as in coronary artery atheroma, i.e. anticoagulants, clofibrate, aspirin, sulphinpyrazone and other anti-platelet drugs and carotid artery surgery. No definite advantage has been shown consistenly for any one intervention; results of surgery depend on the surgeon.

Treatment of an acute stroke is largely the control of complications, but active interventions are under investigation. Controlled trials of management in specialist stroke units suggest these may be beneficial[16], as may active rehabilitation programmes in the minority of patients able to undertake them[17]. Patients with subarachnoid haemorrhage who are young with accessible aneurysms may benefit from early surgery to prevent recurrent bleeds.

References

1. World Health Organization Meeting on Community Control of Stroke and Hypertension. *Control of stroke in the community: methodological considerations and protocol of WHO Stroke Register.* CVD/S/73.6. Geneva: WHO, 1973.

2. World Health Organization. *International Classification of Diseases. Ninth revision 1975.* Geneva: WHO, 1977.

3. Heasman MA, Lipworth L. *Accuracy of certification of cause of death.* Studies on medical and population subjects. No 20. London: General Register Office, 1966.

4. Fulton M, Adams W, *et al.* Regional variations in mortality from ischaemic heart and cerebrovascular disease in Britain. *British Heart Journal* 1978; **40**: 563–8.

5. World Health Organization. *World Health Statistics Annual.* Geneva: WHO, 1979, 1980, 1981.

6. Soltero I, Liu K, *et al.* Trends in mortality from cerebrovascular diseases in the USA, 1960–75. *Stroke* 1978; **9**: 549–58.

7. Acheson R, Sanderson C. Strokes: social class and geography. *Population Trends* 1978; **12**: 13–17.

8. Yates PO. A change in the pattern of cerebrovascular disease. *Lancet* 1964; **i**: 65–9.

9. Office of Population Censuses and Surveys. *Mortality Statistics. Review of the Registrar General on deaths in England and Wales, 1977.* London: HMSO, 1979.

10. Kuller L, Anderson H, *et al.* Nationwide cerebrovascular disease morbidity study. *Stroke* 1970; **1**: 86–99.

11. Matsumoto N, Whisnant JP, *et al.* Natural history of stroke in Rochester, Minnesota, 1955 through 1969, an extension of a previous study 1945 through 1954. *Stroke* 1973; **4**: 20–9.

12. Weddell JW, Beresford SAA. *Planning for stroke patients. A four-year descriptive study of home and hospital care.* Department of Health and Social Security. London: HMSO, 1979.

13. Aho H, Harmsen P, *et al.* Cerebrovascular disease in the community: results of a WHO collaborative study. *Bulletin of the World Health Organization* 1980; **58**: 113.

14. Department of Health and Social Security. Office of Population Censuses and Surveys. *Hospital Inpatient Enquiry Main Tables 1975.* London: HMSO, 1978.

15. Kannel WB, Gordon T, Dawber TR. Role of lipids in the development of brain infarction: the Framingham study. *Stroke* 1974; **5**: 679–85.

16. Garraway WM, Akhtar AJ, *et al.* Management of acute stroke in the elderly; preliminary results of a controlled trial. *British Medical Journal* 1980; **ii**: 1040–3.

17. Sheikl K, Smith DS, *et al.* Methods and problems of a stroke rehabilitation trial. *British Journal of Occupational Therapy* 1978; **41**: 262–5.

Chapter 10 · The Leukaemias

R J BERRY

The leukaemias cover a wide clinical and pathological spectrum. Although they are amongst the least frequent of the malignant diseases their impact on the community is disproportionately great because of the relatively high proportion of very young patients with some leukaemias. The underlying disease mechanism is a failure of the normal body controls on proliferation of haemopoietic cells. This can occur in any of the differentiation lines, but the majority of leukaemias which present clinically are either myeloid or lymphoid in origin, with monocytic leukaemia being a particularly unpleasant third variant. Leukaemias are described as being either 'acute' or 'chronic', depending on the mode of presentation and the length of time for which the disease is present. The terms are relative: 'chronic' myeloid leukaemia may be as rapidly progressive as 'acute' lymphocytic disease. Another type of malignant haemopoietic proliferation is of plasma cells, which results in solitary plasmacytomata or multiple myelomata, which are not considered here.

Leukaemia most commonly presents with non-specific early symptoms, lassitude, low-grade or relapsing fevers, and glandular or abdominal organ enlargement. At this stage the disease is often confused with glandular fever, even after tests at a laboratory. The disease is systemic from the onset, is characterized by remissions and relapses, and death commonly occurs from failure to overcome intercurrent bacterial or other infection. Whereas myelocytic leukaemia occurs at all ages, acute lymphocytic leukaemia is largely confined to childhood. Chronic lymphocytic leukaemia, a disease of long natural history, often covering tens of years, is usually a disease of advanced age.

Known carcinogenic agents

Ionizing radiation is implicated in the induction of leukaemias, particularly myelocytic leukaemia. Alice Stewart and Kneale[1] and MacMahon[2] have demonstrated a correlation between antenatal X-ray exposure for pelvimetry and a high risk of leukaemia in childhood. However, as these studies are all retrospective it is difficult to exclude the possibility that those mothers whose obstetric condition required pelvimetry may have a higher than normal risk of producing a leukaemic child. In adults, radiation exposure, particularly to the majority of the bone marrow, is associated with an increased risk of the development of leukaemia. Leukaemias had a high incidence in radium dial painters who unwittingly ingested radium salts from their paint brushes. Dose-related increase in leukaemia incidence was seen in the survivors of the nuclear explosions at Hiroshima and Nagasaki[3]. An increased incidence of leukaemia was reported in British patients treated with X-irradiation of a major part of the spine for ankylosing spondylitis[4].

The only chemical carcinogen widely associated with leukaemia is benzene.

Viruses are capable of causing leukaemias in other animal species and for this reason it is widely believed that human leukaemogenic viruses must exist. There is as yet no direct evidence to support this hypothesis.

There may be a genetic predisposition to the development of leukaemia. The disease is clearly associated in frequency with a number of specific chromosomal abnormalities, in particular Down's syndrome (see Chapter 34).

Sources of information

England and Wales

Mortality data for leukaemia are now tabulated separately for acute and chronic myelocytic leukaemia, acute and chronic lymphocytic leukaemia, acute and chronic monocytic leukaemia and unspecified leukaemias. However, until the 8th Revision of the World Health Organization's International Classification of Disease (ICD) was introduced in 1968, all leukaemias were coded together. This makes the assembly of serial mortality data for different types of leukaemia impossible.

Morbidity data on leukaemia have been available from Cancer Registries nationally since 1952. The completeness of registration varies between National Health Service regions. The proportion of leukaemias registered as myeloid during the 1970s increased, possibly owing to a decrease in the number of 'other and unspecified' leukaemias. Registrations are usually coded at the 3 digit ICD level and therefore do not separate acute from chronic presentations. Registration data are also available in several other countries; these are of variable reliability and in most registries acute and chronic leukaemias are not distinguished.

Incidence and prevalence

Mortality

With the exception of chronic lymphocytic leukaemia, mortality data give a good measure of the impact of these diseases, because their clinical course tends to be short and unremitting. Overall the leukaemias are not common causes of death. Lymphocytic leukaemia accounts for less than 1 % of all cancer deaths and myeloid leukaemia accounts for $1-1.5\%$. However, because acute lymphocytic leukaemia has a high incidence in children the number of potential years of life lost is high, and the impact of the disease is greater than is immediately apparent from the numbers of people affected.

In 1979 there were 3217 deaths due to leukaemia in England and Wales (Table 10.1). The majority of these were caused by the myeloid type. The deaths were equally divided between males and females, yielding roughly equal death rates of 39 per million for males and 36 per million for females. Relatively few deaths from myeloid leukaemia occurred in children under 10.

Just over 1000 deaths were due to lymphatic leukaemia amongst these the chronic type occurred more frequently than the acute type. The overall death rate for males (30 per million) was higher than for females (20 per million). However, 28% of the deaths from acute lymphatic leukaemia occurred in children under 10 years of age.

Table 10.1. Death from leukaemia in England and Wales 1979, and percentage aged under 10 years at death.

Type	Males		Females		Total	
	Deaths	% under 10 years	Deaths	% under 10 years	Deaths	% under 10 years
Acute lymphatic	239	29	143	26	382	28
Chronic lymphatic	385	0	271	0	656	0
Acute myeloid	647	4	637	2	1284	3
Chronic myeloid	263	1	286	0	549	1
Monocytic	49	6	41	2	90	4
Other and unspecified	138	2	118	1	256	2
All	1721	6	1496	3	3217	5

The age- and sex-specific death rates for all leukaemias are shown in Fig. 10.1. It is often said that leukaemia has a bimodal distribution with age; however, this is not strictly true. The bimodality is only apparent when all leukaemias are considered together and when the 0–4 year age group is split into those under 1 year and 1–4 year-olds. Death rates tend to be low until the age of 60 years; thereafter they rise steeply with increasing age. In all age groups the male death rate exceeds that for females. The different types of leukaemia show different age-specific mortality patterns. The lymphatic leukaemias show a peak, entirely due to acute cases, in the 5–9 year-olds and high rates in the over 60s, comprising chronic cases. By contrast there is no peak in incidence amongst young children for myeloid leukaemia.

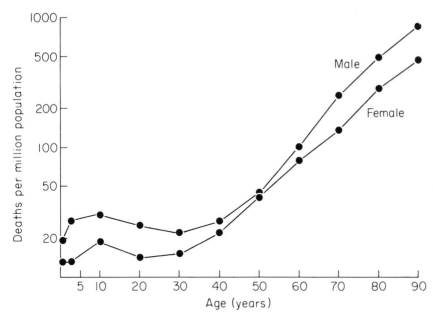

Fig. 10.1. Age-specific death rates from all leukaemias, England and Wales, 1979 (note the log scale).

Time trends

The change in ICD coding has made it impossible to assess time trends in mortality for leukaemias of particular histological types. For leukaemias as a whole there was a 3-fold increase in the age-standardized death rate between 1930 and 1960. This is partly explained by improved diagnosis. Leukaemia is still increasing in incidence in the older age groups, but has remained fairly stable in the young. This is largely because there has been a continuing rise in incidence in chronic lymphocytic leukaemia in the older age group.

Social class

There is no clear variation in leukaemia incidence with social class. The standardized mortality ratio ranges from 120 in Social Class I to 90 in Social Class V for lymphocytic and myeloid leukaemias in males. For other leukaemias, where the numbers of patients are very small, the opposite pattern is seen. There are no clear correlations between occupation and the incidence of leukaemia.

Morbidity

Morbidity data show patterns similar to those shown by mortality data. A total of 3625 new cases of leukaemia were registered in England and Wales in 1973. Of these, 1630 were myeloid and the remaining 1550 lymphocytic. Registrations of lymphocytic leukaemias showed a peak incidence in children aged 1–4 years with a rate of nearly 70 per million. There was another peak in the elderly, with a rate of 500 per million over the age of 85.

Age-standardized incidence rates are available for a number of other countries. In Western Europe the rates for both myeloid and lymphocytic leukaemia are each around 30 per million in males with incidence in females somewhat lower, as in the United Kingdom. Lower rates have been recorded in India (Bombay, 15 per million males) and Japan (20 per million males for myeloid, 8 per million males for lymphocytic leukaemia). Incidence in females is generally lower. Childhood leukaemias are reported as being rare in Africa[5].

Special features

The treatment of leukaemia has undergone great changes in the last decade with the technical improvement of radiotherapy and the advent of multiple cytotoxic drug regimes. This has been reflected in the dramatic improvements in survival that have been recorded by United Kingdom Cancer Registries[6]. For all leukaemias, patients registered in 1959 had a 5 year survival rate of 3.6 % for males and 5.6 % for females. By 1964–66 this had risen to 6.8 % in males and 8.0 % in females, and by 1971–73 it was 14 % in both sexes. Most of the deaths occur in the first year. The apparent improvements in survival could be accounted for by changes in proportions of the different forms of leukaemia or better follow-up data, as well as real improvements in the effectiveness of treatment.

Survival varies dramatically with the age of the patient. For lymphocytic leukaemia in children under 10 years of age, the 5 year survival rate ranges from 35 to 50 %. At all other ages it tends to be around 20 %. Overall 5 year survival rates vary with histology. In 1971–3 lymphocytic leukaemia had a 25 % 5 year survival rate, myeloid 6 %, monocytic 4 % and others 7 %.

Prognosis and treatment

Acute leukaemias are characterized by episodic outbursts of disease with remissions between, some of which may be spontaneous and may last for weeks or months. The most common cause of death is either uncontrolled infection or from haemorrhage. Typically, only 25 % of patients diagnosed as having acute leukaemia survive 3 months, although children (unless under 1 year of age at presentation) survive better than adults. The success of treatment of acute leukaemias declines with age, particularly over 65 years. This is due to the decreased tolerance of aggressive cytotoxic therapy.

The prognosis for acute lymphocytic leukaemia is somewhat better than that for acute myelocytic leukaemia. In children, 50 % of those presenting with acute lymphocytic leukaemia now survive 5 years, with a median survival of 4 years. This is clearly the result of the intensive cytotoxic chemotherapy which has been used in the last decade. In older patients, about 50% will achieve some clinical remission, but the course is still rapidly fatal. Of the chronic leukaemias, chronic myeloid leukaemia often progresses to an acute form which presages the terminal event. 50% of patients will survive $2\frac{1}{2}$ years, but the use of multiple cytotoxic drugs has been less rewarding in this condition than in the acute leukaemias. Treatment is often directed to the palliation of symptoms such as the reduction of size of an enlarged spleen by local radiotherapy, the relief of thrombosis and the correction of anaemia. The best prognostic group is comprised of patients who develop chronic lymphocytic leukaemia, of whom 50% will survive 5 years or more. The range of treatments employed include local radiotherapy to enlarged nodes and spleen, low-dose total body radiotherapy or low-dose maintenance chemotherapy, using the orally administered nitrogen mustard Chlorambucil.

References

1. Stewart A, Kneale GW. Radiation dose effects in relation to obstetric X rays and childhood cancers. *Lancet* 1970; **i**: 1185–8.
2. MacMahon B. Prenatal X-ray exposure and childhood cancer. *US Journal of the National Cancer Institute* 1962; **28**: 1173–91.
3. Japan Radiation Research Society. A review of thirty years study of Hiroshima and Nagasaki atomic bomb survivors. Supplement to *Japan Radiation Research Society. Journal* 1975; **16**.
4. Court Brown WM, Doll R. *Leukaèmia and aplastic anaemia in patients irradiated for ankylosing spondylitis.* M.R.C. Special report series 295, London: HMSO, 1957.
5. Fleming AF. Epidemiology of the leukaemia in Africa. *Leukemia Research* 1979; **3**: 51–9.
6. Office of Population Censuses and Surveys. *Cancer Statistics, Survival 1971–1973 registrations.* Series MB1 No 3. London: HMSO, 1980.

Chapter 11 · Anaemia

W E WATERS AND P C ELWOOD

Causes

Anaemia is widely considered to be an important health problem, particularly in developing countries, in many of which large proportions of the population are affected[1]. By far the most common cause of anaemia is iron deficiency. Whether this is due directly to a dietary deficiency of iron, or to a relative deficiency consequent on an increased blood loss, it leads to a microcytic, hypochromic blood picture. On the other hand, folate and B_{12} deficiency lead to a macrocytic, megaloblastic blood picture. However, these latter types are rare and do not constitute a major problem of any size in the Western world. In this chapter, only iron deficiency anaemia will be considered.

Definition

Anaemia is defined as a concentration of haemoglobin in the blood (expressed as g/dl) below a particular value. For example, the World Health Organization (WHO)[1] has defined anaemia as the occurrence of a haemoglobin level below 12 g/dl in adult non-pregnant women, or below 13 g/dl in adult males. An alternative definition is given in terms of packed cell volume, and in much population survey work a haematocrit, often estimated by a micro method, has been found to be eminently suitable as it correlates highly with circulating haemoglobin level[2]. However, the use of the term 'anaemia' is most unsatisfactory because it ignores cause completely. A microcytic and a macrocytic anaemia have nothing in common other than a low circulating haemoglobin level. Therefore, in this chapter the term anaemia will refer only to an iron deficiency state in which the haemoglobin level is low.

The main difficulty, ignored by the use of a diagnostic criterion such as that proposed by WHO, is that community surveys have shown that levels of circulating haemoglobin have a continuous distribution, with a slight negative skewness and kurtosis (Fig. 11.1). This makes the definition of anaemia by reference to a single level of haemoglobin rather meaningless, implying a dichotomy of 'normal' and 'anaemic'. Garby[4] approached this problem by determining the proportion of subjects in a community whose response to iron therapy showed a rise in circulating haemoglobin level (or haematocrit), whatever their initial level. He found that, in these terms, the prevalence of iron deficiency is about twice as high as that suggested by the simple application of the

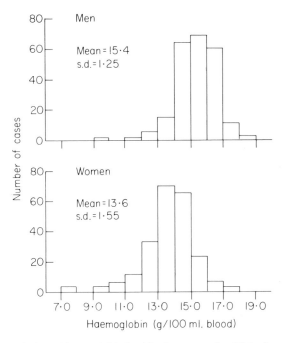

Fig. 11.1. The distribution of haemoglobin level in the community, Wales.[3]

WHO criterion of anaemia. Moreover, many subjects with levels above the WHO criterion showed a rise, while many below did not. However, anaemia is still defined in terms of a set level of circulating haemoglobin in many studies.

Prevalence

Since iron deficiency is difficult to diagnose clinically, the epidemiological picture of anaemia can only be inferred from the pattern of haemoglobin levels in the community.

After the first 10 years of life, mean haemoglobin levels are significantly higher in males than in females[5]. Following an initial dramatic fall after birth, the haemoglobin level rises steadily during childhood. After adolescence, mean haemoglobin levels remain steady throughout adult life (Fig. 11.2). There is, however, a steady fall in men[6] which is probably physiological as most men have considerable iron stores at post mortem examinations[7]. In women mean haemoglobin levels are about 2 g/dl lower than in men, and there is very little change with age, other than perhaps a slight fall at advanced ages[6]. It is often stated that anaemia is common in women of child bearing years and in the elderly of both sexes. The epidemiological evidence gives remarkably little support to such statements and the fall in mean levels seems to occur only at very advanced

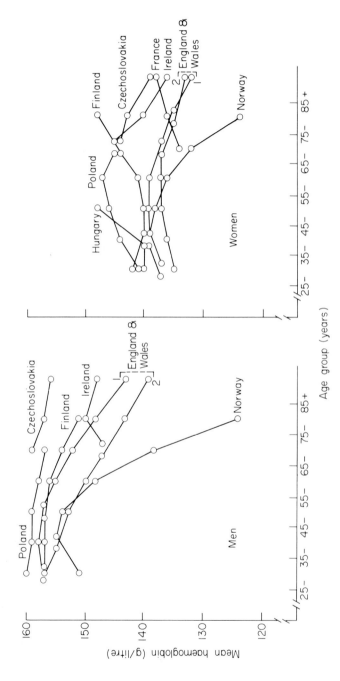

Fig. 11.2. Mean haemoglobin levels at various ages.[6]

ages. Other groups within our community which are believed to be especially vulnerable to anaemia are immigrants. Yet one cannot generalize about immigrants as studies of some have detected a high prevalence of low haemoglobin levels but studies of others have not[8].

Importance to health

Clinical impressions of the frequency of anaemia differ greatly from those derived from epidemiological investigations based on representative population samples. This is undoubtedly because patients with anaemia who consult doctors are either likely to be severely affected by the anaemia or to have complications, or another underlying condition. Ultimately the importance of a condition must be judged from direct measurements of its effects on health and function. Appropriate studies are difficult but those which have been done indicate that anaemia of a degree which impairs health is rather uncommon in developed countries.

Any lowering of haemoglobin level will reduce the oxygen carrying capacity of the blood. It is reasonable therefore to expect anaemia to cause symptoms such as fatigue, breathlessness, dizziness, palpitations and general malaise. But these occur to some extent in most subjects. Anaemia is likely, therefore, to be used frequently as a 'scape-goat' to explain such symptoms, particularly in women or elderly patients. Yet surveys based on representative population samples have failed to detect a significant association between symptoms and circulating haemoglobin level[9]. Furthermore, randomized controlled trials of the effect of treatment have given evidence suggestive of benefit in terms of an improvement in symptoms only when anaemia is fairly severe, say, around 8 or 9 g/dl or lower.

Other effects of anaemia can occur, such as cardiac failure, but these too, almost certainly, only occur as a consequence of a very severe reduction in haemoglobin level and, therefore, are exceedingly rare in our community. Some of these effects, including possible effects on psychomotor function, cholesterol level and blood pressure were reviewed by Elwood[10].

Any association between haemoglobin level and work output is clearly of tremendous importance. Early studies of this association were laboratory based and although some evidence emerged indicating that the circulating haemoglobin level could be a limiting factor, it appeared that this only operated at maximal, or near maximal, work outputs[11]. More recent work in 'real life' situations in developing communities based on sugar workers in Guatemala, latex tappers in Java, weeders in Indonesia and tea pickers in Sri Lanka[12], has suggested that there is a beneficial effect from iron therapy. The benefit, however, does not appear to be derived solely from a change in haemoglobin level and it may be that the direct tissue effects of iron deficiency, which may be to some extent independent of circulating haemoglobin level, are important. It has also been suggested that iron therapy may increase the appetite of a subject with iron deficiency and his intake of a wide range of nutrients may increase.

While these studies on work output are of immense importance, particularly in developing countries, their relevance to Western communities, where general nutrition is good, and work outputs are far from maximal, is unknown.

Screening for anaemia has often been encouraged on the argument that often, particularly in hospital practice, it leads to the identification of a serious underlying disease. Such arguments are only reasonable if the underlying disease detected can be effectively treated and this is probably seldom the case. In one epidemiological study[13] in which over 1000 women were seen, there was little evidence that those below 12 g/dl more frequently had detectable pathology. In this study, those women with concentrations of less than 10 g/dl, and not already under treatment, were referred to hospital out-patients for further examination and investigation, and in only one case was there evidence of serious disease and this turned out to be virtually untreatable. Results such as these give little encouragement for *ad hoc* community screening for anaemia.

An overall assessment of the importance to health of a condition such as anaemia can be obtained from long-term follow-up studies in which the haemoglobin level is related to subsequent mortality. This approach is crude and necessitates very large numbers. Two such studies[14,15] showed only a very slight increase in deaths in subjects with anaemia (and in neither study was this statistically significant), but both detected a considerable increase in mortality in subjects with higher haemoglobin levels, above about 15 g/dl.

In any assessment of the importance of anaemia, possible beneficial effects must not be ignored, nor should be the possible harmful effects of a high haemoglobin level. While none of these have been adequately worked out, they do merit careful study. They include a possible advantage of marginally lowered haemoglobin levels in relation to mortality from cardiovascular disease and a well established raised mortality in subjects with high haemoglobin levels[14,15]. Other findings, including a greater frequency of electrocardiographic abnormalities in patients with iron overload, a positive correlation between haemoglobin and cholesterol levels and a greater number of coronary anastomoses in anaemic subjects, all of which are consistent with causal relationships but none of which has yet been fully worked out (see Elwood[10]).

Iron balance

Iron balance is normally maintained by regulation of the gastro-intestinal absorption of iron. Absorption is usually now envisaged on the basis of the 'two pool model' of Hallberg and others. This postulates that both endogenous and exogenous iron in the diet enters two pools within the gastro-intestinal tract, one of inorganic iron salts, the other of organic bound iron. All absorption occurs from these 2 pools. Absorption of the inorganic iron (whether from food or from fortification iron added to food) is modified by the size of the pool, the presence of factors which may enhance absorption (such as ascorbic acid and certain amino acids) and factors which inhibit absorption, including cereals and eggs.

As a result of the interplay of these and other factors relevant to iron absorption, the iron uptake from a diet is difficult to predict. Detailed nutrition studies have either demonstrated no association, or at best only a very weak association between dietary iron intake and any measure of iron balance.

Prevention

Ultimately iron balance is largely dependent on iron intake and if this is raised sufficiently, then almost no case of iron deficiency should occur. This line of thought is behind the attempts which are being made, or have been proposed, to reduce the prevalence of iron deficiency by the fortification of staple foodstuffs with iron. Extensive studies of iron deficiency have been conducted in the United Kingdom, and flour has been fortified with iron for many years. Experience gained in this country may be valuable in the planning of preventive measures for other parts of the world. In the United Kingdom, white bread and flour products provide about 25 % of the total average daily intake (11–12 mg per person). Approximately 60 % of the iron in white flour is endogenous and the remainder is added to comply with the Bread and Flour Regulations. This added iron supplies to the average person just over 1 mg of extra iron per day, or about 8 % of the average total dietary iron intake. Despite a fairly steady fall in the consumption of white bread there is still evidence that white bread plays an important dietary role and makes a substantial contribution to iron intake, particularly in large households, households with several children and low income households.

The absorption of various forms of iron added in fortification programmes has been well investigated. Results indicate that powdered iron which has been widely used as an alternative to Reduced Iron BP is very poorly absorbed. Absorption of ferrous sulphate and ferric ammonium citrate from bread is fairly good. True 'reduced iron' is absorbed about half as well as most iron salts[16].

The results of laboratory work are an inadequate basis for a national nutritional measure. Yet very few realistic community based trials have been conducted. In a randomized controlled trial in South Wales, women with anaemia were supplied with bread fortified with an iron salt sufficient to give an increase in the dietary iron level of about 3 mg per person per day. There was a very small rise in their circulating haemoglobin levels over the course of a year, consistent with an absorption of about 3 % of the iron added to the bread[17]. In another trial, an extra 15–22 mg iron per person per day, given in bread to 221 elderly anaemic subjects in Boston (Mass.) in the USA, had no significant effect.

In a trial, as yet unpublished, 15 mg iron given daily in bread rolls to Yugoslavian school children gave no convincing evidence of benefit. The value of iron fortification of foodstuffs is also questioned in a study of several European countries with differing food fortification practices (Damberg, personal communication). Despite very marked differences in dietary iron intakes, there appears to be a remarkably similar prevalence of anaemia (Table 11.1).

Table 11.1. Iron supply and the prevalence of anaemia in some European countries.

	Sweden	Denmark	England & Wales
Natural food iron mg Fe per person per day	19	19	14
Fortification iron mg Fe per person per day	6.5	5	1.6
Tablet iron mg Fe per person per day	6.6	2.7	2.0
Total iron intake mg Fe per person per day	32	27	18
Percentage subjects anaemic			
Women < 12 g/100 ml Hb	7	8	7
Men < 13 g/100 ml Hb	6	6	6

References

1. World Health Organization. *Nutritional anaemias.* Technical report series. No 503. Geneva: WHO, 1972.
2. Department of Health Education and Welfare. Mean blood hematocrit of adults. *Vital and Health Statistics.* Series II No 24. Washington: US Government Printing Office, 1967.
3. Campbell H, Greene WJW, *et al.* Pilot survey of haemoglobin and plasma urea concentration in a random sample of adults in Wales 1965–66. *British Journal of Preventive and Social Medicine* 1968; **22**: 41–49.
4. Garby L. The normal haemoglobin level. *British Journal of Haematology* 1970; **19**: 429–34.
5. Department of Health, Education and Welfare. *Haemoglobin and selected iron related findings of persons 1–74 years of age: United States, 1971–74.* Advance data, National Center for Health Statistics. No 46. Washington: US Government Printing Office, 1979.
6. Elwood PC, Hughes J, *et al.* An international haematological survey. *Bulletin of the World Health Organization* 1976; **54**: 87–95.
7. Charlton RW, Hawkins DM, *et al.* Hepatic storage iron concentrations in different population groups. *American Journal of Clinical Nutrition* 1970; **23**: 358–71.
8. Elwood PC, Burr ML, *et al.* Nutritional state of elderly Asian and English subjects in Coventry. *Lancet* 1972; **i**: 1224–7.
9. Elwood PC, Waters WE, *et al.* Symptoms and circulating haemoglobin level. *Journal of Chronic Disease* 1969; **21**: 615–28.
10. Elwood PC. Evaluation of the clinical importance of anaemia. *American Journal of Clinical Nutrition* 1973; **26**: 958.
11. Viteri FE, Torun B. Anaemia and physical work capacity. *Clinics in Haematology* 1974; **3**: 609–26.
12. Edgerton VR, Gardener GW, *et al.* Iron deficiency anaemia and its effect on worker productivity and activity patterns. *British Medical Journal* 1979; **ii**: 1546–9.

13. Elwood PC, Waters WE, *et al.* Evaluation of a screening survey for anaemia in adult non-pregnant women. *British Medical Journal* 1967; **iv**: 714–7.
14. Waters WE, Withey JL, *et al.* Ten year haematological follow-up: mortality and haematological changes. *British Medical Journal* 1969; **iv**: 761–4.
15. Elwood PC, Waters WE, *et al.* Mortality and anaemia in women. *Lancet* 1974; **i**: 891–4.
16. Ministry of Health. *Iron in Flour.* Reports on public health and medical subjects. No 117. London: HMSO, 1968.
17. Elwood PC, Waters WE, *et al.* The haematinic effect of iron in flour. *Clinical Science* 1971; **40**: 31–7.

Further reading

Garby L, ed. Anaemia and hypoxia. *Clinics in Haematology* 1974; **3** (3).

Hardisty RM, Weatherall DJ. *Blood and its Disorders.* Oxford: Blackwell Scientific Publications, 1974.

International Nutritional Anaemia Consultative Group. *Guidelines for the eradication of anaemia.* New York: INACG. The Nutrition Foundation Inc., 1978.

World Health Organization. *Nutritional anaemias.* Technical report series. No 503. Geneva: WHO, 1972.

SECTION 3 · CHRONIC RESPIRATORY DISEASES

Chapter 12 · Chronic Non-specific Lung Diseases (CNSLD) and Asthma

J R T COLLEY

Definitions

Recognition of the importance of chronic non-specific lung diseases as a cause of mortality and morbidity stimulated research in the 1950s into this group of diseases. The often large differences in respiratory mortality between countries were thought to be due in part to suspected differences in the meaning of terms such as chronic bronchitis, emphysema and asthma. Fig. 12.1 illustrates the wide variation in mortality from pneumonia and bronchitis in European

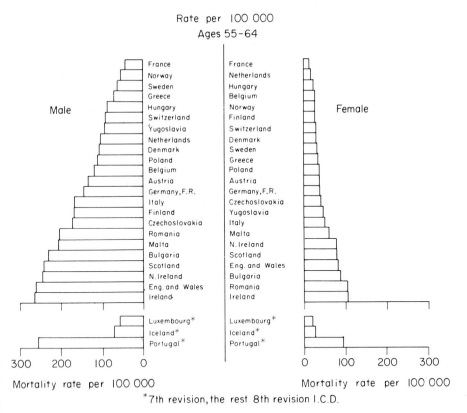

Rate per 100 000
Ages 55–64

Male

France
Norway
Sweden
Greece
Hungary
Switzerland
Yugoslavia
Netherlands
Denmark
Poland
Belgium
Austria
Germany, F.R.
Italy
Finland
Czechoslovakia
Romania
Malta
Bulgaria
Scotland
N. Ireland
Eng. and Wales
Ireland

Luxembourg*
Iceland*
Portugal*

Female

France
Netherlands
Hungary
Belgium
Norway
Finland
Switzerland
Denmark
Sweden
Greece
Poland
Austria
Germany, F.R.
Czechoslovakia
Yugoslavia
Italy
Malta
N. Ireland
Scotland
Eng. and Wales
Bulgaria
Romania
Ireland

Luxembourg*
Iceland*
Portugal*

300   200   100   0

Mortality rate per 100 000

0   100   200   300

Mortality rate per 100 000

*7th revision, the rest 8th revision I.C.D.

Fig. 12.1. Mortality from pneumonia and bronchitis for European countries, 1969. (World Health Organization. *Respiratory disease in Europe.* Geneva: WHO, 1974.)

countries. It is not known how far these differences are simply a result of variations in diagnostic habits between physicians in these various countries or reflect true differences in incidence. In 1959, at a CIBA guest symposium, proposals were made on the definition and classification of chronic bronchitis. These gained wide acceptance among chest physicians and epidemiologists, but have probably had little influence in standardizing diagnoses on death certificates. In the proposals it was suggested that patients be classified according to 3 types of disorder:

1   chronic or recurrent excessive secretion of bronchial mucus (chronic bronchitis);
2   intermittent obstruction to bronchial air flow (asthma);
3   persistent obstruction to bronchial air flow.

Since 1959 increased knowledge of these conditions has led to a gradual evolution of this classification[1]. Linked with this development was the construction in 1960 by a Medical Research Council Committee of a standardized questionnaire to record the presence of respiratory symptoms, including cough, phlegm, wheeze and shortness of breath, as well as smoking habits. This has proved an invaluable tool for field studies of chronic respiratory disease all over the world. Instead of the need to attach a diagnosis to persons seen in population studies, the presence of symptoms, and changes in measures of ventilatory function, such as peak expiratory flow rate and forced expiratory volume (FEV), can be used to define persons with a range of disease severity and type. The production of this questionnaire has been a major contribution to present understanding of this group of respiratory diseases.

Chronic non-specific lung diseases (CNSLD)

Routine mortality statistics data

Analysis of mortality, in spite of the above reservations regarding diagnostic precision, has provided information about the distribution of these diseases, as well as clues to possible aetiological factors. Mortality data are inevitably limited by the constraints imposed by the World Health Organization's International Classification of Diseases (ICD). The appropriate categories that cover CNSLD include bronchitis, pneumonia and emphysema. The data that follow have been abstracted from various sources and the reader will note the mixture of diagnostic groupings.

Age, sex and time trends

Mortality data, using various combinations of diagnoses, all show a characteristic age and sex pattern; mortality has a *J* or *U* shaped age distribution with consistently higher rates for adult males. In England and Wales since the early 1950s there has been a marked and consistent decrease in bronchitis mortality in women; the pattern in men has changed little at older ages (Table 12.1). Cohort analysis* of mortality rates (Fig. 12.2) indicates that for successive cohorts bronchitis mortality has decreased, suggesting circumstances in early life which influence subsequent mortality from bronchitis.

Table 12.1. Annual death rates per 100 000 for the periods 1951–53, 1961–63 and 1971–73 for chronic and unqualified bronchitis, England and Wales[2].

Year	Age group (years)	Males	Females	Male/female ratio
1951–53	25–44	4.0	2.0	(2:1)
	45–64	113.8	30.4	(3.7:1)
	65–74	446.8	137.5	(3.2:1)
	75+	903.3	456.0	(2:1)
1961–63	25–44	2.9	1.7	(1.7:1)
	45–64	114.3	21.0	(5.4:1)
	65–74	550.2	108.0	(5.1:1)
	75+	1071.0	334.0	(3.2:1)
1971–73	25–44	1.5	0.9	(1.6:1)
	45–64	72.4	19.0	(3.8:1)
	65–74	416.2	70.0	(5.9:1)
	75+	1017.0	209.6	(4.8:1)

As well as these long-term trends in bronchitis mortality, there are marked seasonal variations. Both in the United Kingdom and the USA bronchitis mortality is higher in the winter than in the summer. Deaths from pneumonia as well as bronchitis show this pattern. In years when there are winter influenza epidemics, bronchitis and pneumonia mortality may be higher than usual. This could reflect a true increase in bronchitis and pneumonia or some imprecision in certification; some bronchitis or pneumonia deaths may be certified as due to influenza and vice versa. The extent of such diagnostic shift is unknown.

Occupation and social factors

In the United Kingdom mortality rates have shown large differences between men working in different occupations. In addition mortality has a consistent and large social class gradient. It is low in Social Class I, rising to a maximum in Social Class V. Over the 40 years spanned by Table 12.2 the gradient has

* Cohort is the term used to describe a segment of the population born around the same time period, labelled by the central year around which the subjects in it were born. This enables changes in the mortality rate from one generation to another to be displayed, and sometimes these can be related to different exposures to aetiological factors.

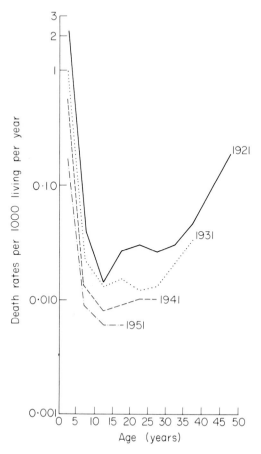

Fig. 12.2. Bronchitis death rates in male generations born in 1921, 1931, 1941, and 1951, England & Wales. (Hull D, ed. *Recent advances in paediatrics 5*. London: Churchill Livingstone, 1976: 230.)

persisted. The reasons for these marked social class differences in bronchitis mortality are not wholly clear.

Geographic variations

Mortality from bronchitis varies within the United Kingdom, both by region and population density. For example, the standardized mortality ratio (SMR) for bronchitis and emphysema in areas of different population density in 1973 ranged from 75 in rural areas to 118 in large conurbations. Comparable SMRs for women ranged from 79 to 119. Southern England, including East Anglia, has

Table 12.2. Bronchitis mortality by social class for men aged 20–64, United Kingdom[2].

Social Class	Standardized mortality ratio		
	(1921–23)	(1949–53)	(1959–63)
I	26	34	28
II	55	53	50
III	94	98	97
IV	121	101	116
V	177	171	194

a low bronchitis mortality in comparison with that in South Wales, the Midlands and Northern England. These geographic variations in mortality are thought most unlikely to be due to differences in certification practice. Weather may play some part in explaining the regional differences, but the main reasons could be a concentration of lower social class in the urban areas, undue occupational exposure, and higher prevalence of smoking.

Routine morbidity statistics data

These are of limited use in describing the epidemiology of these groups of diseases. Hospital admissions and discharges, for which data are available in England and Wales, are insufficiently sensitive indicators of incidence for comparative studies. Morbidity statistics from General Practice are available only for a small number of selected practices. Certified sickness absence has been used to study the geographic and occupational patterns of bronchitis and its association with air pollution, as well as time trends. However, these data only refer to the working population and then not all of them. The precision of the diagnostic information on these medical certificates is also suspect. In spite of these reservations, sickness absence trends do tend to correspond with those for deaths and suggest that morbidity from bronchitis has fallen in women and not in men.

Epidemiological studies

The world literature on the epidemiology of CNSLD is large. The major areas of study have been into the effects of air pollution, smoking and occupational exposure. Higgins[3] provided an extensive review of the world literature up to 1974. Other reports that may be consulted for more recent references include those by Speizer and Tager[4] and the Royal College of Physicians of London report on Smoking or Health[5].

Factors in aetiology

Cigarette Smoking

This appears to be the major factor in the aetiology of bronchitis. There is a close relationship between cigarette smoking habits and subsequent mortality from chronic bronchitis. Fig. 12.3, taken from Doll and Hill's follow-up study of British doctors, demonstrates the increasing risk of death from bronchitis with the number of cigarettes smoked. In field surveys a similar relationship is found between the prevalence of symptoms, such as persistent cough and phlegm, and current smoking habits. Differences in smoking habits probably explain the higher bronchitis mortality in men. The review[5] published in 1977 by the Royal College of Physicians of London should be consulted for further discussion of this aspect of aetiology.

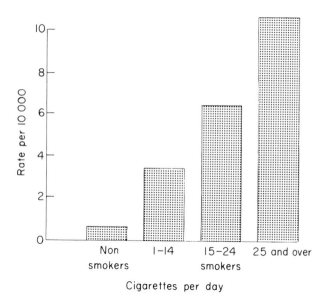

Fig. 12.3. Mortality from chronic bronchitis in British doctors. (Doll R, Hill AB. Mortality in relation to smoking. *British Medical Journal* 1964; **i**: 1399.)

Air pollution

Short term exposure to high levels of general air pollution have been associated with a high rate of deaths, most notably in London in December 1952 when some 4000 excess deaths occurred mostly in middle-aged and elderly adults already suffering from chronic cardiovascular or respiratory diseases.

    The role of longer term exposure to lower levels of general air pollution in the aetiology of chronic bronchitis is less clear. Evidence from the United Kingdom suggests that after allowing for differences in smoking habits and age, populations living in air polluted areas have a higher prevalence of bronchitic symptoms. One national study found that among non-smokers age-adjusted morbidity ratios (%) were 41 in the lowest air pollution exposure group against 71 in the highest, while the ratios for smokers in the same areas were 121 and 209, the population mean being 100 %. The effect of air pollution on bronchitis morbidity in this population was less than that of cigarette smoking.

The Clean Air Acts in the 1950s have resulted in major reductions in smoke levels in the United Kingdom but not in sulphur dioxide levels. Over this same period, bronchitis mortality has tended to fall, especially in areas where smoke pollution has diminished greatly. Taken with the other evidence on associations between respiratory disease and air pollution, these changes are suggestive of a causal relationship. Another report[6] from the Royal College of Physicians of London, published in 1970, reviews evidence on health effects of air pollution.

Occupation

Studies of men working in dusty occupations, for example, coal miners and foundrymen, have provided evidence for some effect of occupational exposure in increasing the risk of chronic bronchitis. Interpretation is bedevilled by uncertainty, for example, on how far cigarette smoking habits in these occupational groups could account for the differences found rather than inhalation of dust.

Social class

Striking social class gradients in mortality from chronic bronchitis in the United Kingdom are seen in both men and women, and are thus unlikely to be due mainly to occupational exposures. They may reflect differences in smoking habits and in general and domestic environmental exposure between the social classes.

Childhood experience

Evidence is suggestive that respiratory illness in childhood may contribute to the evolution of chronic bronchitis in adult life. Lower respiratory tract illness under the age of 2 years increases the risk at the age of 20–25 of chest symptoms such as cough and phlegm.

Familial and genetic factors

A rare familial emphysema in which the onset is in early adult life has been found to be associated with a deficiency of α1-antitrypsin. Apart from this condition almost nothing is known about possible genetic influences in CNSLD.

Atopy

The relationship between asthma and CNSLD is not clear. Wheeze is a common symptom in the absence of asthma and may be associated with CNSLD. Whether this indicates an atopic component in CNSLD is uncertain.

Natural history

As with many chronic diseases with evolution extending over many years, the knowledge of natural history of CNSLD is incomplete. Furthermore, the clinical spectrum is wide, both in terms of severity and rate of progression. Studies of the pathology of CNSLD indicate a range of possible structural changes. These include mucous gland hypertrophy concentrated in the more central bronchi; stenotic and inflammatory lesions of the small conducting airways (typical of chronic bronchitis); centrilobular and panlobular emphysema characterized by localized destructive changes in respiratory and terminal bronchioles, and destructive changes in supporting lung connective tissue framework.

These changes are associated with corresponding clinical and functional abnormalities. A current view is that two major syndromes can be distinguished; one characterized by chronic phlegm production, the other by chronic airflow obstruction[7]. Either condition may be present without the other, although a mixed picture is not uncommon. There is evidence that the hypersecretory syndrome may be reversible, for example, where a smoker gives up the habit, whereas the obstructive syndrome is not. Serial $FEV_{1.0}$ measurements on samples of adults have been used to study the evolution of CNSLD. The findings suggest that most adults show a steady loss of $FEV_{1.0}$ of about 20–30 ml/year. In cigarette smokers the decline may be up to 60–80 ml/year, a rate at which disabling chronic obstructive lung disease becomes apparent in middle age. Ceasing to smoke may result in a slowing of the rate of decline.

Prevention

Primary prevention

Susceptibility to CNSLD cannot yet be measured. On the other hand exposure to smoking can be readily estimated and theoretically at least such exposure could be removed or reduced. Thus the major preventive measure for an individual would be to give up cigarette smoking.

A more difficult primary preventive approach is the continuing reduction of general air pollution. The specific components which need attention and the levels to which they should be reduced are at present uncertain. As childhood respiratory illness is probably a contributing factor in adult disease, measures to reduce the risk of chest infections and their severity in early life could be of benefit.

Secondary prevention

In established chronic obstructive airways disease, ceasing to smoke may only retard progression as the pathological changes are irreversible. Those in whom phlegm production is the major feature will often find that ceasing to smoke results in a reduction or even cessation of phlegm. In contrast to the apparent benefits of giving up smoking medical treatment has a very limited role in the secondary prevention of CNSLD.

Asthma

Mortality and morbidity data

Age and sex

Mortality ascribed to asthma has a characteristic pattern. The rates in childhood and early adult life are low and then rise progressively from the mid-20s throughout the rest of life. This can be seen in Table 12.3 where data for England Wales in 1978 are given. Overall mortality tends to be higher in females than in males.

Table 12.3. Asthma (ICD 493) death rates per million by sex, 1978, England and Wales[8].

Age (years)	Male	Female	Age (years)	Male	Female
All	19	28	35–44	19	12
< 1	0	0	45–54	21	29
1–4	7	4	55–64	26	50
5–14	4	3	65–74	55	70
15–24	6	8	75–84	89	95
25–34	11	8	85+	101	98

Time trends

Examination of the time trends in asthma mortality in England and Wales during the 1960s revealed a striking rise and subsequent fall in mortality (Fig. 12.4). The reasons for this epidemic are even now not agreed. It is unlikely that changes in diagnostic habits, coding practices, or in the incidence and severity of asthma can account for the sudden increase in mortality. The increased use of pressurized aerosols was proposed as the most likely cause, and this view gained support when asthma mortality fell with their reduced use. However, other countries, for example the USA, where these aerosols were also used, did not see this epidemic. It is thought that in the USA, unlike in England and Wales, the high dose aerosol

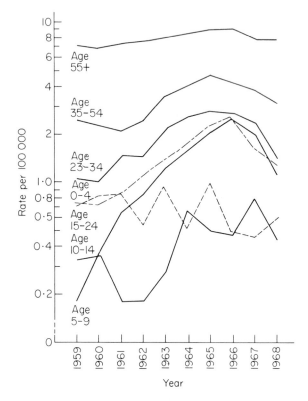

Fig. 12.4. Mortality from asthma (ICD 241) in England & Wales, expressed as annual age-specific rates per 100 000 living, 1959–68. (Inman & Adelstein. *Lancet* 1969; **ii**: 279–85.)

nebulizers were not used, and that this accounts for the difference in mortality experience.

Asthma mortality in England and Wales shows a seasonal pattern. Quarterly data for asthma and other respiratory diseases in the epidemic years 1959–68 are given in Fig. 12.5 for persons aged 5–34 years. The peak mortality from asthma occurs in the third quarter coinciding with troughs of mortality for other respiratory diseases.

Geographic variation

Mortality rates ascribed to asthma vary between countries. How far these represent differences in certification and coding practices or indicate true differences in incidence or in case fatality is unclear.

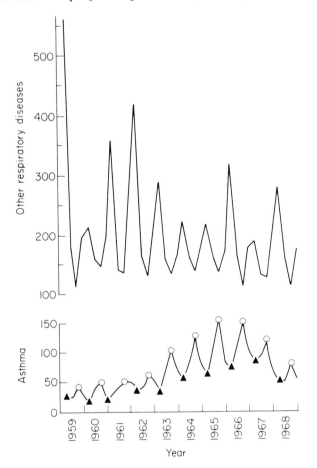

Fig. 12.5. Numbers of quarterly deaths from asthma (ICD 241) and from other respiratory diseases (ICD 470–527) among people aged 5–34, England & Wales. ▲Winter deaths (Jan.– Mar.); O Summer deaths (July–Sept.). Other respiratory diseases include: acute upper-respiratory tract infections (ICD 470–75), influenza (ICD 480–3), pneumonia (ICD 490–3), bronchitis (ICD 500–2) and other diseases of the respiratory system (ICD 510–527). (Inman & Adelstein. *Lancet* 1969; **ii**: 279–85.)

Social factors

In men in England and Wales mortality from asthma tends to be low in Social Class I and higher in Social Class V; in contrast the pattern is reversed in children, with mortality being higher in Social Class I than in the other classes.

Routine morbidity statistics

The same comments in relation to CNSLD can be made in respect of asthma.

Epidemiological studies

Age and sex

Most of the epidemiological investigations into asthma have been conducted among children. Almost all have been prevalence studies employing a variety of methods and definitions of asthma. It will be no surprise that wide differences have been found in the prevalence of asthma in these studies. In the United Kingdom among secondary school children reported prevalence rates have varied between 0.9% and 4.8% in different studies.

Although mortality data suggest that the incidence of asthma increases sharply with age (Table 12.3) the absence of reliable morbidity data on incidence necessitates reliance upon prevalence data which may, in a disease of long duration, provide reasonable estimates of the extent of the disease. Prevalence data from the USA National Health Survey suggest that asthma currently affects 2.2% and 4.2% of the adult population and that there is no consistent relationship with age. This suggests that case fatality increases markedly with age, particularly after 35 years.

In children, males show a higher prevalence of asthma than females, and tend to suffer a more severe form of asthma, although mortality rates in boys and girls are broadly similar. In adults, prevalence of asthma tends to be higher in women than men. This difference is also seen in their pattern of mortality.

Factors in aetiology

Familial and genetic factors

Twin studies suggest a genetic component in the aetiology of asthma. Studies in the United Kingdom on national samples of children have found the risk of developing asthma where one or both parents had had the disease to be almost twice that of children whose parents never had asthma.

Atopy

An association between eczema and asthma, found in children attending hospital for asthma, has been confirmed in studies in the general population. The major component in the aetology of the disease seems to be an as yet not fully understood disturbance of the immune system. Although children may be sensitive to a wide variety of allergens, the house-dust mite (*Dermatophagoides pteronyssinus*) is probably the most important cause of allergic asthma.

Occupational exposure

Allergic sensitivity to various dusts, for example wood dust, may result in asthma. These are not common causes of asthma.

Natural history

There have been few longitudinal studies on asthmatics derived from well-defined populations. It is thus not possible to make any clear statement about its natural history. What evidence there is suggests that most asthmatic children will be free of the disease by early adult life. Asthma starting in adult life is thought to carry a far worse prognosis, but evidence on outcome is almost wholly lacking.

Prevention

Primary prevention

Lack of understanding of the underlying causes of asthma have hampered attempts at prevention. Immunologists have suggested contact with antigens in the first few months of life may be a factor in the aetiology of both eczema and asthma. The effects of antigen avoidance in early life on subsequent risk of asthma are currently being investigated.

Secondary prevention

In house-dust-sensitive asthmatic children, studies involving avoidance of exposure to the house-dust mite and its products suggest that some improvement in asthma may occur. Most of these studies have not been well controlled and their findings should be viewed with caution.

Adequate medical treatment can result in most asthmatic children leading a normal life with little or no disability. The main problem is to be sure that they take their medication and that the treatment is adequate.

References

1. Fletcher CM. Terminology in chronic obstructive lung diseases. *Journal of Epidemiology and Community Health* 1978; **32**: 282.
2. Office of Health Economics. *Preventing Bronchitis No 59*. London: Office of Health Economics, 1977.
3. Higgins ITT. The epidemiology of chronic respiratory disease. *Preventive Medicine* 1973; **2**: 14–33.
4. Speizer FE, Tager IB. Epidemiology of chronic mucus hypersecretion and obstructive airways disease. *Epidemiological Reviews* 1979; **1**: 124.
5. Royal College of Physicians of London. *Smoking or health*. London: Pitman Medical, 1977.
6. Royal College of Physicians of London. *Air pollution and health*. London: Pitman Medical, 1970.
7. Fletcher C, Peto R, *et al. The natural history of chronic bronchitis and emphysema*. Oxford: Oxford University Press, 1976.
8. Office of Population Censuses and Surveys. *Routine Mortality Statistics, Cause 1978*. Series DH 2. No 5. London: HMSO, 1980.

Further reading

Gordis L. *Epidemiology of chronic lung diseases in children*. Baltimore: The John Hopkins University Press, 1973.

Chapter 13 · Industrial Lung Diseases

G KAZANTZIS

A wide variety of respiratory disorders have been shown to be associated with exposure to noxious agents encountered in the working environment[1]. The causal agents may be vapours, gases or dusts that are inhaled into the respiratory tract. For aerosols to be capable of inhalation into, and deposition in the lower

Table 13.1. Principal pulmonary reactions and causal agents.

Pulmonary reactions	Causal agents
Pulmonary fibrosis	Silica, coal dust, Fibrous silicates – asbestos, talc Non-fibrous silicates – mica
Extrinsic allergic alveolitis	Mouldy hay (micropolyspora), other mouldy vegetable produce Other fungal spores, mouldy bagasse Avian antigens
Asthma	Platinum complexes Isocyanates Flour and grain dusts Laboratory animal urine Certain wood dusts Formaldehyde Cotton, flax, hemp, (byssinosis) Epoxy resin curing agents
Pulmonary oedema	Oxides of nitrogen, ozone, phosgene Ammonia, sulphur dioxide
Specific infections Tuberculosis Anthrax Q fever Ornithosis	*Myobacterium tuberculosis* *Bacillus anthracis* *Coxiella burneti* Chlamdia
Cancer	Asbestos Radon daughters Haemitite mining, processes involving exposure to chromite ores and to certain nickel compounds ?Arsenic, ?cadmium, ?beryllium Polycyclic hydrocarbons in coal gas manufacture
Other	Cadmium, bauxite (emphysema) Beryllium (granuloma)

respiratory tract, they have to be finely particulate, with a mass median aerodynamic diameter of less than about 5 μm.

The principal pulmonary reactions and the more important agents that give rise to them are listed in Table 13.1. The pulmonary fibroses discussed in this chapter are silicosis, coal workers' pneumoconiosis and asbestosis caused by the inhalation of mineral dusts. Some inhaled dusts produce no discernable pulmonary reaction but may accumulate in the lung parenchyma and if they contain elements of high atomic number will produce opacities on a chest X-ray which may mimic a pulmonary fibrosis.

Alveolar reactions result from inhalation of a variety of fungal spores from mouldy vegetable produce or particulate matter of animal origin. The disease in this group that has been most carefully studied is Farmers' lung. A variety of both organic and inorganic agents can cause asthma. Acute pulmonary oedema can be precipitated by inhalation of certain fumes and gases. The occupational exposures giving rise to increased mortality from cancer of the lung are dicussed in Chapter 14.

Some occupations are associated with an increased risk of certain infections, or with an altered clinical course. For example, medical and allied workers carry an increased risk of pulmonary tuberculosis. Workers exposed to silica dust who acquired a tuberculous infection have developed a rapidly progressive and often fatal form of silico tuberculosis.

Chronic industrial lung diseases are sometimes loosely referred to as 'pneumoconioses'. This term has a precise meaning in Britain for the purpose of industrial injury benefit; it is defined as 'fibrosis of the lungs due to silica dust, asbestos dust or other dust, and including the condition of the lungs known as dust reticulation'; this latter term describes a radiological abnormality only.

Clinical and pathological features

The pneumoconioses

Most pneumoconioses are chronic conditions that present insidiously with exertional dyspnoea. This may slowly progress to respiratory failure or right heart failure. Other symptoms, such as cough and sputum may be due in part to an associated chronic bronchitis. Silica particles in the lung evoke a focal fibrosis which produces an opacity in the chest X-ray with firm nodules which may be felt in the parenchyma. The presence of coal dust with silica modifies the fibrotic response. Where coal dust is present without silica, the fibrotic reaction is minimal. In simple pneumoconiosis multiple small opacities are present on the chest X-ray (Fig. 13.1). In the absence of chronic bronchitis these are not associated with symptoms or with significant abnormality on the respiratory

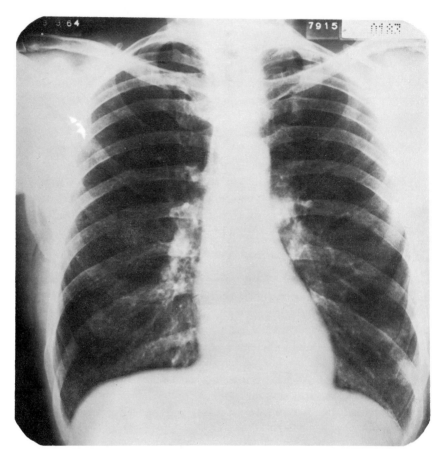

Fig. 13.1(a). Radiographs illustrating the International Labour Organization (ILO) U/C International Classification of Radiographs of the Pneumoconioses, 1971. Category 1 type p: small rounded opacities definitely present but few in number, up to about 1.5 mm diameter; category A large opacities also present.

function tests. Thus radiological abnormality usually precedes symptoms and functional abnormality in silicosis and in coal workers' pneumoconiosis. However, symptoms may be present in more advanced cases.

Where the small fibrotic nodules coalesce to form large fibrous masses, the condition is known as progressive massive fibrosis (PMF) or complicated pneumoconiosis. There is a relationship between the length of exposure, or more precisely, the amount of dust inhaled, and the stage of the disease. However, in cases where there is existing tuberculosis, or where there is a rheumatoid diathesis, massive fibrosis occurs earlier than otherwise. It is believed that an

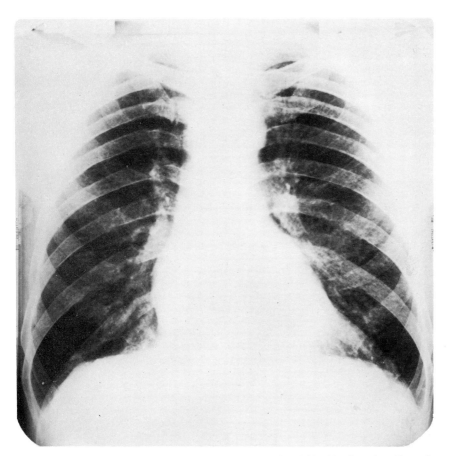

Fig. 13.1(b). Radiographs illustrating the ILO U/C International Classification of Radiographs of the Pneumoconioses, 1971. Category 2 type q: numerous small rounded opacities between about 1.5 mm and 3 mm diameter.

immunological factor is involved. Where fibrosis produces distortion of the surrounding parenchyma which results in focal emphysema, the translucent spaces so formed make the fibrotic nodules appear less opaque on the X-ray, thus the stage of the disease in such cases may be underestimated. Focal emphysema of this type may be found in coal workers' pneumoconiosis. Silicosis and coal workers' pneumoconiosis are diagnosed on a history of exposure, exclusion of other disease and on the chest X-ray. Parenchymal opacities are essential for the diagnosis.

The fibrosis produced by the inhalation of asbestos dust is interstitial rather than focal in distribution and futhermore pleural fibrosis encases the lung and

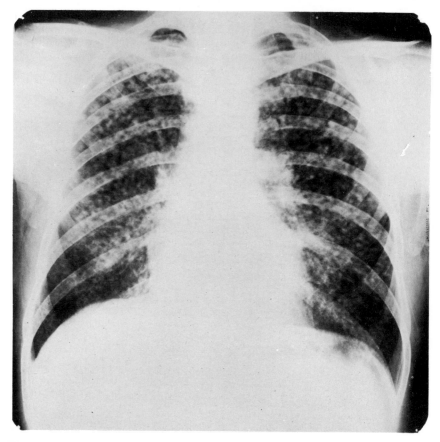

Fig. 13.1(c). Radiographs illustrating the ILO U/C International Classification of Radiographs of the Pneumoconioses, 1971. Category 3 type r: very numerous small rounded opacities between about 3 mm and 10 mm diameter.

restricts its expansion. This results in a diminution of the subdivisions of the lung volume. The diffuse interstitial fibrosis impedes gas transfer at an early stage, giving rise to functional abnormality when radiological features of asbestosis may be minimal. Another radiological feature indicative of asbestos exposure, but not necessarily of asbestosis, is pleural plaque formation. The diagnosis of asbestosis is made on a history of exposure, the presence of basal crepitations, the pattern of impairment on respiratory function tests and the chest radiograph.

Allergic alveolitis

The inhalation of a variety of organic dusts of vegetable, microbial or avian origin, may give rise to an immunologically determined inflammatory response

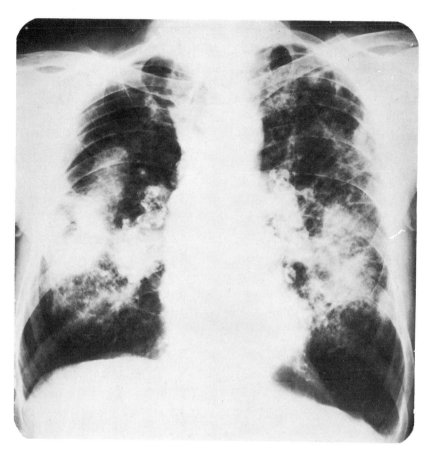

Fig. 13.1(d). Radiographs illustrating the ILO U/C International Classification of Radiographs of the Pneumoconioses, 1971. Category C w.d.: well-defined large opacities whose combined area exceeds one-third of the area of the right lung.

of the peripheral gas-exchanging tissue of the lung, probably mediated by precipitating antibody. Where sensitization occurs, an acute respiratory illness with breathlessness develops some hours after exposure, which usually subsides rapidly but recurs with re-exposure. With repeated attacks, the patient may develop progressive pulmonary fibrosis ending in cardio-respiratory failure. Farmers' lung is the commonest form of extrinsic allergic alveolitis seen in Britain. The condition is diagnosed on the history of exposure, the presence of precipitating antibody, the restrictive ventilatory defect with impaired gas transfer, and the chest radiograph. However, precipitating antibody has been found in surveys in 15–20% of farm workers without the disease and may be absent in a similar percentage of patients with Farmers' lung.

Sources of mortality and morbidity data

Morbidity and mortality data on the pulmonary fibroses of occupational origin
are more complete than for many other chronic diseases but some important
limitations remain. For a long time, occupational disease in Britain has entitled
the worker to financial benefit from the State. Initially, this was covered by the
Workman's Compensation Acts, but since 1948 it has been covered by the
National Insurance (Industrial Injuries) Act. The pneumoconioses, as legally
defined, are now covered under Part 2 of the Social Security (Industrial Diseases)
(Prescribed Diseases) Regulations 1975, in which there is a schedule of occupations where it is recognized that these diseases may be contracted. Farmers'
lung, mesothelioma of the pleura, tuberculosis and anthrax resulting from
occupation, beryllium and cadmium lung, and lung cancer associated with
certain processes where there is exposure to nickel, are prescribed diseases under
Part 1 of the 1975 regulations.

A worker who believes he may have one of these conditions has to initiate a
claim with his local Social Security Office. A claimant for silicosis or coal
workers' pneumoconiosis in the first instance has a chest X-ray. If this shows
evidence of the disorder he is referred to a pneumoconiosis panel where he is
assessed clinically and with physiological tests. A claimant for asbestosis is
referred to the panel without having a preliminary chest X-ray. If his claim is
refused, he has recourse to a complex appeal procedure. As industrial death
benefit to dependants is also payable, a person who dies from a suspected or
confirmed industrial lung disease has a post mortem examination during which
the lungs are scrutinized by a pathologist with specialist knowledge. Thus,
these cases are well documented, and mortality data is likely to be comprehensive.

Despite the notification and investigative procedures, data from pneumoconiosis panels, with certain exceptions, tend to give only an approximate guide
to incidence or prevalence rates. A variety of factors determine whether a claim is
initiated at all; these include awareness of the legislation on the part of claimant
and medical adviser. Furthermore, while for certain occupational groups it may
be possible to estimate the size of the population at risk, for others such
information is not available. Incidence rates can only be obtained in occupational groups by means of carefully planned field studies. Such studies are being
performed by the National Coal Board Medical Service on miners and in a
variety of large groups exposed to asbestos, by the Medical Research Council
(MRC) and by academic and other organizations in a number of countries
throughout the world.

Survey methods

Because of the insidious onset of some of these diseases there are difficulties in the early ascertainment of cases, which is necessary in order to estimate incidence in relation to exposure, and to describe the natural history of the disease. Most investigations rely on regular screening, using standardized methods for clinical evaluation, assessment of radiological abnormality and respiratory function.

The MRC questionnaire on respiratory symtoms[2] is an invaluable and widely used tool for clinical evaluation.

The role of the chest radiograph in the diagnosis of pneumoconiosis has already been made clear. Full size films of good quality are required. The interpretation of these films is subject to both inter and intra-observer variation. To compensate for this, each film should be read by at least 2 observers on more than one occasion with appropriate controls in a design that can be subjected to statistical analysis. The International Labour Organization's International Classification of Radiographs of Pneumoconioses (1971) uses standard films for limits of normality and classifies opacities in terms of size, shape, profusion and situation. The extent of pleural involvement is also recorded. Sets of standard films issued by the International Labour Organization (ILO)[3] are available to readers and now widely used on an international basis (Fig. 13.1). On this system, the earliest abnormality is designated category 0 whilst the presence of a few small opacities in the lung fields is designated category 1. More numerous small opacities which may partly obscure lung markings form category 2, and very numerous small opacities partly or totally obscuring lung markings form category 3. Massive opacities are designated by the terms A, B and C.

Respiratory function tests require careful standardization of instruments and technique. The simplest test which can be performed in the field, is the estimation of peak flow rate and the forced vital capacity (FVC) with its timed subdivisions. These tests are especially valuable in studies on environmental factors which might give rise to occupational asthma. Determination of peak flow rates before and after a work shift, on successive days in the week, may demonstrate a variety of patterns of ventilatory impairment. For example, where there is incomplete recovery from one day to the next, a stepwise decline may be seen through the working week. More elaborate tests such as estimation of residual volume, transfer factor and compliance may be performed in a physiological laboratory.

Biological investigation of the workers needs to be accompanied by environmental measurement of dust concentration or of chemical contaminants. Personal samplers worn by the workers measure the concentration of contaminant in the breathing zone and static samplers give information on its evolution and distribution through the work place. Dust particles can now be identified, sized and counted and the data interpreted by industrial hygienists, with the necessary training in the physical sciences and in statistical methods. In this way estimates can be made of exposure levels and cumulative exposures over time for the calculation of dose–response relationships.

Silicosis

Incidence and causation

Silicosis occurs wherever free silica in particles of respirable size is released into the working environment. Hippocrates in his *Epidemics* described the metal digger as a man who breathes with difficulty. Agricola, in *De re metallica*, published in 1556, observed: '. . . some mines are so dry that they are entirely devoid of water and this dryness causes the workmen even greater harm, for the dust, which is stirred and beaten up by digging, penetrates into the lungs and produces difficulty in breathing . . . . In the mines of the Carpathian Mountains women are found who have married seven husbands, all of whom this terrible consumption has carried off to a premature death.'

Charles Thackrah in his monograph, *The effects of the principal arts, trades and professions . . . on health and longevity*, published in 1831, wrote of the cutlery grinders of Sheffield: 'the fork-grinders, who use a dry grindstone, die at the age of 28 or 32, while the table-knife grinders, who work on wet stones, survive to between 40 and 50.' Almost certainly these workers died of silico-tuberculosis. Free silica in a respirable size range is released into the breathing zone whenever silica-containing minerals are worked either by hand or by mechanized tools. Thus miners, including gold, tin and haematite miners, as well as coal miners who drill through siliceous rock strata, are high risk groups. Other high risk groups are stone masons who fashion sandstone or granite, potters who may handle powdered flint, boiler scalers, slate quarriers, metal grinders, iron and steel foundry workers and sand blasters. Foundry workers clean their castings of adherent sand in a process known as fettling. The fractured sand particles are in a respirable size range and give rise to silicosis when inhaled. Sandblasters are exposed in a similar way and are normally protected with a helmet and external air line. Despite such protection a group of sandblasters in New Orleans in the 1970s developed silico-tuberculosis with a high fatality rate[4].

Silicosis has occurred predominantly in men. However, women have also been occupationally exposed to free silica. For example, a group of young women domestics developed rapidly progressive silicosis after using a scouring agent containing powdered silica for cleaning baths.

It is clear from the above that silicosis, probably with tuberculosis, could be a rapidly fatal disease in the younger adult age groups, with a duration measured in months rather than years. During the present century, with increasing control of both dust exposure and tuberculous infection, silicosis has become a more chronic disease which affects an older age group. Progression may occur even after cessation of exposure, when massive fibrosis may develop, probably as a result of an immunological reaction.

The relative importance of silicosis, in terms of numbers of new cases diagnosed in each of the 5 years 1972–76, compared with coal miners' pneumoconiosis and asbestosis, can be seen from Table 13.2. The table is derived from the number of examinations made by the pneumoconiosis medical panels at which pneumoconiosis and byssinosis were first diagnosed (i.e. category 2 pneumoconiosis and above). The age distribution of the new cases diagnosed by the medical panels in 1976 is shown in Table 13.3. Very few diagnoses were made below the age of 40.

Table 13.2. Number of examinations made by the British pneumoconiosis medical panels at which pneumoconiosis and byssinosis were first diagnosed, by attributable industry, 1972–76[5].

Disease	Year 1972	1973	1974	1975	1976
Pneumoconiosis	919	792	788	981	935
Asbestos	125	143	139	161	189
Coal mining	626	515	539	683	575
Mining and quarring (other than coal)	42	31	24	41	76
Foundry workers	40	34	30	31	35
Pottery manufacture	24	16	15	24	17
Other industries, including steel dressers and refractories	62	53	41	41	43
Total other than asbestos and coal mining	168	134	110	137	171
Byssinosis	48	32	126	156	102

Table 13.3. Age distribution of cases diagnosed as pneumoconiosis in 1976 as set out in Table 13.2, in asbestos, coal mining and other industries.

Age group (years)	Asbestos Number	%	Coal mining Number	%	All others Number	%
< 30	0	0	0	0	0	0
30–39	4	2	9	2	5	3
40–49	38	20	37	6	16	9
50–59	56	30	213	37	54	32
60–69	72	38	219	38	75	44
70+	19	10	97	17	21	12
Total	189	100	575	100	171	100

Prevention

The pneumoconioses are all preventable provided the inhalation of respirable particles over a working lifetime is kept below the minimum required to give rise to the disease. Guidelines for exposure to dust in the working environment are set out by the American Conference of Governmental Industrial Hygienists

(ACGIH). These have been adopted by Western industrial countries including the Health and Safety Commission in Britain[6]. The guidelines are based on a set of Threshold Limit Values (TLV). For dusts these are expressed in terms of millions of particles per cubic foot (mppcf) or as a respirable mass in mg/m³. The TLVs are not sharp dividing lines between safe and dangerous concentrations, and are revised, often in a downward direction, as new data become available. The Health and Safety Commission adopts the policy that while exposure should in any case be kept within the TLV by the application of suitable engineering controls, exposure should also be kept as low as is reasonably practicable below the TLV. Where necessary, suitable respiratory equipment should be provided which should be regarded as providing a backup for other techniques that aim to control the risk at source rather than a first line of defence. TLVs for silica are given separately for quartz, cristobalite, tridymite, fused silica and amorphous silica. As in practice a worker inhales a mixture of mineral dusts, formulae are available for calculating the TLV from the composition of the mixture.

While the measures taken to prevent inhalation of free silica at the workplace have greatly reduced the risk of silicosis, the figures shown in Table 13.2 are still appreciable and show little recent change. However, it should be borne in mind that 90 % of these newly diagnosed cases occurred in workers over the age of 50 who may have been exposed many years previously in industries in which there was then inadequate environmental control.

Coal workers' pneumoconiosis

This remains by far the most common form of industrial lung disease (Table 13.2). The annual numbers must be interpreted in relation to the size of the population at risk. Manpower in the coal mining industry was a little over 540 000 in the period 1959–62, with the reshaping of the industry, this had fallen to 200 000 by 1973–77. The publicity given to the Pneumoconiosis Compensation Scheme, introduced in 1974, led to an increase in retired and ex-miners applying for certification. This is in part responsible for the increase in numbers of cases seen in 1975.

A high proportion of men, about 90 %, avail themselves of the National Coal Board's Periodic X-ray Scheme started in 1958–59. Men are advised to apply for certification on a 'clinical reading' of their films and most in fact do so. In this way, the cases certified by the medical panels (category 2 and above) can be used for the calculation of approximate incidence rates. These are the only incidence rates available to the National Coal Board, and for the years 1974–76 were, respectively, 2.2, 2.8 and 2.4 per 1000 men employed[7]. In 1976, the average age at diagnosis was 61 years compared with 53 years in 1951.

Over the last 20 years the National Coal Board's Periodic X-ray Scheme made it possible to obtain prevalence rates for pneumoconiosis, and to study regional differences. Chest X-rays were initially taken every 5 years. In 1974, this interval was changed to 4 years. Prevalence, expressed as a diagnosis of pneumoconiosis on the chest X-ray (all categories) as a percentage of all men examined, fell steadily from 13.4% in 1959–60 to 7.6% in 1974–77. There were large regional differences throughout this period, with a low of 2.8% in the Scottish area, contrasted with a high of 20.0% in South Wales over the latter period. These differences may, in large part, be related to differences in both physical and chemical properties and in concentration of inhaled dust.

Changes in prevalence could be explained by the selective departure of men with pneumoconiosis from the coal mining industry. To overcome such difficulties in interpretation the National Coal Board Medical Service instituted an additional epidemiological study taking a subsample of men working at the coal face, who had been X-rayed on 2 successive occasions. The pairs of films were read according to a design amenable to statistical analysis. An index was derived summarizing the changes in the pairs of films, known as the progression index, which is considered to reflect an increase in dust retention. The index can be used only as a means of ranking collieries in terms of the proportion of miners showing X-ray changes. The progression index has fallen each year. It is important to note that there was no correlation between prevalence and progression. Thus in South Wales the progression index was only a little above the national average in 1977–78.

With regard to prognosis in coal workers' pneumoconiosis, a 20 year mortality study of men in the Rhondda Fach[8] found that miners and ex-miners with simple pneumoconiosis survive as well as those without, a finding supported by observations elsewhere. Furthermore, the survival rate of those with category A complicated pneumoconiosis was also similar, a finding which conflicts with clinical observation. More detailed analysis showed a compensatory lower mortality in this category from ischaemic heart disease, which may account for the finding. It should be pointed out however, that the standardized mortality ratio (SMR) of the miners as a whole was substantially higher than the SMR of the non-miners in the same community.

As has been made clear, certification of pneumoconiosis in coal miners is assessed on the chest X-ray, not on the symptoms, such as those associated with chronic bronchitis. The role of inhaled dust in causing chronic bronchitis has been a contentious point for many years. The Industrial Injuries Advisory Council in 1973, after reviewing the evidence then available, concluded that bronchitis and emphysema should continue to be excluded from the definition of pneumoconiosis.

In the past, it was not possible to unravel the separate effects of cigarette smoking and dust exposure. A number of studies showed that cigarette smoking and other social factors were more important determinants than dust exposure in giving rise to respiratory symptoms. For example, one study[9] showed a higher prevalence of chronic bronchitis in miners' wives than in wives of non-miners. However, a long term prospective study in miners[10] has shown a progressive reduction in forced expiratory volume (FEV), with increasing cumulative exposure to airborne dust. Furthermore, increasing severity of bronchitic symptoms was associated with a reduction in FEV, which was greater than that expected from the effects of smoking and dust exposure as measured.

Asbestosis

The first case of asbestosis was diagnosed in 1900, and it was not until 1928 that a survey found pulmonary fibrosis in one-third of a group of asbestos workers who were examined. The association between asbestosis and lung cancer was first recognized in 1935, and the association between asbestos exposure and mesothelioma of the pleura and peritoneum was first described in 1964.

About 200 000 tons of asbestos are now imported into the United Kingdom each year, mainly from Canada and South Africa. Asbestos is a generic title for a group of fibrous silicates, the most important of which are chrysotile, amosite (brown asbestos), anthophyllite and crocidolite (blue asbestos). Asbestosis has been seen only in those occupationally exposed, the principal groups at risk being in mining, asbestos factories, the fire insulation industry, shipbuilding, lagging and in the stripping of old lagging, in the building industry, the asbestos cement industry, in processes involving the cutting or processing of asbestos sheet, board or other products which may involve small groups of workers in many diverse occupations.

Table 13.2 shows a small but consistent increase in the number of cases of asbestosis diagnosed annually by the medical panels. With asbestosis, the preliminary scrutiny of the chest X-ray does not apply and all claimants are examined. As with the other pneumoconioses, asbestosis is a disease of the later years of life, with fewer cases diagnosed below the age of 40 years, but a rather higher proportion in the 40 to 50 age group (Table 13.3). Incidence and prevalence figures cannot be derived from the medical panel's data because of difficulties in defining the denominator, and recourse must be made to epidemiological studies designed to provide such answers. In Britain, exposure to asbestos was likely to have been heavy before the introduction of the first Asbestos Industry Regulations in 1931. With the exception of the war years the implementation of the regulations brought about a progressive reduction in dust exposure. In 1969 new asbestos regulations set the permissible limit for exposure at 2 fibres/cm^3 of air. In a cohort (a segment of the population born around the same time period) study of workers in an asbestos textile factory[11] a ratio of observed to expected deaths of 3.6 was found for non-malignant respiratory diseases in the cohort exposed for 10 or more years before 1933. This ratio fell to 1.5 for the cohort first exposed between 1933 and 1950.

A morbidity study of dose–response relationships in an asbestos textile factory showed that 6.6 % of the workers first employed after 1950 had possible asbestosis with an average exposure of 5 fibres/cm^3 and an average length of follow up of 16 years. There was a significant fall in FEV and FVC with exposure, and a smaller fall in transfer factor. The cumulative dose was calculated from the data, and it was concluded that possible asbestosis would occur in not more than 1 % of men after 40 years exposure at concentrations of between 0.3 and 1.1 fibres/cm^3. Possible asbestosis was defined as the presence of basal crepitations, radiological changes of varying degree, a falling gas transfer factor and restrictive changes in ventilatory capacity. 50 % of these cases were certified by a pneumoconiosis medical panel within 3.5 years. The investigators concluded that there should be no complacency over the 1969 2 fibre/cm^3 standard.

A large scale study of asbestosis in civilian employees in United Kingdom naval dockyards is now in progress. Initially, in 1965, a radiological survey of a 10 % sample of the dockyard population showed that 4.5 % had radiographic abnormalities of the lung or pleura attributable to asbestos. Chest radiography has since been extended to every civilian employee (a total of over 40 000 workers) and the data used for estimating prevalence of asbestos related disease. A subsample of men aged 30–59 years chosen for more detailed study[12] showed that smoking played a large part in increasing prevalence rates of radiographic, clinical and physiological abnormalities. Most of this group had only intermittent exposure to asbestos, although in the past mixed exposure to chrysotile, amosite and crocidolite had occurred.

Another large scale mortality study is in progress in the chrysotile producing industry in Quebec, Canada. This cohort study includes all subjects born over a 30 year period from 1891–1920 who worked in the industry for a minimum period of 1 month. Within this study, a subgroup of ex-employees was examined to assess whether radiological progression might occur after withdrawal from exposure[13]. The interval between radiographs varied between 11 and 25 years. A substantial proportion of men showed an increase in parenchymal small opacities, but these increases were confined to those who had the heaviest past exposure.

The United Kingdom Advisory Committee on asbestos of the Health and Safety Commission[14] has reviewed the risks to health posed by exposure taking account of a wealth epidemiological data. Their more important recommendations are summarized in Chapter 14.

Farmers' lung

There were 17 certified cases of Farmers' lung under the Prescribed Diseases Regulations in 1975. The condition is likely to be considerably underdiagnosed in clinical practice and where diagnosed, claims for benefit are less likely to be made by a farming than by an industrial community. The number of cases diagnosed under the Prescribed Diseases Regulations are therefore likely to represent a considerable underestimate of the incidence of the disease.

Respiratory symptoms were elicited using the MRC Questionnaire, precipitin tests were performed and peak flow rates estimated in surveys of random samples of the farming population of Devon and Wales[15]. On the basis of relevant chest symptoms, a prevalence rate was found of 177 per 1000 in Devon and 129 per 1000 in Wales. The prevalence rate for a positive serological test was 87 per 1000 in Devon and 302 per 1000 in Wales. However, a combination of relevant symptoms with positive serological tests reduced the prevalence rates to 22 per 1000 in Devon and 54 per 1000 in Wales. In spite of both false positive and false negative results, the precipitin test, especially if used with a wide range of antigens, remains of great value in diagnosis. The authors of this study commented on the ease with which the prevalence rates could be manipulated according to the standard used, but pointed to the similarity of their results with a Scottish study which found a prevalence of 36 and 43 per 1000 on the basis of clinical criteria and positive precipitin tests. Chronic bronchitis was a confounding variable in the population studied.

It is of interest that several such studies have now found an increased proportion of positive serological tests in non-smokers. In the study quoted above, there was a suggestion that peak expiratory flow rate in non-smokers was lower in those who had positive precipitin tests.

References

1. Parkes WR. *Occupational lung disorders.* London: Butterworths, 1981.
2. Medical Research Council. *Questionnaire on respiratory symptoms.* 2nd ed. London: MRC. 1976.
3. International Labour Organization. *ILO U/C International Classification of Radiographs of the Pneumoconioses, 1971.* Occupational safety and health series. No 22 (revised). Geneva: ILO, 1972.
4. Bailey WC, Brown M, *et al.* Silicomycobacterial disease in sandblasters. *American Review of Respiratory Disease* 1974; **110**: 115–25.
5. Health and Safety Executive. *Health and Safety Statistics 1976.* London: HMSO, 1979.
6. American Conference of Governmental Industrial Hygienists. *Threshold Limit Values for Chemical Substances in Workroom Air.* Adopted by ACGIH for 1980.
7. National Coal Board Medical Service. *Annual Report* 1975–76; 1976–77; 1977–78. ISSN: 0307–9899. London: National Coal Board.
8. Cochrane AL, Haley TJL, *et al.* The mortality of men in the Rhondda Fach, 1950–70. *British Journal of Industrial Medicine* 1979; **36**: 15–22.
9. Higgins ITT, Cochrane AL. Chronic respiratory disease in a random sample of men and women in the Rhondda Fach in 1958. *British Journal of Industrial Medicine* 1961; **18**: 93–102.
10. Rogan JM, Attfield MD, *et al.* Role of dust in the working environment in development of chronic bronchitis in British coal miners. *British Journal of Industrial Medicine* 1973; **30**: 217.
11. Peto RL, Doll R, *et al.* A mortality study among workers in an English asbestos factory. *British Journal of Industrial Medicine* 1977; **34**: 169–73.
12. Rossiter CE, Harries PG. United Kingdom Naval Dockyards Asbestosis Study: survey of the sample population aged 50–59 years. *British Journal of Industrial Medicine* 1979; **36**: 281–91.

13. Becklake MR, Liddell FDK, *et al.* Radiological changes after withdrawal from asbestos exposure. *British Journal of Industrial Medicine* 1979; **36**: 23–8.

14. Health and Safety Commission Advisory Committee. *Asbestos. Vols I & II.* London: HMSO, 1979.

15. Morgan DC, Smyth JT, *et al.* Chest symptoms in farming communities with special reference to farmers' lung. *British Journal of Industrial Medicine* 1975; **32**: 228–34.

Chapter 14·Neoplasms of the Respiratory System

G KAZANTZIS

Classification, clinical features and pathology

Neoplasms of the respiratory system may arise in the nose, pharynx, larynx, the epithelium of the bronchial tree, the lung parenchyma, or the pleural membrane.

Nasopharyngeal tumours often present with enlargement of the upper deep cervical lymph nodes, or with symptoms involving the nose, ear or eye. The majority of malignant growths are squamous cell carcinomata. Adenocarcinoma is uncommon. In the oropharynx, neoplasms present with discomfort or ulceration of the throat. Tumours in this area are often benign. The most commonly occurring malignant lesion is a poorly differentiated squamous cell carcinoma, with lymph node metastases present by the time it is diagnosed. The condition is seen most commonly in men over the age of 50 who are heavy drinkers and cigarette smokers. Neoplasms of the larynx present with hoarseness or discomfort in the throat. These may be benign, but malignant tumours, which are not uncommon, are usually squamous cell carcinomata of a vocal cord, with wide variation in their degree of differentiation. Cancer of the larynx is most often seen in middle-aged and elderly men who have been heavy smokers and moderately heavy or heavy drinkers.

The most common malignant neoplasm arising from the respiratory tract is carcinoma of the bronchus. It presents in many different ways, either with thoracic symptoms or with distant effects which may be metastatic, biochemical or endocrine in origin. Altogether the extrathoracic manifestations account for more than 10% of all presentations. About 5% of all cases are first discovered in asymptomatic persons on routine chest radiography. Squamous cell tumours are the most common, accounting for more than half of all bronchial carcinomata. Undifferentiated growths, which may be pleomorphic or oat cell, account for nearly 40% of the total, and adenocarcinoma for less than 10%, although these are becoming more common, especially in women.

The adenocarcinomata can be distinguished by their site and clinical course, tending to be peripheral in origin and to grow more slowly. As a result they are more often first recognized on chest radiography. Adenocarcinoma was thought not to be related to environmental factors, but some authorities now consider all histologic types to be associated with cigarette smoking. Alveolar cell or bronchiolar carcinoma which may be multicentric in origin, accounts for about 1% of bronchial cancers. Carcinoma of the bronchus has a bad prognosis which has been little altered as a result of treatment with surgery, radiotherapy or chemotherapy. Overall survival at 5 years is less than 7%. In some selected surgical series, 1 year survival rates may be over 60% and 5 year rates over 25%, compared with 14% and 0.3% respectively in untreated cases.

Mesothelioma of the pleura, which was a rare tumour in the earlier years of the century, is now progressively increasing in frequency. It usually presents with chest pain, pleural effusion and increasing breathlessness with a course which is almost uniformly fatal. The condition may be suspected on chest radiography and confirmed on cytological examination of the pleural fluid. It is seen some 20–40 years after exposure to asbestos.

Neoplasms of the respiratory tract are of great importance because of their frequency and high mortality and because of the implication of environmental factors in their aetiology. These environmental factors, cigarette smoking, atmospheric pollution and occupational exposure, all have behavioural, sociological, economic and political interactions, particularly in industrialized communities. While a causal relationship between bronchial carcinoma and environmental exposure, in particular with cigarette smoking, has been demonstrated in many epidemiological studies, no clear relationship to genetic factors has yet been shown.

Sources and quality of data

The relatively short clinical course and lethal nature of bronchial carcinoma makes it likely that mortality data provide a good approximation to the incidence of the disease. With the better prognosis of some cancers of the upper respiratory tract, in particular cancer of the larynx originating on the vocal cords, incidence data are required to give a truer picture. The relative accessibility of respiratory tract neoplasms to direct observation, and in particular to histological verification from exfoliative cytology or biopsy, means that a clinical diagnosis can in most cases be readily confirmed during life. However, the protean clinical presentations of bronchial carcinoma must imply that where modern diagnostic methods are not available to the whole population, the diagnosis will in many cases be missed. It is in such communities too, that diagnosis by post mortem examination is less likely to be made. Therefore, comparisons in bronchial cancer mortality between countries with different standards of medical care must be made with caution.

It has been postulated that bronchial carcinoma has always been a common disease, but that in the past it was misdiagnosed. Chest radiography, bronchoscopy and cytology have certainly increased the accuracy of diagnosis, but within the United Kingdom improved diagnostic methods are unlikely to have played a significant part in the steep rise in mortality ascribed to bronchial carcinoma since the inception of the National Health Service in 1948. The differential increase in mortality between sexes and at different ages cannot be explained by better diagnosis or treatment and could have resulted only from real changes in the incidence of the disease.

There is no special legislation in the United Kingdom governing notification of neoplasms of the respiratory tract. However, certain neoplasms are associated with occupation and are covered by the Social Security (Prescribed Diseases) Regulations, 1975. Notifications for this purpose provide an additional source of data. The relevant tumours are carcinoma of the nose or associated air sinuses in workers in factories where nickel is produced by decomposition of a gaseous nickel compound, or in workers 'in or about a building where wooden furniture is manufactured'; primary carcinoma of the lung associated with nickel production in the occupations described above; and mesothelioma of the pleura in workers handling or working with any form of asbestos. There are other pulmonary neoplasms associated with occupational exposure which are not covered by the above regulations.

Lung cancer mortality

Malignant neoplasms of the trachea, bronchus and lung (World Health Organization International Classification of Diseases (ICD) 162, 1975 revision) now account for more than one-quarter of all cancer deaths in England and Wales. In 1978 the total was over 34 000, 112 per 100 000 men and 30 per 100 000 women. About a third of all lung cancer deaths occurred below the age of 65. The number of deaths continue to rise annually for both sexes although the rate of increase in women is much greater than in men (Fig. 14.1).

In a cohort (segment of the population) born between 1891 and 1895, (Fig.14.2) lung cancer mortality up to the age of 65 rose much faster in men than in women, with a male to female ratio as high as 10:1. However, in the cohort born between 1921 and 1925, this ratio had fallen to just over 3:1. During the 1970s there has been a decline in lung cancer mortality in men below the age of 65, but the mortality rate in women above the age of 45 has been rising steeply. In Britain and the USA lung cancer is the leading cause of death from cancer in men. It has been estimated that if the present trend continues during this decade, it will also become the leading cause of death in women, exceeding even deaths from breast cancer.

Aetiology of respiratory tract cancers

Extensive studies have been performed in a number of countries over the last 40 years to determine the aetiology of the 20th century increase in lung cancer. With progress in experimental carcinogenesis, it is not surprising that suspicion should fall on inhaled environmental agents. Tobacco smoking was first suggested as a cause of lung cancer in the 1920s. Later, atmospheric pollution and certain

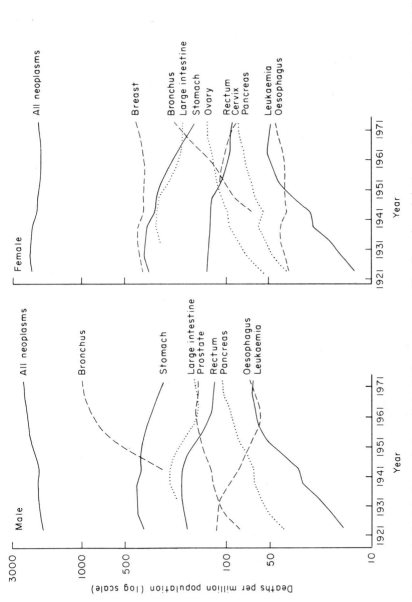

Fig. 14.1 Age-standardized death rates for bronchial and other carcinoma and for all neoplasms in both sexes, England & Wales, 1921–74. Office of Population Censuses and Surveys. *Trends in Mortality 1957–75*. London: HMSO, 1978)

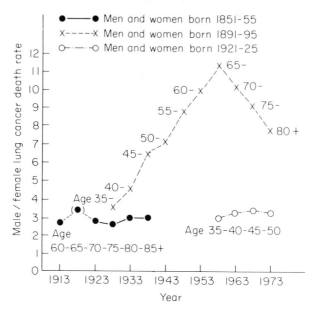

Fig. 14.2. Male/female ratios for lung cancer mortality in 3 cohorts of people born 1851–55, 1891–95, 1921–25 England & Wales[1].

occupational exposures were implicated. It has been estimated that occupational exposures account for not more than 15 % of lung cancer deaths. Studies on the association between environmental agents and lung cancer in particular are considered in more detail below. Reference is also made to mesothelioma of the pleura and to carcinoma of the larynx.

Smoking

The evidence incriminating cigarette smoking as the major cause of lung cancer was reviewed by the Royal College of Physicians in the United Kingdom in 1962, 1971 and 1977[1], and by the Surgeon General of the USA in 1964 and 1979[2]. More than 50 retrospective studies and at least 9 major prospective studies in several countries have shown an association between tobacco smoking and the subsequent development of lung cancer. This consistency is important in the assessment of the validity of the observations with regard to causation.

In 1950, Doll and Bradford Hill published a preliminary report in Britain on their now classical case–control study on smoking and carcinoma of the lung. In the same year the results of a similar study were published in the USA. In the British study, hospital patients with lung cancer were asked about their smoking habits and were compared with a non-cancer control group of general hospital patients, matched for sex and age. The study originally carried out in the London region was later extended to other parts of the country with a more detailed enquiry on smoking habits[3]. The study showed not only a great excess of smokers in the lung cancer group, but also evidence of a dose–response relationship of approximately linear form, with the increase in lung cancer in simple proportion with the number of cigarettes smoked.

Subsequent studies amply confirmed these findings, expanding the observations on dose to include not only the number of cigarettes smoked but also ways of smoking, such as inhalation, number of puffs, length of cigarette smoked and tar and nicotine content of cigarettes, all of which can increase the exposure of the bronchi to carcinogens present in tobacco smoke (Fig. 14.3). In addition the total period of exposure was found to be a relevant variable, those starting to smoke early in life having a much greater risk. These studies have also shown an increased lung cancer risk associated with cigar and pipe smoking, but substantially less than that associated with cigarettes.

A causal association with cigarette smoking can explain the remarkable trend in lung cancer mortality in Britain and other countries during this century. Standardized death rates (which allow for population changes) for lung cancer in the period 1901–20 were 1.1 per 100 000 in males and 0.7 per 100 000 in females. In 1936–39 these figures were 10.6 and 2.5 respectively. Cigarette smoking amongst men increased in popularity towards the end of the last century, but women only took up the habit during the First, and to a much greater extent the Second, World War (Fig. 14.4). Since then there have been brief downward trends for smoking in men, with a more consistent decrease in men in younger age groups, but in women the steady upward trend has continued. While the steep increase in lung cancer mortality in women has followed their increasing cigarette consumption, the decline in mortality from lung cancer in younger men can be attributed not only to less smoking, but also to the increasing use of filter tipped cigarettes, and to cigarettes with a lower tar and nicotine content.

The attribution of a causal role to an association can be materially strengthened if it can be shown that modification of the suspected causal factor will produce a change in the observed effect. This has been convincingly demonstrated in a 20 year prospective study on male British doctors[4]. The distinctive features of this study were the completeness of follow-up and the accuracy of death certification. Doctors as a whole heeded the evidence on the health effects of smoking and reduced their cigarette consumption over the years of the study (Fig. 14.5). Lung cancer death rates in doctors have progressively reduced and are now far below the national rates. Mortality from other cancers has not changed in the same way. This and other similar studies have shown that the relative reduction in risk becomes apparent within a few years of stopping smoking, so that after about 10 years abstention, the ex-smokers' risk approaches that of non-smokers.

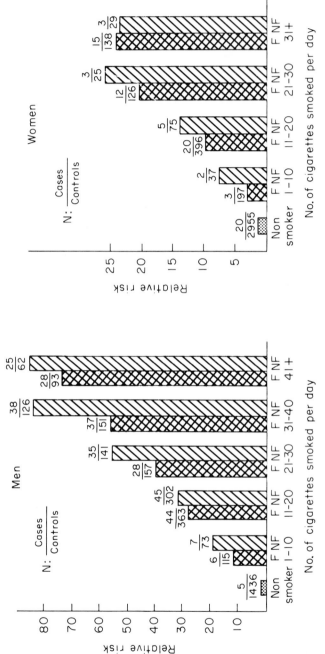

Fig. 14.3. Relative risk of lung cancer for men and women, by number of cigarettes smoked per day and long-term use of filter (F) or non-filter (NF) cigarettes.[2]

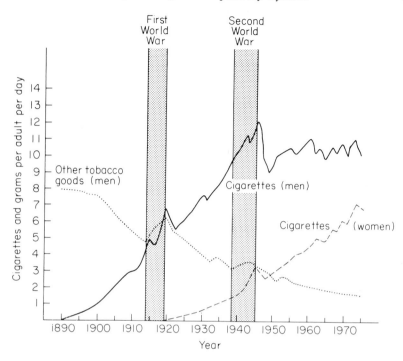

Fig. 14.4. Tobacco consumption in the United Kingdom, 1890–1975, showing changing smoking habits in men and women[1].

The retrospective studies have been criticized on the grounds that smoking histories obtained by recall are likely to be biased, especially in patients with lung cancer. All the studies have been criticized on the grounds that they were not carried out on strictly random samples. Some years ago an alternative hypothesis was advanced. This postulated that the association between smoking and lung cancer had a genetic rather than a direct causal basis, and thus that both the desire to smoke and the liability to lung cancer were inherited through genes sufficiently similar to account for the association. However, the data do not fit this hypothesis, in particular with regard to the temporal changes in lung cancer mortality and the different mortality rates between the sexes. The evidence against the genetic hypothesis is considered further in the Royal College of Physicians 1977 report[1]. A study on twins with different smoking habits supported the hypothesis of a causal relationship between smoking and lung cancer, although the number of deaths from lung cancer was low[5].

The relative risk of lung cancer from cigarette smoking varies in different countries where studies have been made. It is lower in Canada than in Britain, and lower still in Japan. The scarcity of cigarettes in Japan during the war years may have been in part responsible for the lower mortality from lung cancer there.

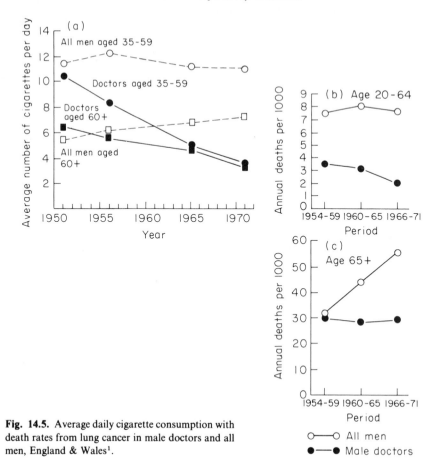

Fig. 14.5. Average daily cigarette consumption with death rates from lung cancer in male doctors and all men, England & Wales[1].

There are also marked differences in sex ratio for lung cancer in different countries, which remain unexplained[6]. There are synergistic effects between cigarette smoking and certain occupational exposures and possibly also with air pollution in the causation of lung cancer. Synergistic effects between cigarette smoking and alcohol in the causation of cancer of the larynx have also been demonstrated. While cigarette smoking is likely to be the most important cause of lung cancer, it must not be assumed that it is the only cause of this disease.

In the assessment of the evidence for smoking as a cause of lung cancer it is important to take into account data from other sources which support or refute the epidemiological findings. Experimental animal models have been developed in which lung cancer can be produced by tracheo–bronchial implantation of tobacco extracts or by inhalation of cigarette smoke or of aerosols of its constituents. Carcinogenic substances have been isolated from cigarette smoke, although the precise carcinogens responsible for lung cancer in man are unknown. Pre-malignant changes are present in the bronchial epithelium of smokers who have died of other diseases, these decrease in frequency after giving up smoking. Recently, the urine of heavy smokers has been shown to exhibit evidence of mutagenic activity. All the evidence from experimental sources supports the epidemiological findings.

Cigarette smoking is also an important cause of carcinoma of the larynx. Here, too, experimental data support the epidemiological observations, and a dose–response relationship has been demonstrated. The long term use of filter tipped cigarettes reduces the laryngeal cancer risk substantially and again there is a gradual reduction in risk after cessation of smoking. Both heavy alcohol ingestion and asbestos exposure appear to have a synergistic effect. One difference from lung cancer is that pipe and cigar smokers have an equally high risk of developing laryngeal cancer.

Strategies for the prevention of respiratory tract cancers caused by smoking are based on the education of the public on the harmful effects of smoking, on attempts to discourage smoking, especially by children, and on attempts to produce a less harmful cigarette. If the effects of health education and of attempts to discourage smoking are judged by the pattern of cigarette consumption then these measures have so far been inadequate, except perhaps for the reduction in smoking seen in persons in Social Class I. The success rate in smoking withdrawal clinics has not been high. Examples of attempts made to discourage smoking are warning notices, the limitation of tobacco sales promotion, taxation on tobacco and the institution of non-smoking areas in public places. Perhaps the most successful measures to date have been the promotion of filter tipped cigarettes and of cigarettes with a low tar and nicotine content.

Up to the present there has been careful consideration of the rights of the smoker. However, the non-smoker also has his right to an atmosphere unpolluted by tobacco smoke. In this respect Britain lags behind other countries in the provision of smoke-free areas in restaurants, places of entertainment and public transport. Further consideration on the prevention of lung cancer and other smoking related diseases is given in the reports of the Royal College of Physicians and of the Surgeon General of the USA[1,2].

Air pollution

Specific occupational exposures cannot account for the consistently higher mortality from lung cancer in urban than in rural areas. Large conurbations have the highest mortality rates and these rates decrease with decreasing size of the towns. The internal consistency seen in the mortality pattern in Britain and in other countries, in particular the USA, suggests the presence of an urban factor in the causation of lung cancer. Differences in smoking habits between town and country dwellers could account for part of this difference. The prospective study on British doctors already referred to confirmed the higher mortality from lung cancer in urban than in rural dwellers even amongst people with similar smoking habits. There is an association between urbanization and general atmospheric pollution including the products of the combustion of hydrocarbon fuels which include known carcinogens. These might well play a causal role. However, there is no consistent increase in lung cancer mortality in groups with the highest exposure, such as policemen, bus conductors or garage mechanics. Furthermore, a similar urban–rural gradient is seen in countries such as Norway, where there has been low urban air pollution over a long period.

While atmospheric pollution may be in part responsible for the greater lung cancer mortality seen in urban areas, even where differences in smoking habits are taken into account, the data suggest the presence of an additional urban factor. Both the USA and Britain show a similar trend of increasing mortality with increasing urbanization, but the British figures are almost twice as high as the American ones. This suggests the presence of a further, as yet obscure 'British factor'. British migrants to South Africa and other countries with lower mortality than that in Britain show a lung cancer mortality between the rates prevailing in the indigenous population and those in Britain, even when account has been taken of their smoking habits. British born residents in Britain, American born residents in the USA and Norwegians born in their own country have shown age-standardized lung cancer death rates of 151, 72 and 31 per 100 000 respectively. Comparable rates in British and Norwegian migrants to the USA have shown 94 and 48 per 100 000 respectively. These rates have thus been highest for Britons and lowest for Norwegians in their own country, with rates for US residents from all three ethnic groups coming in between[18]. It is not known whether this is explained by exposure to high levels of air pollution in infancy and childhood or by a persistent behavioural pattern.

Asbestos

Asbestos exposure is associated with increased mortality from both bronchial carcinoma and mesothelioma of the pleura. There is also evidence for a causal relationship between asbestos exposure and laryngeal cancer. An increased frequency of bronchial carcinoma was first observed in histological studies of the lungs in asbestosis. In one early study, the relationship was particularly striking because 41 % of the cases occurred in women, at a time when the male/female ratio for primary cancer of the lung was 4:1. All the cases occurred in workers with a history of heavy exposure to asbestos. Mesothelioma of the pleura was rare until 20 years ago when it was first associated with asbestos amongst the inhabitants of the asbestos mining areas in Cape Province, South Africa. Here small townships had grown around the asbestos workings, where children played on the asbestos dumps from mine and mill. Since then the association has been amply confirmed in several countries in asbestos miners and quarriers, in factory process and shipyard workers, and in a few cases in the wives of asbestos workers and in people living near asbestos factories. In contrast to bronchial carcinoma, asbestos has only been identified in a minority of these cases.

Although exposure to all varieties of asbestos carries an increased risk of developing bronchial carcinoma, it is greater following exposure to the amphiboles crocidolite or amosite, than to chrysotile. The cases of mesothelioma in Cape Province were all associated with exposure to crocidolite, or South African blue, asbestos and subsequent observation elsewhere has confirmed a relatively high increased risk. However, exposure to amosite also increases the risk of mesothelioma, as shown in studies of American insulation workers, whilst after chrysotile exposure the risk appears to be small. Mesothelioma develops clinically many years after the initial exposure to asbestos dust, which may give rise to difficulties in individual cases in identifying the nature of past exposure. Where tissue is available it is now possible to identify and count the mineral fibre content of the lung, thus adding to the accuracy of exposure data in epidemiological studies. However, the physical attributes of the fibre with regard to length and diameter have also to be taken into account with regard to their carcinogenic activity.

Studies in occupational groups, in which attempts have been made to compute the cumulative dose of inhaled asbestos dust, have shown an increase in the risk of developing bronchial carcinoma with an increasing dose of dust. Within the range of dust levels studied there is no evidence of a threshold below which there is no increased risk. In a study of Quebec chrysotile miners and millers a linear dose–response relationship has been demonstrated[7]. The risk of mesothelioma also appears to increase with dose. In contrast with bronchial carcinoma, however, more cases have occurred following exposure to low doses, both in terms of concentration and length of exposure. The estimation of dose in retrospective studies presents considerable difficulty and leaves a wide margin of uncertainty. While the length of exposure may be fairly accurately determined, techniques for estimating levels of dustiness, in terms of numbers of fibres per cubic centimeter, which were crude in the past, have improved over the last decade because of the more general use of personal sampling and fibre rather than total particle counting.

The mortality from mesothelioma has increased over the past decade in industrial countries: 292 deaths were reported in Britain in 1976, the majority in men in the older age groups. The increasing uses of asbestos over recent years makes it likely that the number of new cases will continue to rise to reach a peak during the last part of this century. The geographical distribution of cases of mesothelioma is remarkable: cases are clustered in cities with shipyards. Thus the ratio of observed to expected cases, based on Canadian incidence as a standard, was 27 for Manville, New Jersey, 22 for Wilhelmshaven and 14 for Plymouth[8]. In

Britain, the concentration in areas with naval shipyards is striking, and likely to be related to the use of crocidolite in marine insulation, with high exposures in confined spaces over many years. However, of the global total of 4539 cases reported between 1960 and 1975, only two-thirds were associated with a definite or probable history of exposure[8]. It is likely that the history of asbestos exposure in these cases was incompletely ascertained, but also probable, from estimates of basic annual incidence in different countries, that there is a low background incidence of mesothelioma not associated with asbestos exposure.

A number of studies have shown an interaction between asbestos exposure and cigarette smoking in increasing mortality from bronchial carcinoma. Smoking habits were ascertained in a cohort of asbestos factory workers of both sexes. Those who had been heavily exposed and who were cigarette smokers had a highly significant greater mortality from lung cancer[9]. The data supported a hypothesis of 2 carcinogens acting together to give a multiplicative risk rather than acting independently to give an additive risk. The greater risk of lung cancer in asbestos workers who smoke has been estimated as approximately 90-fold.

The finding of pleural plaques and of cases of mesothelioma following domestic contact or neighbourhood exposure to asbestos, the presence of asbestos fibres in the lungs of persons with no known exposure to asbestos, the increasing useage of asbestos-containing products and the presumed linear form of the dose–response relationship, with no evidence of a threshold for both bronchial carcinoma and mesothelioma, provide powerful grounds for questioning a possible public health hazard associated with asbestos exposure. Contamination of ambient air in cities and in buildings, of public water supplies and of food have all been demonstrated, but measurements are few up to the present time. The concensus opinion at present is that as far as exposure to chrysotile is concerned it is unlikely that there is any appreciable increased risk of either bronchial carcinoma or mesothelioma at the population level. The position with regard to crocidolite or amosite, or to mixtures containing both is less certain. It is likely that there is a small increased risk of both bronchial carcinoma and mesothelioma in persons exposed in buildings contaminated with these materials and in those living in areas where these amphiboles are handled industrially.

Strategies for prevention are based on limitation of exposure to asbestos dust, especially with regard to the amphiboles, both in occupational and population groups. The Asbestos Regulations (1969) imposed limits on occupational exposure to asbestos and the asbestos industry stopped the import and use of crocidolite in Britain in 1970. However, substantial quantities are present in the insulation of buildings, in pipe lagging and in a variety of asbestos-containing products, and both occupational and environmental contamination may occur when insulating materials and other products are damaged or broken up.

The Health and Safety Commission's Advisory Committee on asbestos recommended in 1979[10] that crocidolite and products containing crocidolite should be statutorily banned from importation into the United Kingdom. Where work with crocidolite imported in the past is unavoidable, as in the demolition of buildings, a control limit of 0.2 fibres/ml should be enforced. Control limits for amosite and for chrysotile should be reduced to 0.5 and 1.0 fibre/ml respectively, representing what the Advisory Committee described as the first stage of a continuing effort to reduce exposure. Controls have also been proposed for dust emissions into the atmosphere, for the transport of asbestos and for waste disposal. One of the 41 recommendations in the report was that all people whose work is liable to expose them regularly to asbestos dust should be advised to refrain from smoking.

Chromium

Since the 1930s workers engaged on the production of chromates from the raw material, chromite or chrome iron ore have been known to have an increased mortality from lung cancer. Epidemiological studies have been undertaken in Germany, USA, Britain and Russia. In the British study the increased risk was computed at a little over 3 times that expected[11], but in other studies 40 times the expected increased risk was observed. The highest incidence of the disease is in people in their early 50s, that is, about 5 years younger than in heavy smokers. The time interval between first exposure to chromate dusts and the development of cancer is of the order of 20 years.

An increased mortality from lung cancer has also been demonstrated in workers producing zinc chromate pigments. However, no such effect has been seen in chrome alloy production, chromium plating or in other industries using chromium. The increased risk appears to be related to exposure to partly soluble hexavalent compounds but the precise nature of the carcinogen is not known.

Nickel

A highly significant excess of both lung cancer and of cancer of the nasal sinuses has been found in nickel refinery workers in several countries. In the Mond nickel works in South Wales where exposure occurred in the past to nickel carbonyl gas, a 10-fold increase in mortality from lung cancer and a 900-fold increase in mortality from nasal cancer was found amongst men first employed before 1914. Some increased risk continued until 1930, after which major changes had occurred in the refinery processes[12].

At first it was thought that highly poisonous nickel carbonyl gas was a specific carcinogen, but this theory was discarded when a similar risk was found in nickel refinery workers in Canada, where an electrolytic process had been used. As with chromium, no excess mortality has yet been demonstrated in nickel alloy manufacture or in nickel plating, although adequate epidemiological studies have not yet been performed. Although dose–response data are lacking, it is clear that exposure under the old nickel refinery conditions had been heavy. From the fall in cancer mortality as exposure was progressively reduced, it seems unlikely that the very much lower levels of exposure encountered in nickel plating would constitute a hazard.

The time interval between first exposure to nickel and the diagnosis of cancer is long, averaging about 25 years, with a range of 10–40 years. Epithelial tumours of the lung have been most frequent, but anaplastic and pleomorphic growths have also been seen. Routine cytological screening, using nasal biopsy, which was introduced recently in Norway, has revealed presymptomatic cases of nasal cancer and a high rate of epithelial dysplasia. Sputum cytology has shown malignant cells and epithelial dysplasia in workers without clinical or radiological evidence of cancer.

Haematite mining

Haematite miners in Cumberland in the United Kingdom have lung cancer mortality significantly higher than expected from national or regional mortality data[13]. An increased lung cancer mortality has also been observed in the iron miners of Kiruna in Sweden, in Lorraine (France) and in Minnesota (USA). Some iron foundry workers have also been shown to have had an increased lung cancer mortality. In one study almost all the cases also had silicosis but there is no evidence that silicosis alone is associated with lung cancer. Haematite miners and foundry workers may be exposed to a number of potential carcinogens. In the Cumberland miners there is exposure to radio activity in the form of radon, and foundry workers may be exposed to polycyclic hydrocarbons. Smoking histories have not been taken into account in the above studies and furthermore there is no data on a dose–response relationship. While it is difficult to conceive of an element as ubiquitious as iron, with its major role in metabolism, as a carginogen, the possibility that it may have such a role when inhaled as an oxide has to be considered.

Arsenic

An increased mortality from lung cancer has been found in chemical process workers engaged in the production of inorganic arsenicals, in smelter workers, in sheep dip workers and in vineyard workers who used a pesticide spray containing arsenic. In all these studies exposure to arsenical-containing aerosols has been heavy. Smelter workers, who have been most extensively studied, are exposed predominantly to arsenic trioxide, but exposure patterns are mixed, other suspected carcinogens are frequently present and sulphur dioxide levels may be high. Some evidence of a dose–response relationship has been observed. For example, in one study on copper smelter workers, a time weighted index of total lifetime exposure to arsenic trioxide was linearly related to lung cancer mortality, with a standardized mortality ratio (SMR) of 111 at the lowest exposure to 833 at the highest[14]. As with the other metals considered, the interval between first exposure and the diagnosis of cancer has ranged up to 40 years. The significance of epidemiological observations can be strengthened if supporting data can be obtained by other methods of study. It is of interest, but not necessarily relevant, that arsenic is the only example of a possibly carcinogenic metal in man which has not given rise to experimental tumours.

Ionizing radiation

The metal mines of Schneeberg and Jachymov have been notorious since medieval times for their unhealthy atmosphere. Paracelsus referred to the fatal disease of miners as the 'mala metallorum'. More recently this has been recognized as lung cancer. While a number of metallic ores including arsenic and cobalt were recovered from these mines they are distinguished by their high level of radioactivity. Indeed it was from here that the Curies obtained the pitchblende from which radium was first isolated. An increased lung cancer mortality has now been found in the uranium miners of the Colorado plateau, and this has been attributed to air borne radiation from radon and daughter products[16]. The study included 3415 miners, in whom there were 22 deaths from lung cancer where 5.7 were expected with no greater mortality from cancer at other sites. A dose–response relationship between air borne radiation and lung cancer was found.

How convincing is the case for causation? The strength of the association is not great, with a 4-fold increase in lung cancer compared with the 10-fold increase found in asbestos workers. Air borne radiation has been found to be associated only with lung cancer, and this specificity of association increases its significance. While a dose–response relationship has been demonstrated, calculation of the accumulated dose involved a number of approximations. The consistency of the association is strengthened by the findings of an increased mortality from lung cancer in fluorspar miners in Newfoundland, also exposed to radon daughters. The presence of air borne radiation in the Cumberland haematite mines has already been referred to. Furthermore, animal experiments have shown that pulmonary tumours may follow the inhalation of radio-nuclides. It seems likely, therefore, that the long term inhalation of radioactive particles can give rise to lung cancer.

Coal carbonization

A 12 year prospective study on the mortality experience of gas retort house workers has confirmed greater risk of lung cancer[17]. The men most at risk worked on 2 jobs in particular, as top men and as hydraulic mains attendants where heavy exposure to gas fumes occurred before the extraction of tar and other products. Extremely high concentrations of benzpyrene and other polycyclic hydrocarbons were found in the fumes from the horizontal retorts which have since been dismantled.

References

1. Royal College of Physicians. *Smoking or health.* London: Pitman Medical, 1977.
2. Department of Health, Education and Welfare. *Smoking and health, a report of the Surgeon General.* DHEW No (PHS)79–50066. Washington: US Government Printing Office, 1979.
3. Doll R, Hill AB. A study of the aetiology of carcinoma of the lung. *British Medical Journal* 1952; **ii**: 1271–86.
4. Doll R, Peto R. Mortality in relation to smoking: 20 years observations on male British doctors. *British Medical Journal* 1976; **ii**: 1525–36.
5. Cederlof R, Friberg L, Lundman T. The interactions of smoking, environment and heredity and their implications for disease aetiology. A report of epidemiological studies in the Swedish twin registries. *Acta Medica Scandinavica* 1977; **612** (Supplement): 1–128.
6. Belcher JR. World wide differences in the sex ratio of bronchial carcinoma. *British Journal of Diseases of the Chest* 1971; **65**: 205.
7. Liddell FDK, McDonald JC, Thomas DC. Methods of cohort analysis: appraisal by application to asbestos mining. *Royal Statistical Society. Journal* Series A: General. 1977; **140**. 469.
8. McDonald JC, McDonald AD. Epidemiology of mesothelioma from estimated incidence. *Preventive Medicine* 1977; **6**: 426–46.
9. Berry G, Newhouse ML, Turok M. Combined effect of asbestos exposure and smoking in mortality from lung cancer in factory workers. *Lancet* 1972; **iii**: 476.
10. Health and Safety Commission Advisory Committee. *Asbestos. Vols I & II.* London: HMSO, 1979.
11. Bidstrup PL, Case RAM. Carcinoma of the lung in workmen in the bichromates-producing industry in Great Britain. *British Journal of Industrial Medicine* 1956; **13**: 260–64.
12. Doll R, Matthews JD, Morgan LG. Cancers of the lung and nasal sinuses in nickel workers: a reassessment of the period of risk. *British Journal of Industrial Medicine* 1977; **34**: 102–5.
13. Boyd JT, Doll R, *et al.* Cancer of the lung in iron ore miners. *British Journal of Industrial Medicine* 1970; **27**: 97–105.
14. Pinto SS, Enterline PE, *et al.* Mortality experience in relation to a measured arsenic trioxide exposure. *Environmental Health Perspectives* 1977; **19**: 127–30.
15. Lemen RA, Lee JS, *et al.* Cancer mortality among cadmium production workers. *Annals. New York Academy of Science* 1976; **271**: 273–9.
16. Wagoner JK, Archer VE, *et al.* Radiation as the cause of lung cancer among uranium miners. *New England Journal of Medicine* 1965; **273**: 181.
17. Doll R, Vessey MP, *et al.* Mortality of gas workers – final report of a prospective study. *British Journal of Industrial Medicine* 1972; **29**: 394.
18. Royal College of Physicians. *Air pollution and health.* London: Pitman Medical, 1970.

SECTION 4 · DISEASES OF THE DIGESTIVE SYSTEM

Chapter 15 · Peptic Ulceration

B G GAZZARD AND P LANCE

Peptic ulcers occur in those parts of the gastro-intestinal tract that are exposed to gastric acid and pepsin. Therefore, the vast majority are in the stomach and in the first part of the duodenum; those found at other sites such as the oesophagus, post-surgical anastomoses and Meckel's diverticulum will not be considered further. Chronic gastric and duodenal ulcers in which erosion extends through the muscularis mucosa, leading to fibrosis and permanent scarring, must be distinguished from the acute variety where only the superficial mucosa is involved and healing leaves no trace. Gastritis is an invariable accompaniment of chronic peptic ulceration. In gastric ulceration it is often atrophic and in duodenal it is usually confined to the antrum. It is extremely unusual for benign gastric ulcers to become malignant; malignant change never occurs in duodenal ulceration.

There are no clinical symptoms that clearly distinguish gastric from duodenal ulcers. In addition to dyspepsia patients may present with the complications of the disease. These include pyloric stenosis, gastro-intestinal haemorrhage and perforation.

Diagnosis

A firm diagnosis cannot be made from the history and clinical examination; it is usually established by barium meal or fibro-optic upper gastro-intestinal endoscopy. Radiological accuracy has improved considerably since the introduction of double-contrast techniques in the late 1960s but the findings are still often equivocal. Some enthusiasts regard endoscopy as an infallible diagnostic tool, but even in the best hands up to 10 % of gastric and duodenal ulcers may be missed. The combination of endoscopy and barium meal is claimed to detect nearly all, but there is no definitive yardstick for comparison.

Types of study

Estimates of incidence, prevalence and complication rates are usually little better than informed guesses. Sources of information about peptic ulcer disease relevant to epidemiological studies fall into the following categories: mortality statistics, hospital records, post mortem studies, and population surveys.

Mortality statistics

Quite apart from the general limitations of crude mortality figures, such as the inaccuracy of certification, they tell little of the natural history of a disease which is said to affect 10–15 % of the population of the Western world at any time. The disease only accounts for 1 % of all deaths in England and Wales[1].

Hospital records

Only a minority of patients with gastric or duodenal ulcers are referred to hospital. Thus material derived from the hospital in-patient enquiry (HIPE) is a highly selected source of information. The analysis of secular trends of HIPE data is probably more affected by changes in treatment than true changes in incidence. The introduction of potent drugs such as carbenoxolone and cimetidine for the management of uncomplicated ulcers, coupled with a greater reluctance to confine otherwise fit people to bed in hospital has almost certainly reduced the numbers of patients referred.

A fertile area for study has been perforation rates, on the assumption that in the developed world virtually every patient whose ulcer perforates will reach hospital and that then an unequivocal diagnosis can be made at laparotomy. Clearly this begs the question of the proportion of ulcers which perforate.

Post mortem studies

There have been some large and painstaking studies of the incidence of chronic peptic ulcers as an incidental finding at post mortem, but they must be interpreted with caution. Duodenal ulcer disease predominantly affects a much younger age group than the population dying in hospital and therefore likely to come to post mortem. Furthermore, all patients coming to post mortem form a highly selected group, depending largely on the local zeal for post mortem examinations. Finally, whereas the findings of a perforation at operation does provide sure evidence of peptic ulcer disease, necropsy studies are not so reliable, because features such as scarring without a definite ulcer crater depend on a subjective interpretation by the examining pathologist.

However, even after more than 20 years the Leeds (England) 1960 Necropsy Study[2] has scarcely been bettered for the detail of its information about ulcer prevalence. 86 % of patients dying between 1930 and 1949 in the University hospital had autopsies providing sufficient detail for a retrospective analysis of gastric and duodenal ulceration. Both active and inactive ulcers were included but only if they were found incidentally and thought not to have contributed to death.

Population surveys

There are few well-constructed prospective population studies. Those that have already been completed were mainly conducted before the days of endoscopy and double-contrast barium studies. There are two approaches to the population survey. Some workers have studied all patients in a defined locality developing gastric or duodenal ulcers, whereas others have taken a random sample. An important example of the latter is still in progress in Copenhagen County[3,4] which is a mixed urban and rural area. This is a prospective study of 1905 patients with peptic ulcers, representing a random 50 % sample of all new cases diagnosed during a 5 year period beginning 1 January 1963.

Although data from closed communities are often more complete than in the population at large, investigations based upon closed communities suffer from their very concentration on highly selected groups. For example, soldiers, who have been studied by various workers, are all young men in whom physical fitness is a prime requisite. Both of these factors are likely to bias the pattern of peptic ulcer disease.

These surveys only reflect the incidence and prevalence of peptic ulceration causing symptoms severe enough to take the patient to his doctor. Because the threshold of symptoms may differ from person to person they are unlikely to give the 'true' figures for the population as a whole.

Incidence and prevalence

Compared with cardiovascular disease and lung cancer, peptic ulceration is a rare cause of death in England and Wales. The average annual age- and sex-specific death rates for 1973–77 are shown in Fig. 15.1 The trends in mortality between 1951 and 1977 are shown in Fig. 15.2.

The annual incidence rates of peptic ulceration are much lower than the prevalence rates because the disease tends to have a relatively long natural history. Gastric ulceration has an incidence of 0.5 per 1000 amongst men and 0.3 per 1000 amongst women. The incidence of duodenal ulceration that has been calculated in most European studies is higher, 2–5 per 1000 in men and 0.5–1 per 1000 in women.

Prevalence figures from the Leeds (England) Necropsy Study are shown in Table 15.1.

Risk factors

From the above surveys and other data it is possible to draw conclusions on possible risk factors.

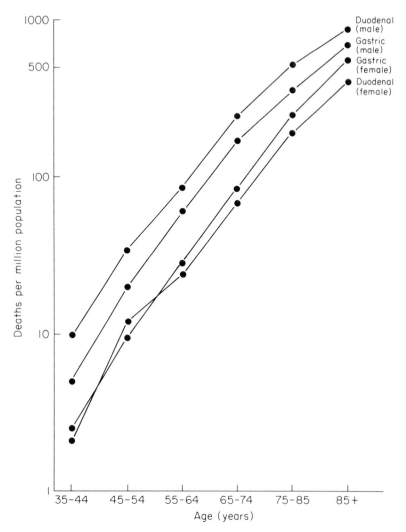

Fig. 15.1. Average annual age- and sex-specific death rates for gastric and duodenal ulcers, England and Wales, 1973–7 (log scale).

Age and sex

Duodenal ulceration is rare before the age of 20 years but the incidence then rises steadily throughout early adult life and middle age. Gastric uleration tends to be more a disease of old age. Mortality rates are roughly equal although the indicence of duodenal ulcers is probably 3 or 4 times that of gastric ulcers.

Duodenal ulceration is 4 or 5 times more common in men than in women but

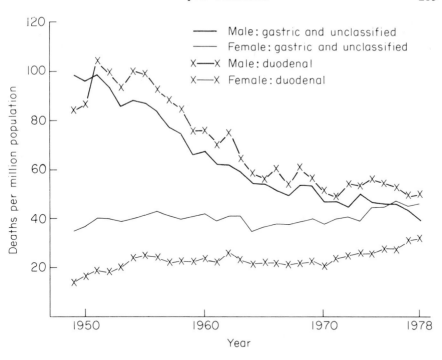

Fig. 15.2. Crude death rates from duodenal and gastric (including unclassified peptic) ulcers, England and Wales, 1949–78.

Table 15.1. Percentage of patients having chronic ulcers at autopsy, Leeds Necropsy Study[2].

Type of ulcer	Men	Women
Gastric	3.9	2.9
Duodenal	11.6	4.8
Gastric & Duodenal	2.3	1.1
Total	17.8	8.8

the male/female ratio for gastric ulceration is less than 2. Sex ratios fall steadily for both with increasing age.

Social class

In the United Kingdom mortality rates from gastric ulceration have always been highest in unskilled workers and this difference is now becoming apparent in duodenal ulceration. Perhaps more important, particularly in view of the low mortality rates even in classes most at risk, is that similar changes have been shown in the incidence of morbidity from duodenal ulcer, so that both gastric and duodenal ulcer now have highest prevalence rates in social classes IV and V.

Genetics

People with blood group O are more susceptible to duodenal ulceration than the rest of the population. It has been claimed that if in addition they are non-secretors of the ABO (H) blood group substances, the ulcer disease is especially liable to complications or recurrence. Blood groups other than O are more common amongst patiensts whose duodenal ulcers develop before the age of 20[5].

An elevated level of serum popsinogen I acts as a marker of gastric acid hypersecretion. This characteristic has been shown to be inherited as an autosomal dominant in the families of some duodenal ulcer patients[6]. There is a significant association between human leucocyte antigen (HLA)-B5 and duodenal ulceration, which is stronger than the combination of blood group O and non-secretor status, the relative risks being 2.9 and 1.3 respectively[7].

Trends

Duodenal ulcers were rare until the end of the 19th century whereas gastric ulcer complicated by perforation was relatively common, particularly in women. Throughout this century, duodenal ulcer has predominated. It has been suggested that the incidence of gastric and duodenal ulceration peaked in the 1950s and has been declining slowly since. The HIPE data between 1958 and 1972 show considerable reductions in the numbers of admissions for uncomplicated ulcers (Table 15.2).

The rather flimsy data for uncomplicated ulcers are strengthened by corresponding reductions in the numbers of perforations, at least for gastric ulcer in England and Wales (Table 15.3) and also for duodenal ulcer in Scotland where admission rates fell by about one quarter between 1951 and 1971.

Geographical variations

Both the HIPE data and the reported perfoation rates imply that duodenal ulcer is more common in Scotland and in the north of England than it is in the south of England. There is no such clear pattern for gastric ulcers. Gastric ulcers appear to be less common in Canada and the USA than in Western Europe. There is general agreement that duodenal ulceration is much more common in southern rice-eating India than in the north of that country, where unrefined wheat is the staple diet. The pattern is changing in Africa where it used to be stated that duodenal ulceration was common in the West but uncommon in the East and South. The incidence of duodenal ulcers is increasing dramatically amongst

Table 15.2. Percentage reduction in the number of hospital admissions for uncomplicated ulcers 1958–72, England & Wales[8].

Type of ulcer	Men	Women
Gastric ulcer	44	32
Duodenal	14	19

Table 15.3. Perforation rates of ulcers in England and Wales[8].

Type of ulcer	Year 1959–62	1963–66	1967–70	1971–74
Gastric	2567	1887	1700	1478
Duodenal	5430	5271	5259	4853

urban Blacks and Indians of Durban and Johannesburg (South Africa), providing further evidence against the old contention that duodenal ulceration is a disease of the higher socio-economic groups.

Aetiology

The complex interaction between genetic and environmental influences which causes peptic ulcers and their resulting epidemiology is poorly understood. Not only are there many differences between gastric and duodenal ulcers, but each is itself probably a heterogeneous condition, although the old aphorism of 'no acid, no ulcer' still holds. Broadly, gastric ulceration is associated with hyposecretion of gastric acid and duodenal ulceration with hypersecretion.

Specific factors

It is well established that smoking delays the healing of gastric ulcers and there is also some evidence that it has a minor role in the development of the disease. In a prospective study of American College students a small but significantly higher incidence of peptic ulcers was found in smokers compared to non-smokers[9]. American doctors with peptic ulcers were shown to have smoked more, and those with duodenal ulcers to have started younger than controls[10]. Coffee consumption was more strongly associated with ulcer disease than cigarette smoking in American College students.

Aspirin-containing analgesics have been blamed for the increased incidence of gastric ulcer and its complications in Australian women and this has been supported by case–control studies[11]. There was a similar though small risk amongst heavy consumers of aspirin in the Boston Collaborative Drug Enquiry.

The chances of developing an ulcer in heavy consumers of aspirin was estimated as 10 per 100 000 per year[12].

From a review of 42 controlled trials of corticosteroid therapy for various diseases it was suggested that steroids played no part in the aetiology of their ulcer in 38 of 2985 patients; 18 of the 2346 controls had ulcers[13]. Many still suggest that corticosteroids may cause, exacerbate or delay the healing of peptic ulcers but it seems that the risk, if any, is small.

Associated diseases

Of the many diseases which have at one time or another been said to predispose to ulcer, the most likely and well-substantiated candidates are cirrhosis, chronic renal failure and massive small bowel resection[14]. Hyperparathyroidism, cardiovascular disease, chronic bronchitis and tuberculosis have fallen out of favour in this context.

Natural history

In a Scandinavian study a cohort of 227 patients was followed up 14 years later by which time 154 were available for assessment[15]. 50 had died from unrelated causes and 23 were untraceable. Of the remainder, 37 % were free of symptoms, 29 % had occasional symptomatic recurrences which were easily controlled and 34 % had either had operations or were likely soon to need surgery because of the severity of symptoms. About 50 % of patients with gastric ulcers eventually have operations.

Screening, prevention and treatment

Except for research purposes, screening for peptic ulcer has no place. Even tobacco smoking is not a major aetiological factor and there is, therefore, no preventive measure which can be recommended at the moment.

There are numerous trials that demonstrate that the great majority of ulcers can be healed medically. These include trials of simple antacids, if taken in sufficient quantities frequently enough, and of carbonoxolone sodium and cimetidine. However, once therapy is withdrawn, there is no lasting influence on the natural history of the disease and, for example, about 80 % of duodenal ulcers recur within 6 months of completing a healing course of cimetidine.

The role of cimetidine in the long-term management of ulcer disease has yet to be defined. Most clinicians do not recommend that it should be taken indefinitely because firstly the majority of patients are young or middle aged and otherwise fit, secondly the nature and frequently of side effects are not fully known, and lastly, the cost would be enormous. Surgery remains the treatment of choice when the disease is incapacitating or complications supervene.

References

1. The Registrar General. *Statistical Review of England and Wales for 1973.* London: HMSO, 1975.
2. Watkinson G. The incidence of chronic peptic ulcer found at necropsy. *Gut.* 1960; **1**: 14–31.
3. Bonnevie O. The incidence of gastric ulcer in Copenhagen County. *Scandinavian Journal of Gastroenterology* 1975; **10**: 231–9.
4. Bonnevie O. The incidence of duodenal ulcer in Copenhagen County. *Scandinavian Journal of Gastroenterology* 1975; **10**: 285–393.
5. Lam SK, Ong GB. Duodenal ulcers: early and late onset. *Gut* 1976; **17**: 169–79.
6. Rotter Jerome I, Sones James Q, *et al.* Duodenal ulcer disease associated with elevated serum pepsinogen I. *New England Journal of Medicine* 1979; **300**: 63–6.
7. Rotter Jerome I, Rimoin David L, *et al.* HLA-B5 associated with duodenal ulcer. *Gastroenterology* 1977; **73**: 438–40.
8. Brown RC, Langman MJS, Lambert PM. Hospital admissions for peptic ulcer during 1958–72. *British Medical Journal* 1976; **i**: 35–7.
9. Paffenberger RS, Wing AL, Hyde RT. Chronic disease in former college students. *American Journal of Epidemiology* 1974; **100**: 307–15.
10. Manson RR. Cigarette smoking and body form in peptic ulcer. *Gastroenterology* 1970; **58**: 337–44.
11. Gillies MA, Styming A. Gastric and duodenal ulcer. The association between aspirin ingestion, smoking and family history of ulcer. *Medical Journal of Australia* 1969; **2**: 280–5.
12. Levy M. Aspirin use in patients with major upper gastro-intestinal bleeding and peptic ulcer disease. *New England Journal of Medicine* 1974; **290**: 1158–62.
13. Conn HO. Blitzer BL. Non-association of adreno-corticosteriod therapy and peptic ulcer. *New England Journal of Medicine* 1976; **294**: 473–9.
14. Langman MJS, Cooke AR. Gastric and duodenal ulcer and their associated diseases. *Lancet* 1976; **i**: 680–3.
15. Griebe J, Bugge P, *et al.* Longterm prognosis of duodenal ulcer. *British Medical Journal* 1977; **ii**: 1572–74.

Further reading

Langman MJS. *The epidemiology of chronic digestive disease.* London: Edward Arnold, 1979: 9–39.
Watkinson Geoffrey. Peptic ulcer. Epidemiological aspects In: Truelove SC. and Willoughby CP, eds. *Topics in gastroenterology 7.* Oxford: Blackwell Scientific Publications, 1979: 3–34.
Wormsley KG. *Duodenal ulcer. Vol 2.* Edinburgh: Eden Press Inc. (Churchill Livingstone), 1979: 2–6.

Chapter 16 · Malignant Disease of the Upper Gastro-intestinal Tract

B G GAZZARD AND P LANCE

Carcinoma of the oesophagus

Neoplasms of the oesophagus usually arise from the squamous epithelium, but occasionally they arise from the mucus glands. Lesions at the lower end of the oesophagus are commonly adenocarcinomas. Most of these are primary tumours of the stomach which spread into the gullet.

Nearly all patients present with progressive dysphagia and rapid weight loss. Their survival is very short and therefore death rates should give a good guide to incidence rates. However, a recent study found that the clinical diagnosis on the death certificate was in agreement with that at autopsy in only 70 % of cases[1].

Incidence and prevalence

The incidence of oesophagus carcinoma rises steeply with age (Fig. 16.1). Therefore one of the factors which affects the frequency of the disease is the age structure of the community. In order to determine possible risk factors age-specific incidence rates are required but are not available for all parts of the world.

In countries where serial data are available there is no remarkable secular trend in death rates.

Geographical variations

Most European countries have rates similar to those shown in Fig. 16.1. However, there is a 300-fold variation in incidence across the world. This is probably a greater variation than for any other tumour and strongly suggests the existence of important, but as yet unknown, environmental factors in its aetiology.

A very high incidence has been recorded in sub-Saharan Africa, in Brazil and around the southern borders of the Caspian Sea. The epidemiology of the condition on the Caspian littoral has been extensively studied by Kmet and Mahboubi[2]. In the western province, Gilan, comparatively low age-standarized incidence rates are found for men (0–26.7 per 100 000, standardized to world population). This rate rises dramatically towards the east, and in parts of Mazandaran reaches 108 per 100 000 standard population. The range in incidence amongst women is even greater.

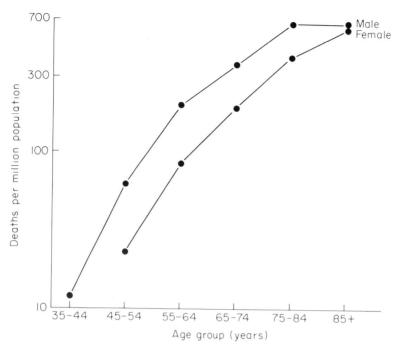

Fig. 16.1. Carcinoma of the oesophagus: age- and sex-specific death rates, England and Wales, 1977 (log scale).

There are striking differences between the provinces in climate, the high incidence area being semi-desert with predominantly saline soils, whereas the low incidence area is in a humid rainbelt with a non-saline soil. The main population group in the high incidence region is Turkoman who eat mostly bread and drink very hot tea. This, and the relatively low calorie and protein intake, together with multiple vitamin deficiencies, may be important aetiological factors. More than half of the population over the age of 35 regularly smoke opium in the high incidence region. The aetiological significance of these observations is not known. However, no correlation has been found there between alcohol or tobacco consumption and oesophageal carcinoma, which have been implicated as aetiological agents in many other parts of the world.

Risk factors

An association between wine drinking and carcinoma of the oesophagus was first noted by Sir Arthur Hurst in 1939. This relationship has been confirmed by many subsequent investigators. This is probably the most important explanation of the male predominance of the tumour in the Western world. Calvados drinkers in France and maize-beer drinkers in Kenya have a much higher incidence than people who drink similar quantities of alcohol but in different types of drink. This suggest that the congeners in the alcohol may be of importance.

Tobacco consumption appears to be associated independently with an increased risk of oesophageal neoplasms. The risk is directly proportional to the amount smoked. In recent reports of doctors' mortality in relationship to smoking, Doll and Peto[3] showed a drop in incidence of carcinoma of the oesophagus following cessation of smoking.

There is an increased incidence of the tumour amongst persons in Social Classes IV and V which is independent of smoking and alcohol consumption.

Two relatiavely uncommon conditions, achalasia of the oesophagus and tylosis, are associated with an increased incidence of oesophageal cancer. The association between cricoid-web, upper oesophageal carcinoma and iron deficiency anaemia is well recognized, although the reasons are not clear.

Carcinoma of the stomach

Virtually all tumours of the stomach are adenocarcinomas. About 30% arise from areas of intestinal metaplasia, which is usually considered to be a pre-malignant condition. The initial clinical presentation is often vague, with anorexia, vomiting and weight loss frequently occuring after the tumour has metastasized.

Incidence

The 5 year survival rate of carcinoma of the stomach is so low that mortality rates provide a relatively accurate guide to the incidence. The latest year for which both cancer registration and death rates are available is 1973. In that year in England and Wales the death rate was 29.7 per 100 000 for men and 20.1 for women: the corresponding registration rates were 28.8 per 100 000 for men and 17.7 for women. The male/female ratio is similar in most countries of the world. Like carcinoma of the oesophagus the incidence of the tumour increases exponentially with age in all countries where it has been studied (Fig. 16.2). This suggests repeated exposure to a small dose of carcinogen throughout life, or a failing host protective mechanism.

In the United Kingdom the incidence in Social Class V is nearly 4 times as great than in Social Class I. However, there are no obvious occupational differences. The relationship with socio-economic class holds good for areas of both high incidence (e.g. Japan) and low incidence (e.g. USA).

Geographical variations

There is considerable geographical variation in frequency, although to a lesser extent than that found for oesophageal cancer. Japan and Russia are high

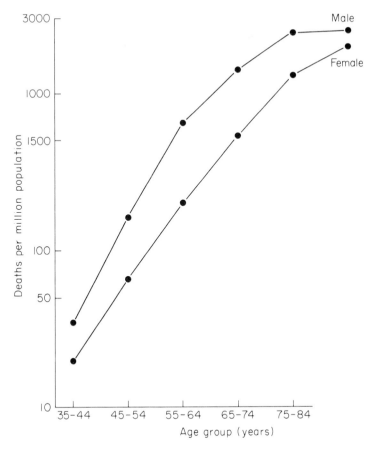

Fig. 16.2. Carcinoma of the stomach: age- and sex-specific death rates, England and Wales, 1977 (log scale).

incidence countries, whereas the disease is rare in rural Southern Africa[4]. The incidence in Western Europe and America is intermediate between these two extremes. White North Americans have a lower incidence than other races in the country. The incidence varies widely within the continent of South America, with high incidences in Argentina, Brazil and Chile, but low incidence in Gautemala, Mexico and Peru. There is also a wide variation in incidence within individual countries. Thus in the Netherlands and in the United Kingdom there is a 100-fold difference between high and low incidence areas.

Secular trends

In most countries where it has been studied the mortality from this tumour has been steadily declining in recent years, with the exception of Poland and Russia[5].

The trend has not been seen amongst the elderly, possibly because of less accurate certification of cause of death in this age group. As there has been little radical change in the methods of diagnosis or treatment this is likely to represent a genuine change in incidence and must be accounted for in any satisfactory aetiological theory of carcinoma of the stomach.

Risk factors

Exogenous atmospheric pollution

Some studies have shown a positive correlation between high levels of particulate material in the atmosphere and gastric cancer. Such an association has been shown in Great Britain for men but not for women[6].

Diet

At present the most fashionable explanation for the variation in incidence between socio-economic classes and the geographical distribution is diet. Studies of diet are notoriously difficult to interpret because of patients' inability to recall their food intake accurately over long periods. There appears to be an inverse relationship between carcinoma of the stomach and the consumption of meat and fat, but a positive correlation with cereal eating[7]. It has not been possible to show whether it is eating too little fat or meat, or eating too much cereal which is of importance. Studies which have attempted to control one of these factors have failed to show any significance for the other.

Amongst protein foods, it has been suggested that milk products are protective in Japan and India. This has not been confirmed in studies in Africa, America or Iceland. In some countries consumption of certain foods has been shown to be positively correlated with the incidence of carcinoma of the stomach. Thus in Iceland, home smoked ham, which has a high benzyprene content, and in Japan salted fish and pickled vegetables, are associated with a high incidence of carcinoma. There also appears to be a general correlation between high intake of Vitamin C and low incidence of gastric cancer.

Further support for a dietary aetiology is gained by the study of populations migrating from high risk areas to low risk areas. One of the classic studies in this field was in Japanese settlers in Hawaii who have an incidence of gastric carcinoma intermediate between the Japanese (high) and native Hawaiians (low)[8]. A likely cause for this change in risk is a change in diet with succeeding generations.

N-nitroso compounds are possible dietary carcinogens. They have been shown to produce tumours in all laboratory animals studied. Nitrosamines are found in certain foods and can be formed *in vivo*, from nitrates and secondary amines, trace amounts of which are found in the stomach. Normally nitrosation occurs in the presence of an acid pH, but achlorhydria is associated with an increased incidence of gastric carcinoma. However, the chemical reaction can proceed at neutral pH in the presence of certain bacteria, which have been shown to be present in increased numbers in achlorhydric patients. It has been suggested that the N-nitroso compounds may themselves produce gastric atrophy and achlorhydria. Many of these bacteria also have the capacity to reduce nitrates and thus increase the stomach concentration of nitrite, which is more stable at a neutral pH. While the quantities of nitrite are markedly increased in patients with gastric cancer, the more persuasive evidence of finding increased levels of volatile nitrosamine compounds is at present lacking.

If endogenously produced N-nitroso compounds are important in the aetiology of gastric cancer a high incidence of the tumour would be expected in areas of high nitrate consumption. Crude studies in the provinces of Chile, where gastric cancer is common, have shown a close correlation between the amount of nitrate fertilizer used, and thus persumably the amount of nitrate in vegetables, and the mortality rate from the tumour. In the high nitrate use areas there is an increased prevalence of achlorhydria in young people. Similar results in Japan showed a high incidence of gastric cancer in well-water drinkers (high nitrate concentration) compared with municipal water users (low nitrate content). However, the nitrate concentration of food and water in Japan and Chile is much higher than is likely to be found in Britain. Indeed, in Britain, the area of highest nitrate use (East Anglia) has the lowest mortality rate from gastric carcinoma. Thus the epidemiological evidence for nitrates and carcinogenesis is at present inconclusive.

Endogenous

Atrophic gastritis is a histological finding which increases in frequency with old age, and is commonly associated with gastric carcinoma. However, it is a difficult diagnosis to establish, even histologically, and a causal relationship with gastric cancer has not been proved. Likewise achlorhydria is found in 60–80% of all patients with gastric cancer and increases in frequency with age. There is a 4-fold increase in risk of gastric cancer in patients with achlorhydria and 3-to 20-fold increase in patients with pernicious anaemia, who are always achlorhydric. Persons of blood group A have a greater risk of pernicious anaemia and gastric cancer (20% increase), but it has been shown that these are independent associations. 90% of gastric polyps occur in patients with atrophic gastritis and alchlorhydria. Up to 40% of such polyps may undergo malignant transformation[9].

Early diagnosis

One of the reasons for the high mortality of gastric cancer is the frequency with which metastases have already occured at the time of diagnosis, which has led to an intensive search for methods of early diagnosis. This can be attempted either by whole population screening, such as the Japanese studies, or investigation of patients at high risk[10]. The screening of whole populations in Japan has been somewhat disappointing. 70% of the cancers so detected were already symptomatic. Reports from Minnesota indicate that screening programmes improve survival in asymptomatic patients (50% 5-year survival in this group).

High risk groups that have been identified are patients with achlorhydria, pernicious anaemia, gastric polyps or certain histological changes in the gastric mucosa (see below). In Finland screening of patients with achlorhydria has been attempted. Gastric cancer developed in 9 of 116 patients with this condition during a 16–20 year follow-up. Accurate screening for achlorhydria usually requires an unpleasant intubation of the stomach. Attempts have been made to develop an indirect method. Two alternative tests are the Azure test and the concentration of Uropepsin in the urine. 1000 patients found by these methods to have achlorhydria were followed up over 2 years. 2 developed gastric carcinoma compared with none in a controls group of people who produced gastric acid. In a regular follow-up of 123 patients with pernicious anaemia over 13 years, 16 asymptomatic gastric cancers were detected. The 5-year survival in the 14 patients who agreed to surgery was excellent (81%).

Recent histological studies have shown in certain individuals changes called 'early gastric cancer' with dysplasia and microscopic invasion, not through the submucosa. The 5 year survival rate in these cases is excellent. In Japan there is a very large screening programme looking for these lesions, both by double contrast barium meal and fibre-optic endoscopy.

Many authors claim that the diagnosis of early gastric cancer has led to the recent fall in mortality in this condition. However, the incidence has been falling steadily since the 1930s in most developed countries. As there are no long-term longitudinal studies of early gastric cancer, we cannot yet be certain that it always has the same natural history of gastric carcinoma, but this approach seems the most helpful at present in reducing the incidence of this tumour, which is still the most commonly fatal neoplasm in the Western world.

References

1. Heasman MA, Lipworth L. *Accuracy of certification of causes of death*. Studies in medical and population subjects 2. London: HMSO, 1966.
2. Kmet J, Mahboubi E. Oesophageal cancer in Caspian littoral of Iran: initial studies. *Science* 1972; **175**: 846.
3. Doll R, Peto R. Mortality in relation to smoking, 20 years observations on male doctors. *British Medical Journal* 1976; **ii**: 1925.

4. Doll R. *Prevention of cancer. Pointers from epidemiology.* London: The Nuffield Provincial Hospitals Trust, 1967.

5. Case RAM, Coghill C, *et al.* Serial Mortality Tables. *Neoplastic diseases. Vol I.* Division of Epidemiology. London: Institute of Cancer Research, 1976.

6. Stocks P. On the relation between atmospheric polution in urban and rural communities and mortality from carcinoma, bronchitis and pneumonia *British Journal of Cancer* 1960; **14**: 397.

7. Armstrong B, Doll R. Environmental factors and cancer incidence and mortality in different countries with special reference to dietary practices *International Journal of Cancer* 1975; **15**: 617.

8. Haenczel W, Kwitiara M. Studies of Japanese migrants. *US Journal of National Cancer Institute* 1968; **40**: 43.

9. Day DW, Morson BC. Gastric Cancer. In Woolf M, Antony PP, eds. *Recent advances in pathology. Vol 10.* London: Churchill Livingstone, 1978: 159.

10. Nikado N. *Early diagnosis of gastric cancer by mass survey.* Advanced abstracts 4th World Congress of Gastroenterology. Copenhagen, 1970, 274.

Further reading

Langman MJS. *The epidemiology of chronic digestive diseases.* London: Edward Arnold, 1979.

MacDonald J. Epidemiology of gastric cancer. In *Cancer of the gastrointestinal tract* Chicago: Chicago Year Book Medical Publishers, 1967.

Gregor O. Epidemiology of gastric cancer. In *Recent advances in gastroenterology.* 2nd ed. London: Churchill Livingstone. 1976.

Chapter 17 · Inflammatory Disease of the Lower Gastro-intestinal Tract

B G GAZZARD AND P LANCE

The 2 varieties of idiopathic chronic inflammatory bowel disease were first described by Wilkes in 1859 – ulcerative colitis – and Crohn in 1932 – Crohn's disease. However, both diseases must have existed for many hundreds of years. Ulcerative colitis is the condition in which there is inflammation and ulceration of the large bowel, limited to the mucosa and submucosa. The disease may affect the rectum only (proctitis) or extend to involve the whole of the large bowel. Crohn's disease is a chronic granulomatous condition which may affect all coats of the entire length of the bowel but is most commonly seen in the distal small intestine and colon. Ulcerative colitis usually starts with bloody diarrhoea. The presentation of Crohn's disease is more variable, with diarrhoea, small intestinal colic, fistulae, or malabsorption. Both may occasionally present with constitutional symptoms or extra-intestinal manifestations.

Epidemiological studies of the incidence and prevalence of these diseases are difficult for 2 reasons. Firstly, the important observation that Crohn's disease may affect the large bowel has been made only recently[1] and secondly, it has been increasingly recognized that the histopathology of rectal biopsies and radiological findings do not always distinguish between ulcerative colitis and Crohn's colitis. A further difficulty is that acute terminal ileitis has been recognized as probably representing a separate entity. This condition, which is often caused by infection with Yersinia organisms, presents in a very similar manner to acute appendicitis and an acutely inflamed ileum is found at laparotomy. There is only a small chance that such patients will subsequently develop the classic features of Crohn's disease.

None of these conditions is usually fatal, therefore mortality statistics are not a guide to incidence or prevalence. Hospital admission statistics have often been used to measure incidence, but they may be misleading, particularly in ulcerative colitis because a large number of patients have only mild symptoms and may never be admitted to hospital. It has been estimated that only 10% of patients with ulcerative proctitis are admitted. Thus the overall incidence of ulcerative colitis will be underestimated from hospital admission statistics. One study from Denmark estimated that only 40% of new cases of ulcerative colitis are correctly diagnosed in the first year of symptoms and 2% were not diagnosed until 25 years later[2]. This delay in diagnosis will accentuate the tendency to underestimate both incidence and prevalence. From a study in Oxford (England), Evans and Atkinson[3] showed that virtually all cases of ulcerative colitis were diagnosed as hospital patients but this does not overcome the above problem. Although some data can be obtained from the hospital in-patient enquiry (HIPE), it is impossible to measure the numbers of individuals attending as out-patients only.

Reliable information can only be obtained by careful study of a relatively small geographical area when an attempt is made to ascertain all cases by use of hospital in-patient and out-patient data and by inquiry of general practitioners. Such studies have been undertaken in Aberdeen (Scotland)[4], Nottingham (England)[5], Oxford (England)[3], Baltimore (USA)[6] and in various Scandinavian studies, notably Uppsala (Sweden)[7].

Incidence and prevalence

Despite the problems of ascertainment, there is a surprising degree of agreement on the incidence and prevalence of these two conditions in the USA, the United Kingdom and Sweden (Table 17.1). Because of the difficulty of diagnosis in patients under 20, the Baltimore study excluded them. This reduced the incidence by approximately 20%. The annual incidence of ulcerative colitis in the Oxford study is about 5 times greater than that of Crohn's disease and its prevalence is 9 times greater. In these studies, the ranges of incidence for ulcerative proctitis (3–7 per 100 000), ulcerative colitis (3–7 per 100 000) and Crohn's disease (2–4 per 100 000) are very narrow, as are the ranges of prevalence (proctitis 40–80 per 100 000; ulcerative colitis 36–70 per 100 000; Crohn's disease 20–40 per 100 000).

Men and women appeared to be equally affected by Crohn's disease in the Oxford study, although there was a slight excess of women in the Nottingham survey. This was mainly accounted for by the greater number of women with Crohn's disease in the older age group. In both studies of ulcerative colitis there were slightly more women (Table 17.1).

The incidence of both diseases is greatest in young people with a mode at 20 years (Fig. 17.1). At all ages ulcerative colitis is more common than Crohn's disease, particularly in children under 6, possibly because many paediatricians limit their investigations to a sigmoidoscopy which would favour the diagnosis of ulcerative colitis, and miss some cases of Crohn's disease. Most, but not all series, have demonstrated a second slight increase in the incidence of both diseases in older age groups at around 55–60 years. In Norway and Copenhagen (Denmark), this trend is less noticeable and is confined to men. This second apparent peak might be due to misdiagnosis of ischaemic colitis, a disease which is difficult to diagnose positively as there are no pathognomonic histological features. The occurrence of colitis in older age groups is associated with an increase in mortality and less frequent relapses. This suggests the possibility of a different aetiology[8].

Table 17.1. Incidence and prevalence of inflammatory bowel disease in various series.

City	Period	Incidence per 100 000				Prevalence per 100 000	
		Ulcerative colitis		Crohn's disease		Ulcerative colitis Men and women	Crohn's disease
		Men	Women	Men	Women		
Oxford[3]	1951–60	5.8	7.3	0.8	0.8	79.9	9.0
Aberdeen[4]	1955–60	—	—	1.4	1.9	—	32.5
Uppsala[7]	1968–73	—	—	1.8	1.8	—	26.5
Nottingham[5]	1968–72	—	—	2.6	3.7	—	
Baltimore[6]*	1960–63	3.9	5.2	2.5	1.2	42.0	

* Patients under 20 years excluded.

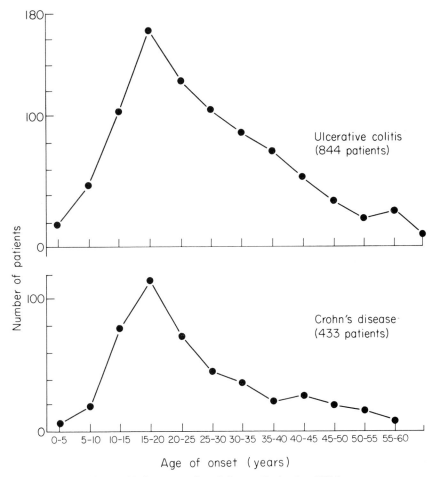

Fig. 17.1. Age incidence of inflammatory bowel disease, England and Wales.

Secular trends

A number of studies over the past 20–30 years have shown a rise in incidence of Crohn's disease[4, 5, 7]. This rise has taken place over the period in which Crohn's colitis has become more generally recognized. Thus part of the increase may be due to reallocation of cases from ulcerative colitis to Crohn's disease. Indeed in the Scottish study the rising incidence of Crohn's disease was largely confined to cases involving the large bowel. In Nottingham the overall rise was 5-fold over a 10 year period, with the incidence in 1958 being 0.73 per 100 000, increasing to 3.6 per 100 000 of the population in 1971. Although the rise was greatest in colonic Crohn's disease there was also a significant increase in patients with small bowel disease only. A report from Sweden, which concentrated on Malmo, a major city with a stable population, showed a rise in incidence from 3.5 per 100 000 to 6.0 per 100 000 when two 8 year periods between 1958 and 1973 were compared. This study specifically excluded an intermediate group, where it was not possible to assign patients either to Crohn's disease or to ulcerative colitis[9].

It is much more difficult to detect time variations in the incidence of ulcerative colitis because comparisons rely on hospital admission rates which will vary with changes in policy with regard to the severity of cases admitted. However, no large changes with time have been observed in England, despite the increased frequency of diagnosis of Crohn's disease. This might suggest some increase in incidence of ulcerative colitis, as the frequency of the disease would be expected to fall as increasing numbers of patients are assigned to the category of Crohn's disease, rather than ulcerative colitis. An increasing rate of diagnosis has been shown in Minnesota, USA, and in Norway, but not in Sweden.

Racial and geographical distribution

Satisfactory epidemiological studies of non-specific inflammatory bowel disease are lacking for most areas of the world, other than the United Kingdom, Scandinavia and the USA. These diseases are thought to be rare in most tropical countries, where acute dysenteric illnesses predominate. This may be due to poor diagnostic and follow-up facilities. Racial differences occur within those countries that have been surveyed. There is said to be a low incidence of Crohn's disease amongst Canadian Eskimos, and amongst Red Indians and Black Americans, and a high incidence in American Jews. The initial reports on American Jews indicated a 2- to 6-fold higher rate over the general population; however, later studies have shown a smaller difference. These differences may be due to varied admission policies, more severe disease amongst the Jews, or a genuinely higher frequency of the condition amongst them.

Similar variations amongst ethnic minorities tend to occur in the incidence of ulcerative colitis. For example, American Jews seem to have a higher incidence of ulcerative colitis than their fellow countrymen. In general this does not seem to be the case in England, although an early study which compared patients discharged from two London hospitals showed a higher than expected proportion of Jews with ulcerative colitis. Ulcerative colitis does not appear to be particularly common in Israel, although in one study the incidence was shown to be higher amongst Western than Oriental Jews. Like Crohn's disease the incidence of ulcerative colitis appears to be lower amongst Black Americans than amongst non-Jewish Whites and another report documented its rarity in New Zealand amongst Maoris. The rest of the population had a similar incidence to that found in Europe. Possible wide variations in the incidence of ulcerative colitis within a country, but not due to ethnic differences, are suggested by one study from India and one from Switzerland.

Mortality

Crude mortality statistics for these 2 diseases are of little epidemiological value as changes with time may reflect differences in diagnosis, incidence or case fatality. The death rate from ulcerative colitis in England and Wales was about 1.5 per 100 000 in 1940 (when records were first available). It dropped to 0.9 per 100 000 in 1947 since when it has remained relatively constant. Death rates for Crohn's disease are less reliable because of its comparative rarity. Combined figures of ulcerative colitis and Crohn's disease in the USA indicate a higher death rate in the White population (1.9 per 100 000) compared with non-Whites, (1.0 per 100 000). Mortality increases with age and is particularly high amongst elderly White men.

The Oxford study showed an overall excess mortality in patients with both ulcerative colitis and Crohn's disease when compared with the general population. With Crohn's disease the mortality rate increases with each year of follow-up, whereas with ulcerative colitis the risk of death is high in the early years and then seems to diminish to some extent. At 5 years the cumulative mortality rate for Crohn's disease is 6.9 % and for ulcerative colitis is 16.7 %, while at 15 years the figures were 21.4 % for Crohn's disease and 29.8 % for ulcerative colitis[10]. The value of such data is limited by the case selection involved in referral to 1 hospital in the Oxford region, although attempts have been made to overcome this by separating groups of patients who attended locally from those who had been referred from elsewhere. The trends in the 2 groups of patients with Crohn's disease appeared similar, although as might be expected the referred patients appeared to have a more severe disease as judged by higher mortality rates.

Risk factors

Socio-economic

In general, no relationship between socio-economic class or occupation has been found for either Crohn's disease or ulcerative colitis. However, the Baltimore study did suggest a high intellectual attainment in those suffering from Crohn's disease and a study from Denmark suggested a much higher incidence of ulcerative colitis amongst wealthy people.

The Baltimore study and the one in Aberdeen both suggested an increased incidence amongst town dwellers as compared with people living in rural areas. Farmers were shown to have a low incidence of inflammatory bowel disease in a series from Chicago. None of these findings have been confirmed by other studies.

Associated diseases

Both Crohn's disease and ulcerative colitis are associated in some cases with large joint arthritis, uveitis, ankylosing spondylitis, skin rashes and with a variety of liver conditions. There is also an association between ulcerative colitis and urticaria, allergic rhinitis and asthma. Some workers have used such associations to suggest an immune aetiology for the disease. The association between carcinoma of the colon and ulcerative colitis is well recognized. A definite although smaller association between Crohn's disease and tumours of the large and small bowel has been demonstrated more recently.

Genetic and familial factors

Inflammatory bowel disease is not inherited in a simple Mendelian fashion. However, a large number of studies have indicated that both diseases tend to cluster in certain families. Usually either condition may occur in the family members with increased frequency, irrespective of the diagnosis in the proband. In some studies only one condition has been found in other members of the family and in these cases it is more likely to be Crohn's disease. As ulcerative colitis is more common than Crohn's disease it is difficult to be certain that family aggregation of this condition is not fortuitous. It has been calculated that if the prevalence of ulcerative colitis is about 1 per 1000 of the population, a family history in the first degree relatives would be expected in about 0.5% of the patients and in 1–1.5% of patients if second degree relatives are also included. Studies from Leeds (England), Chicago (USA) and Cardiff (Wales) have shown rates far in excess of this. The increased incidence appears highest in first degree relatives and then tails off (Table 17.2). In one series a second affected member was found in 95 out of 113 families[12]. This could be explained by either a genetic aetiology or an environmental influence. However, there appears to be only 1 case report of both husband and wife having inflammatory bowel disease, thus any environmental influence is likely to operate at an early stage of life.

Table 17.2. Familial aggregation of inflammatory bowel disease[11].

	Ulcerative colitis (UC)	Crohn's disease (CD)
Total number of cases	103	39
1st degree relative with UC	4	4
1st degree relative with CD	3	7
2nd degree relative with CD or UC	2	2

Recent studies with lymphocytotoxic antibodies suggest an environmental factor. These antibodies are non-specific and are found in a variety of diseases, but are present in about 40 % of patients with inflammatory bowel disease. Such antibodies have been found only rarely in control groups but they have been found in 30 % of the relatives of patients with inflammatory bowel disease, 50 % of spouses and 40 % of household contacts. It is likely that a subtle interplay of environmental and genetic factors determine the undoubted higher incidence of inflammatory bowel disease in families.

Identification of genetic subgroups of the population who are particularly susceptible to inflammatory bowel disease has been attempted, using the frequency of distribution of ABO and rhesus blood groups, but without success. Early studies suggested that there was an association with glucose 6-phosphate dehydrogenase deficiency. This has since been disputed.

Histocompatibility (human leucocyte antigens (HLA) have also been studied, with conflicting results. An increased frequency of HLA-All and A7 and a reduced frequency of A3 have been found in patients with ulcerative colitis. In Crohn's disease a reduction in frequency of A9 was found.

Ankylosing spondylitis (see Chapter 27) occurs in about 2 % of patients with Crohn's disease or ulcerative colitis. In the general population, 90 % of such patients are HLA-B27 positive. In patients with inflammatory bowel disease Morris *et al.*[13] have shown that large joint arthritis is not HLA-associated but that 75 % of patients with inflammatory bowel disease and ankylosing spondylitis were B27 positive. It was calculated that 16 % of B27 positive patients with Crohn's disease and 47 % of those with ulcerative colitis would develop ankylosing spondylitis.

Infection

An attractive aetiological theory is that inflammatory bowel disease is caused by an infective agent. Epidemiological evidence for this is lacking except that the disease is rare in areas where acute infective disease of the bowel is common. Family studies indicate that such an infection would either be acquired early in life or require close contact over a prolonged period. The increasing incidence of Crohn's disease, but not ulcerative colitis, might suggest that the causative organism in the 2 conditions is different.

Any study of possible infective agents in inflammatory bowel disease is bedevilled by the possibility that the organisms isolated are present as a result of secondary infection of damaged tissue rather than being the causative agent. Studies have suggested that cell-wall deficient forms of atypical Mycobacteria or Pseudomonas, or a possible increase in *Escherichia coli* colonization of the colon with patients with inflammatory bowel disease, may be important in the pathogenesis. Viral agents have been cultured from a proportion of patients with Crohn's disease and ulcerative colitis in America and London. These viruses have not yet been positively identified although their cytopathic effects have been shown to be inhibited by Nebraska calf-virus vaccine.

Reports that it is possible after a long latent interval to produce a granulomatous lesion in foot-pads of mice, by injection of cell-free filtrate of material taken from the bowel of patients with ulcerative colitis or Crohn's disease[14], have now come from 3 laboratories.

In rabbits it was possible to show that material from Crohn's patients produced granulomatous lesions in the gut, lymph nodes and liver, whereas that from ulcerative colitis produced a round cell infiltrate. These observations suggest that separate infective agents may be present in Crohn's disease and ulcerative colitis. In some animals (mice) immunological changes induced by these agents are similar (granuloma formation) whereas in rabbits and possibly man, different sorts of reactions are induced by each organism.

If a transmissible agent is responsible for Crohn's disease it might be possible to show evidence of time–space clustering using the technique devised by Knox. Pike and Smith examined diseases with long latent intervals but found no time–space clustering of Crohn's disease.

References

1. Lockhard-Mummery HE, Marson BC. Crohn's disease (regional enteritis) of the large intestine and its distinction from ulcerative colitis. *Gut* 1960; **1**: 87.
2. Iversen E, Bonnevie O, Anthonisen P. An epidemiological model of ulcerative colitis. *Scandinavian Journal of Gastroenterology* 1968; **3**: 593.
3. Evans JG, Acheson ED. An epidemiological study of ulcerative colitis and regional enteritis in the Oxford area. *Gut* 1965; **6**: 311.
4. Kyle J. An epidemiology of Crohn's disease in north-east Scotland. *Gastroenterology* 1971; **61**: 826.
5. Keighley A, Miller DS, *et al.* The demographic and social characteristics of patients with Crohn's disease in the Nottingham area. *Scandinavian Journal of Gastroenterology* 1976; **11**: 293.
6. Monk M, Mendeloff AI, *et al.* An epidemiological study of ulcerative colitis and regional enteritis amongst adults in Baltimore, II. Social and demographic factors. *Gastroenterology* 1969; **56**: 847.
7. Bermar L, Klause U. The incidence of Crohn's disease in central Sweden. *Scandinavian Journal of Gastroenterology* 1975; **10**: 725.
8. Jalan JN, Prescott RJ, *et al.* An experience of ulcerative colitis, III. Long term outcome. *Gastroenterology* 1970; **59**: 589.
9. Biatime F, Lindstom C, Wenckert A. Crohn's disease in a defined population. An epidemiological study of incidence, prevalance and secular trends in the city of Malmo, Sweden. *Gastroenterology* 1959; **69**: 342.
10. Truelove SC, Pena AS. Course and prognosis of Crohn's disease. *Gut* 1976; **17**: 192.
11. Lewkonia RM, McConnell RB. Familial inflammatory bowel disease. Heredity and environment. *Gut* 1976; **17**: 235.
12. Singer HC, Anderson JGD, *et al.* Familial aspects of inflammatory bowel disease *Gastroenterology* 1971; **61**: 413.

13. Morris RF, Metzger AL, *et al.* HLA 27, a useful discriminator in the arthropathies of inflammatory bowel disease *New England Journal of Medicine* 1974; **290**: 117.
14. Mitchell DN, Rees RJN. Agent transmissable from Crohn's disease tissue. *Lancet* 1970; **ii**: 168.

Further reading

Brook BN, Cave DR, *et al. Epidemiology in Crohn's disease.* London: Macmillan, 1977.
Goliger JC, Domhal FT, *et al. Epidemiology in ulcerative colitis.* London: Balliere Tindall and Cassell, 1968.
Mendeloff AL. Epidemiology of inflammatory bowel disease. In Kirsner JB, Sharter RG, eds. Inflammatory bowel disease. Philadelphia: Lea Febiger, 1975.

Chapter 18 · Large Bowel Cancers

B G GAZZARD AND P LANCE

Large bowel cancers are common in the developed world. More than 95 % of them are adenocarcinomas. Other types of malignant tumours do occur (for example, lymphomas, sarcomas, melanomas and carcinoid tumours) but they are rare and their epidemiology is different from adenocarcinomas. They are not considered in this chapter. Large bowel cancers are arbitrarily divided into rectal tumours, which arise within 8 cm of the anus, and colonic cancers which occur elsewhere. However, 70 % of tumours arise in those parts of the sigmoid colon or rectum that make it practically impossible to classify them securely as either rectal or colonic. There is some debate as to whether or not cancers in the 2 sites should be considered as 1 disease entity or 2. Although there are some differences in their sex and geographical distribution they are usually considered as a single entity.

The disease usually presents by a combination of alteration of bowel habit, passing of blood per rectum, abdominal pain and large bowel obstruction. Surgical excision is the only effective form of treatment. The prognosis depends upon the extent of the tumour at the time of presentation (Dukes' system[1] is used to classify the extent of the tumour) and its histological type. The crude 5 year survival rates for colo-rectal cancers treated in district general hospitals in the United Kingdom is between 19 % and 25 %, depending upon the stage at presentation. In some specialist centres 5 year survival rates of over 50 % have been achieved. Rectal tumours have a worse prognosis than colonic tumours.

Incidence

Most of the figures on incidence are from hospital records, cancer registries and death certificates. Implicit in the use of these sources is the assumption that all bowel cancers are symptomatic and therefore will be detected before death or that the disease is universally fatal. However, a study of Japanese in Hawaii demonstrated that some colo-rectal cancers remain asymptomatic and would not be detected without post mortem examination. Clinically unsuspected large bowel cancers were discovered in 13 (3.4 %) of 379 people over the age of 70 years who had an autopsy for other reasons[2]. Furthermore, increasing numbers of large bowel polyps showing severe dysplasia and focal cancer are being removed with fibre–optic colonoscopes and diathermy. These do not normally feature in incidence figures for colo-rectal cancer.

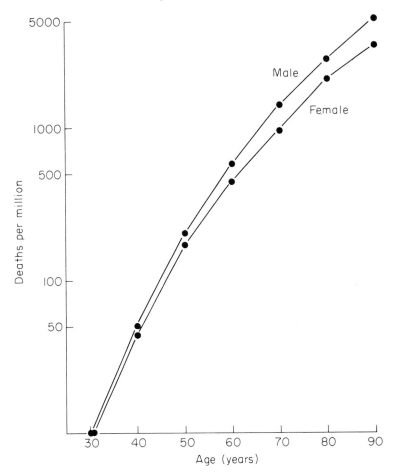

Fig. 18.1. Carcinoma of the rectum and colon: age- and sex-specific death rates, England and Wales, 1979.

The age- and sex-specific mortality rates in England and Wales are shown in Fig 18.1 and the age- and sex-standardized death rates for persons under 65 from 1911 are shown in Table 18.1.

The overall incidence of colo-rectal cancer is roughly equal in men and women but there are some differences in the incidence at the 2 sites. Rectal cancer is more common in men than in women with an overall ratio up to 1.7:1 reported. The incidence is equal at the age of 45, but after 65 years it is twice as common in men. Colonic cancer is more common in women than in men below the age of 60. After 60 the incidence in men and women is equal. There is an exponential rise with increasing age, a picture that is typical of epithelial cancers. The majority of patients who are treated for colo-rectal cancers are in their sixth and seventh decades of life. A small minority of patients, those with familial polyposis syndromes behave quite differently. Most develop large bowel cancer before the age of 40 unless the colon has been removed prophylactically.

Geographical variations

There is a 6- to 8-fold difference in the incidence of colo-rectal cancer in men between the high and low risk parts of the world (Table 18.2). The difference

Table 18.1. Trends in mortality from cancers of the colon and rectum in England and Wales, 1911–70, men and women under 65 years, age-standardized to the standard European population, per 100 000[3].

Period	Colon Men	Women	Rectum Men	Women
1911–15	8.6	9.8	8.7	6.0
1916–20	8.9	10.3	9.1	5.9
1921–25	9.7	10.4	9.4	5.8
1926–30	10.3	10.8	9.2	5.4
1931–35	9:2	9.4	9.2	5.2
1936–40	9.8	10.0	8.8	5.1
1941–45	9.7	10.2	8.4	5.1
1946–50	8.6	9.4	7.4	4.6
1951–55	7.1	7.9	6.0	4.0
1956–60	6.3	7.3	5.2	3.5
1961–65	6.0	6.9	4.8	3.3
1966–70	6.4	6.8	4.7	3.2

Table 18.2. Cancer of the colon and rectum: age-standardized incidence rates in men and women per 100 000[3].

Country	Colon Male	Female	Rectum Male	Female
Japan, Miyagi Perfecture	5.8	5.8	6.9	7.3
Colombia, Cali	4.9	6.2	5.4	4.0
Puerto Rica	7.2	8.9	5.4	5.8
Hawaii: Hawaiian	31.8	19.5	8.6	10.0
Caucasian	28.6	40.8	18.2	14.3
USA, Conneticut	41.0	40.5	24.2	15.8
Canada, Newfoundland	29.1	26.8	16.6	10.9
Quebec	23.1	23.6	15.8	10.7
Yugoslavia, Slovenia	8.2	7.6	12.1	8.8
Finland	9.9	10.9	11.6	9.6
Poland, Warsaw	8.9	10.1	8.1	5.6
Germany, Hamburg	19.1	19.5	16.8	12.7
Norway	18.2	17.6	10.3	7.0
Denmark	24.1	26.6	26.1	15.7
United Kingdom, Birmingham	23.0	22.1	23.9	13.8

increases to between 10- and 20-fold if colonic cancers alone are considered. The range for women is in proportion though numerically smaller. There are no countries where there is a high incidence of rectal cancer and a low incidence of colonic cancer or vice versa.

There is evidence that the incidence in a particular country is approximately proportional to its socio-economic status 30 years previously, which in turn is closely correlated with the consumption of meat and animal fat.

In developed countries different socio-economic groups are equally prone to large bowel cancer. However, in Hong Kong it was found that the mortality rate from large bowel cancer in the highest income bracket was nearly twice that in the lowest[4]. The findings from a study in Cali, Colombia, another low risk area, were similar.

Migrant studies

Two methods of investigating whether geographical differences in the incidence of colo-rectal cancer are due mainly to genetic or to environmental influences, are to study differences between migrant groups and to examine variations in tumour incidence in time. It was found that Jews who migrated to Israel from the Yemen and North Africa had a much lower incidence of large bowel cancer during their early years in Israel than Jewish immigrants from the higher risk areas of Western Europe and Russia[5]. Various workers have shown that with time the incidence in immigrants to the USA gradually converges with that of native Americans. As with stomach cancer, Japanese migrating to Hawaii and the mainland of America have proved rewarding subjects for epidemiologists studying large bowel cancer. The incidence amongst Japanese in America from 1949–52 was intermediate between the rates for the Japanese in their own country and native Americans. By 1959–62, the incidence for the men, both original migrants and their American-born children was almost as high as that for native Americans[6]. There was a similar but less dramatic trend amongst women. The men had mostly given up regular Japanese-style meals.

The incidence of colo-rectal cancer in Miyagi (Japan) has been compared with Japanese and Caucasians in Hawaii. The Japanese immigrants to Hawaii were found to have assumed the incidence of large bowel cancer of their adopted country, which is much higher than in Miyagi. It has been estimated that this change in incidence takes about 2 decades to become apparent.

Aetiological hypotheses

Adenoma–carcinoma sequence

It is widely held that most colo-rectal cancers develop from benign adenomas, whose malignant potential is determined by their histological type, their size and

and the degree of epithelial dysplasia. Of 3 histological types of adenoma, the least common is the villous adenoma which has the highest rate of malignancy (40 %). Malignancy is rare in adenomas of less than 1 cm diameter but, when they reach a size in excess of 2 cm, about 50 % show malignant change. The anatomical distributions of adenomas and colo-rectal cancers are similar but the vast majority of adenomas remain small and benign. The reasons why some grow and become malignant are not known.

Predisposing diseases

Several conditions predispose to large bowel cancer; familial polyposis coli (FPC) and Gardner's syndrome are inherited diseases with an autosomal dominant pattern. Familial polyposis coli is estimated to affect 1 in 8000 individuals and Gardner's syndrome 1 in 14000. Most patients with familial polyposis coli have over 1000 large bowel polyps of varying size. In them, the development of cancer is inevitable by middle age if the colon is not removed prophylactically. Patients with Gardner's syndrome are similarly at risk but they usually have fewer polyps and develop cancer later. Apart from familial polyposis syndromes, of which FPC and Gardner's syndrome are the 2 most important, there is a significant increase in the incidence of colo–rectal cancer among first degree relatives of patients with colo-rectal cancer.

Patients who have had one large bowel cancer removed have an increased risk of developing a second metachronous tumour in any remaining large intestine[7]. The cumulative risk after 25 years is 10 % if, in addition to the cancer, adenomas were found in the original operation specimen.

Patients with ulcerative colitis also have greater risk of developing large bowel cancer[8], but this has been overstated in the past. The group at risk consists of those who have had extensive colitis (disease extending proximally from the rectum to include the hepatic flexure on a double-contrast barium enema) for more than 10 years. In the second decade after diagnosis the estimated risk is 1 carcinoma in 200 patient-years, in other words an individual patient has a 1 in 20 chance of developing cancer over a 10 year period. This risk is considerably greater in the third decade but numbers are small and so figures are likely to be inaccurate.

Dietary and environmental factors

In an attempt to explain the geographical distribution of large bowel cancer and the results from work on migrants there have been numerous studies of the luminal contents of the large bowel and the influence of diet on faecal constituents. The main topics examined include geographical differences in diet, the influence of dietary fibre, the bacterial flora of the large bowel, and faecal concentrations of steroids and bile acids. None of the hypotheses linking differences in tumour incidence with the geographical variations in the contents of the large bowel have been proved.

Dietary differences

In high risk areas the diet tends to be rich in protein and animal fat. Many studies have shown a correlation between the daily consumption of meat and the incidence of colo-rectal cancer. A rise in the consumption of meat was the major difference in dietary habit between Japanese migrants to Hawaii and their compatriots in Japan.

A major problem is that features such as high fat, high cholesterol and low fibre intake are all typical of the Western diet so that there is great difficulty deciding whether a single factor or a particular combination is important. There is a significant correlation between mortality rates from coronary heart diseases and colo-rectal cancer[9]. To test the hypothesis that cholesterol intake is of particular importance, food consumption data from 20 industrialized countries have been studied[10]. The food-balance sheets of the Food and Agriculture Organisation (FAO) in each country for the period 1954–65 were examined. The average daily consumption per person of total fat, saturated, monosaturated and polyunsaturated fatty acids, cholesterol and fibre in each country were calculated. When each was controlled in turn only the partial correlation coefficient between cholesterol intake and the colonic cancer rate was significant.

Dietary fibre

High vegetable-fibre diets are a feature of many low risk parts of the world, such as Africa. A high fibre diet has 3 well substantiated consequences which it has been postulated may explain its inverse relationship with colo-rectal cancer[11]. Bowel transit time is reduced, which might reduce the exposure of the large bowel mucosa to luminal carcinogens. The stool bulk is increased, which might dilute carcinogens. The bacterial flora is altered, which might be advantageous.

Bacterial flora of the large bowel

Comparisons of bacterial counts in faeces from subjects in different countries have shown large numbers of Gram-negative anaerobes in high risk areas and a preponderance of aerobes in low risk countries. High numbers of nuclear dehydrogenating clostridia (NDC) have been reported in patients with cancer of the large bowel whereas two-thirds of healthy adults in the United Kingdom have none of these organisms detectable in their stools. NDC are consistently absent from the faeces of Africans living in Africa. However, a comparison between a high and a low risk area of Scandinavia failed to confirm the correlation between NDC counts and colo-rectal cancers.

Faecal steriods and bile acid

The consumption of a high fat, high meat diet has been shown to increase the steroid content of faeces. The faecal concentrations of steroids and cholesterol conversion products are higher in Western subjects than those from low risk areas. The dihydroxycholanic acids are secondary bile acids probably derived mostly from deoxycholate by the action of intestinal bacteria, and their faecal concentration correlates well with the incidence of colonic cancer. Bile acids have been shown in many animal experiments to promote the induction of colonic cancer by agents such as 1, 2-dimethyl hydrazine.

A unifying theory is that intestinal bacteria, particularly anaerobes, produce a carcinogen or co-carcinogen, perhaps bile acids, in the lumen of the colon from benign substrates such as cholesterol and steroids. To support this, in one study the combination of faecal bile acid concentration and NDC counts provided a better discriminant between patients with colo-rectal cancer and controls than either alone[12]. There is evidence that the concentration of substrate and the biochemical activity of the gut flora can be influenced by diet.

Other factors

Asbestos has been incriminated in several studies[13]. However, it is possible this may be due to diagnostic confusion with mesothelioma of the peritoneum. The findings of an increased incidence of rectal but not colonic cancer in one study of doctors who smoked heavily was probably a statistical quirk and has not been confirmed by any other studies of tobacco smoking[14].

There have been 2 reports of an increased incidence of colo-rectal cancer in men who had a history of heavy beer consumption[15]. Large scale prospective studies amongst brewery workers in Copenhagen and Dublin are in progress.

Screening

If the adenoma–carcinoma sequence applies in practice, by removing adenomas colonoscopically it should theoretically be possible to prevent the development of colo-rectal cancers. Unfortunately the majority of adenomas are asymptomatic. One approach to their early detection is screening for faecal occult blood. The older Guaiac and Orthotoluidine methods had false positive rates approaching 50 % but the Haemoccult test gives only 1 % false positive. In one study of 6579 healthy men and women over the age of 40, 1 % were positive for occult blood and half of these had neoplastic lesions, including 23 with large adenomas and 7 with cancer[16]. Other studies have suggested that 1 or 2 asymptomatic cancers per 1000 subjects screened might be detected. They are likely to have a good prognosis being either polyps amenable to colonoscopic removal or easily resectable cancers without local spread or lymph node involvement.

Screening for colo-rectal cancer in the normal population is in its infancy and it is impossible to quantify either the potential expense or impact on the disease. Screening for early or pre-cancer in ulcerative colitis is on a surer footing. The practice in a number of centres is to recommend prophylactic procto-colectomy when biopsies from patients with extensive or total colitis of more than 10 years' duration show severe dysplasia at multiple sites, either in specimens from more than one place during a single colonoscopy or in a second specimen when colonoscopy is repeated.

References

1. Dukes CE. Cancer of the rectum – analysis of 1000 cases. *Journal of Pathology and Bacteriology* 1940; **50**: 527–39.
2. Stemmerman GN. Cancer of the colon and rectum discovered at autopsy in Hawaiian Japanese. *Cancer* 1966; **19**: 1567–72.
3. Doll R, Muir CS, Waterhouse JAH. *Cancer incidence in five continents. Vol 2*. Geneva: International Union Against Cancer (UICC), 1970.
4. Crowther JS, Drasar BS, *et al*. Faecal steroids and bacteria and large bowel cancer in Hong Kong by socio-economic groups. *British Journal of Cancer* 1976; **34**: 191–8.
5. Doll R, Payne P, Waterhouse JAH. *Cancer incidence in five continents Vol 1*. Geneva: International Union Against Cancer (UICC), 1966.
6. Haenszel W, Kurihara M. Studies of Japanese migrants. *US Journal of the National Cancer Institute* 1968; **40**: 43–68.
7. Heald RJ, Lockhart-Mummery HE. The lesson of the second cancer of the large bowel. *British Journal of Surgery* 1972; **59**: 16–19.
8. Lennard Jones JE, Marson BC, *et al*. Cancer in colitis: assessment of the individual risk by clinical and histological criteria. *Gastroenterology* 1977; **73**: 1280–9.
9. Rose G, Blackburn H, *et al*. Colon cancer and blood cholesterol. *Lancet* 1974; **i**: 181–3.
10. Liu Kiang, Moss Dorothy, *et al*. Dietary cholesterol, fat, and fibre, and colon-cancer mortality. *Lancet* 1979; **ii**: 782–5.
11. Burkitt DP. Epidemiology of cancer of the colon and rectum. *Cancer* 1971; **28**: 3–13.
12. Hill MJ, Drasar BS, *et al*. Faecal bile acids and clostridia in patients with cancer of the large bowel. *Lancet* 1975; **i**: 535–8.
13. Selikoff IJ, Churg J, Hammond EC. Asbestos exposure and neoplasia. *JAMA* 1964; **188**: 22–6.
14. Doll R, Peto R. Mortality in relation to smoking: 20 years' observation on male British doctors. *British Medical Journal* 1976; **ii**: 1525–2536.
15. Enstrom JE. Colo-rectal cancer and beer drinking. *British Journal of Cancer* 1977; **35**: 674–83.
16. Winawer Sidney J, Miller Daniel G, *et al*. Feasibility of fecal occult-blood testing for detection of colo-rectal neoplasia. *Cancer* 1977; **40**: 2616–9.

Further reading

Correa Pelayo and Haenszel William. The epidemiology of large bowel cancer. *Advances in Cancer Research* 1978; **28**: 1–141.

Langman MJS. *The epidemiology of chronic digestive disease*. London: Edward Arnold, 1979: 57–66.
Truelove SC. Lee Emanoel, eds. *Topics in gastroenterology 5*. Oxford: Blackwell Scientific Publications, 1977: 3–99.

Chapter 19 · Carcinoma of the Pancreas

R J BERRY AND D R JONES

The pancreas is the most common site of malignant neoplasia in the gastro-intestinal tract after the large bowel and stomach. Primary malignant tumours of the pancreas can arise from either ductal or glandular structures (the exocrine or endocrine portions of the organ). The most common are adenocarcinomata of the exocrine pancreas. Approximately 60 % of all malignant neoplasms of the pancreas arise in the head of the organ, 25 % in the body, and 15 % in the tail[1]. Insulin-producing tumours of the Islets of Langerhans are clinically interesting because of their metabolic effects but these are rare and are usually benign. Other non-malignant conditions, such as 'malignant pancreatitis' can be confused with invasive pancreatic malignancies, but they too are relatively rare. Secondary tumours of the pancreas are uncommon.

The diagnosis of pancreatic carcinoma is often difficult to establish. It presents with vague upper abdominal symptoms, including central pain which may be related to food and which commonly radiates to the back. Jaundice or weight loss without focal symptoms are also common presentations. Malignancy may arise in existing chronic pancreatitis, and a patient with a long history of alcoholic excess and recurrent bouts of acute pancreatitis may harbour an unsuspected or undetected malignant lesion. Diagnosis has been aided by the development of diagnostic ultrasound and the advent of computerized tomo-graphic scanning. However, tomographic scanning can only detect lesions which cause an expansion of the pancreas, and ultrasonography can be difficult because the pancreas can be obscured by gas in the bowel.

The diagnosis is most commonly made at surgical exploration, but the disease is often indistinguishable from necrotizing pancreatitis with abscess formation. When diagnosed comparatively early as a chance finding arising in pancreatitis, carcinoma of the pancreas is usually already widely disseminated, first via the regional circulation to the liver, and then more distantly to the lungs. The overall surgical cure rate is low, even when radical *en bloc* operation is attempted. The advent of computer assisted tomography (CAT) scanning has allowed the planning of high precision radiotherapy which can give primary tumour local control rates equalling or surpassing those obtained surgically[2].

Incidence and prevalence

Mortality data for carcinoma of the pancreas provide a good measure of the incidence of the tumour. This is because the prognosis is very poor. It is now the seventh most common site of cancers causing death in both men and women. Mortality from pancreatic carcinoma in men is approximately similar to that from carcinoma of the bladder. In 1976 it caused 4.2 % of all male cancer deaths (a crude death rate of 119 per million per year) and 4.7 % of female cancer deaths (a rate of 110 per million per year). There has been a steady and substantial increase in death rates since the turn of the century: for example, for the period 1911–15 the death rates were 18 and 16 per million per year for men and women respectively and were 82 and 66 per million respectively for the 1951–55 period. This change might be due to a combination of better recording of data and better diagnostic skills, and a real change brought about by factors such as the increase in smoking.

In both sexes there is a steady increase in pancreatic cancer mortality with increasing age. The disease is very rare below the age of 40. Death rates rise more rapidly with age in men than in women; in elderly men the mortality rate is about 50 % higher than in elderly women. There is no clear pattern of variation in mortality from pancreatic carcinoma with social class or with geographical area, but rural areas tend to show slightly lower standardized mortality ratios (SMR).

In the USA and countries of Western Europe the picture is broadly similar[3], except that the male/female ratio is about 2 : 1. There are minor racial differences in incidence in the USA, with Blacks having a higher incidence than Whites, and persons of ethnic Jewish lineage having an incidence higher than the national average. The incidence in Maori men and Hawaiian men and women is approximately twice that found in most Western countries[3]. In some African countries and in India the reported incidence rates for carcinoma of the pancreas are far lower, perhaps one-third of the average rate in Western countries, although the reliability of these figures is uncertain.

Special features

A higher risk of the development of malignant tumours of the pancreas, pancreatitis, diabetes and gall bladder disease is correlated with 3 clinical conditions. The correlation with pancreatitis is perhaps not unexpected in that the proliferative response to repeated infection may well precipitate the emergence of a clone of transformed cells which evolve into a gross tumour. It is more difficult to explain why diabetics have twice the incidence in the general population[4]. One mechanism which has been suggested is that the malignant change is a response to the repeated challenge by multiple protein impurities in the insulin they use. However, although immune surveillance has been thought to play a role in the body's defences against malignancy, this mechanism has never been shown conclusively to operate for tumours in any site in man. The incidence of risk of pancreatic malignancy in patients with gall bladder disease is more understandable. It is possibly due to ascending infection and the presence of potentially carcinogenic dietary metabolites in the biliary tree.

Prognosis

The overall prognosis for carcinoma of the pancreas is distressingly poor. The median survival from diagnosis is less than 6 months: the 1 year survival rate is typically around 10 % in unselected series and only about 2 % of patients survive 5 years. Careful case selection, taking full advantage of improved methods of tumour imaging and localization has improved the results of individual surgical and radiotherapeutic series, but at the cost of rejecting as unsuitable the vast majority of patients on presentation. Because carcinoma of the pancreas is common in patients with a history of alcohol or recurrent pancreatitis the immediate operative mortality is high. The disease tends to metastatize early, both locally to the liver and to adjacent lymphatic structures, as well as to the lung. There seems no immediate hope of further significant improvement in early diagnosis.

Aetiology

There are few clues to the aetiology of carcinoma of the pancreas, although at least in part this is because the disease has been relatively little studied. Smoking carries a 2-fold increase in risk of development of carcinoma of pancreas, and the increase in risk is correlated with the number of cigarettes smoked and the length of smoking history[5,6]. This may help to explain the increasing incidence of pancreatic carcinoma, and the widening male/female ratio with age. There is no sex difference in the incidence of carcinoma of the pancreas in non-smokers. Possible mechanisms whereby cigarette smoking influences the development of this cancer are unknown, although there is a suspicion that it may be mediated through effects of smoking on the blood lipids. In the USA the level of dietary fat per capita correlates with the death rates for carcinoma of the pancreas in men, another possible pointer to the importance of blood lipids[6,7]. There is no clear correlation of increased pancreatic cancer risk by occupation, except in chemists and perhaps in individuals known to have been exposed to betanaphthylamine[6,7]. Carcinoma of the pancreas remains an enigma, a distressingly common and invariably fatal one.

References

1. Howard JM, Jordan GL. *Surgical diseases of the pancreas*. Philadelphia: Lippincott, 1960.
2. Wiley AL. *British Journal of Radiology* Supplement No 15. 1981.
3.* Doll R, Muir CS, Waterhouse J, eds. *Cancer incidence in five continents. Vol 2*. Geneva: International Union Against Cancer (UICC), 1970.

* Recommended reading.

4.   Kessler II. Cancer mortality among diabetics. *US Journal of the National Cancer Institute* 1970; **44**: 673–6.

5.* Wynder EL, Mabuchi K, *et al.* Epidemiology of cancer of the pancreas. *US Journal of the National Cancer Institute* 1973; **50**: 645–67.

6.* Wynder EL. An epidemiological evaluation of the causes of cancer of the pancreas. *Cancer Research* 1975; **35**: 2228–33.

7.* Fraumeni JF. Cancer of the pancreas and biliary tract: epidemiological considerations. *Cancer Research* 1975; **35**: 3437–46.

* Recommended reading.

SECTION 5 · DISEASES OF THE GENITO-URINARY SYSTEM AND BREAST

Chapter 20 · Urinary Tract Infections

W E WATERS

The epidemiology of urinary tract infections can be approached from 3 directions. The first is the prevalence and incidence of symptoms and signs of urinary tract infection that patients experience. The second is the frequency of abnormal laboratory findings, particularly those relating to the examination of urine. Unfortunately, the correlation between symptoms and signs and laboratory findings is not particularly good. The interpretation of the results of epidemiological surveys is made more difficult as both symptoms and signs, and laboratory findings often vary considerably over short periods of time. The third starting point is the mortality information that is available from death certificates. In 1978, infection of the kidneys (World Health Organization International Certification of Diseases (ICD) number 590) caused 1000 deaths in women and 500 deaths in men in England and Wales. Mortality has shown considerable fluctuation over the last 30 years, possibly because mortality from infections of the kidney have been confused with deaths from other renal diseases.

Morbidity

Symptoms of urinary tract infections are very common, especially in women and elderly men. Information on prevalence and patterns of referral by general practitioners in the United Kingdom is available from a number of studies including the National Morbidity Studies organized by the Royal College of General Practitioners. The Second National Morbidity Study[1], which involved 53 General Practices, showed that patient consulting-rates for the clinical diagnoses pyelitis, pyelonephritis and pyelocystitis were about 4 times as frequent in women as in men. (Fig. 20.1). In some age groups, particularly the 15–24 year olds, the sex difference was even more marked. However, with increasing age the differences became less. The patient consulting-rates for acute cystitis, (Fig. 20.2) were more than 5 times as high in women as in men and this difference was most marked in the 15–24 year age group. The sex difference decreased with increasing age. As with several other studies reported from General Practice, the consulting rates for women were found to be higher in the younger age group with a maximum rate of 42.3 patients per 1000 consulting over the 1 year period in the age range 25–44 years.

In addition to the data given in Figs. 20.1 and 20.2, there were other

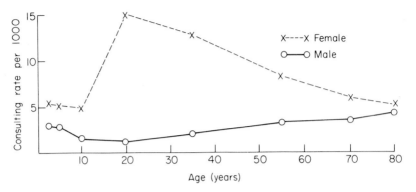

Fig. 20.1. Patient consulting rate for pyelitis, pyelonephritis and pyelocystitis in the Second National Morbidity Study[1].

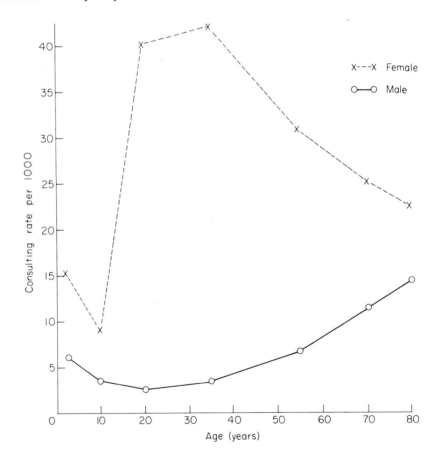

Fig. 20.2. Patient consulting rate for acute cystitis in the Second National Morbidity Study[1].

classification groups in the Second National Study such as chronic cystitis which had patient consulting rate of 0.3 per 1000 for men and 1.5 per 1000 for women, and non-venereal urethritis which had an all-ages patient consulting rate of 0.09 per 1000 for men and 1.0 per 1000 for women. These striking and consistent differences between the sexes are probably related to differences in their anatomy and the fact that in women the pH of urine supports the growth of the commonest organisms producing symptoms better than that in men. Over half of the patients consulting with pyelitis, pyelonephritis and pyelocystitis were investigated outside the practices. About 6 % were referred to out-patient clinics and about 2 % were admitted to hospital. In the case of cystitis, about 43 % were investigated outside the hospital and 4 % were referred to out-patient departments or admitted to hospital. These figures show that patients seen in hospital with these conditions are a small proportion of those with symptoms and may be highly selected.

Patients attending their general practitioner with urinary tract symptoms are, however, also selected. It is known that many women with symptoms of urinary tract infection do not attend any doctor. The first published estimates of the prevalence of women with dysuria in the previous year from a community study in South Wales[2] are shown in Fig. 20.3. Dysuria was defined as 'any pain or burning on passing water' and a prevalence of 21.8 % was found in 2933 women aged 20–65 years. The prevalence in never-married women was 13.9 %, whereas amongst the married-parous it was 23 %. The proportion of women who had dysuria within the previous year did not differ significantly with age. In 9.8 % of all these women the dysuria lasted for a total of 2 weeks or more. Nearly 10 % of all the women, aged between 20 and 65 years, had consulted their doctors during the previous year for dysuria but this proportion was significantly higher in the younger age groups.

It appears that the usual textbook description of a higher prevalence of urinary tract symptoms in younger women is based on those consulting a doctor. However, this finding was not confirmed in an epidemiological study which showed that dysuria in women was approximately equally prevalent at all ages between 20 and 65 years. The clinical significance of such symptoms is at present unclear, but there is some epidemiological evidence that, when they start in childhood, they are more likely to be associated with evidence of impairment of renal function[3]. This increased risk of damage due to infections in childhood is consistent with evidence from other sources. 1.8 % of women dated their urinary tract symptoms back to childhood. However, memory may be poor for such distant events and may introduce bias into the results[2].

It is difficult to establish whether all sufferers from urinary tract symptoms, such as dysuria, have supporting evidence of urinary tract infection. The term 'urethral syndrome' is sometimes given to patients with no bacteriological evidence of infection but obviously much depends on how carefully and how

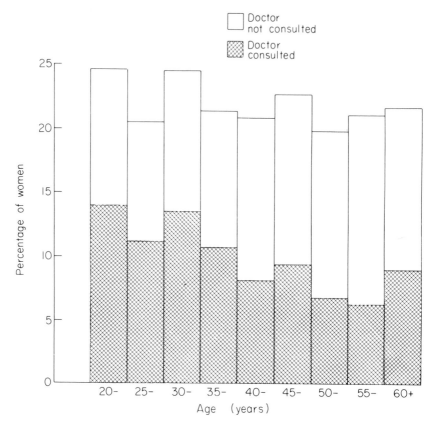

Fig. 20.3. Proportion of women aged 20–64 years with dysuria in the previous year and the proportion who consulted a doctor, South Wales[2].

often this is looked for. It has been suggested that symptoms without bacteriological evidence of infection may be due to nervous tension.

The localization of the site of infection in the renal tract is particularly difficult. High serum antibodies to the O serotype of the infecting strains of *Escherichia coli* have been claimed to correlate well with renal infection. One study in General Practice found evidence of kidney involvement in a quarter of the patients in whom symptoms were confined to the lower renal tract. Other methods of localization of infection require bladder, or even ureteric catheterization and are not suitable for routine epidemiological studies.

Laboratory findings

The pioneering work of Kass[4] in the 1950s showed that quantitive culture of the urine enabled infection in the urinary tract to be distinguished from contamination. Contaminants are added to the urine during or after voiding, but these are few in number if the specimen is cultured immediately (or kept at 4° C to prevent multiplication of organisms). Where there is infection, organisms are present in large numbers due to rapid multiplication in the urine in the bladder. Under standard conditions counts of more than 10^5 organisms per ml of urine indicate infection and this finding is known as 'significant bacteriuria'. Some investigators have stressed the need for 2 consecutive specimens to show counts of 10^5 and have also stipulated that the organism must be the same on both occasions. During the past 25 years the quantitative culture of the urine has been useful both for investigating individual patients and for epidemiological studies. The various techniques have been described by the International Committee for Nomenclature and Nosology of Renal Disease[5]. Significant bacteriuria may often be present for many months or years without symptoms (asymptomatic significant bacteriuria) but is more likely to be present with urinary tract symptoms. Provided the specimen is not contaminated prior to culture, aseptic methods of urine collection (such as suprapubic aspiration) permit the unequivocal diagnosis of urinary infection. These sometimes show lower concentrations of organisms. Bacterial counts lower than 10^5 per ml do occur in cases of true bacteriuria and are sometimes due to dilution in a well-hydrated patient.

Epidemiological surveys of the general population have shown that the prevalence of significant bacteriuria is about 1–2 % in girls and much lower in boys. With an annual incidence of about 0.4 %, at least 5–6 % of girls will have had at least 1 episode of bacteriuria before they leave school[6] and the prevalence increases with age. The prevalence of bacteriuria is low in men until such time as prostatic obstruction and urinary tract instrumentation may give a prevalence of 3.5 % over the age of 70 years. In hospitalized elderly men, a prevalence of 15 % has been reported. The prevalence of significant bacteriuria in women rises with age and with sexual activity[7]. Thus the prevalence of significant bacteriuria in nuns up to 34 years of age is only 0.5 %. Population estimates in several different countries give prevalences of significant bacteriuria in women of up to 5 % or sometimes more. Spontaneous cure of bacteriuria is common and there is a continuous changeover in the affected population with nearly half losing their bacteriuria each year but retaining an increased risk of developing the condition in the future. Short courses of nitrofurantoin and ampicillin for women with asymptomatic bacteriuria were found in a randomized clinical trial to have no significant effect on its prevalence 1 year later nor on the incidence of symptoms reported during the year[8].

The increased risk of acute pyelonephritis in pregnancy in women with asymptomatic significant bacteriuria was demonstrated by Kass[9] and this subject is reviewed by Kunin[6]. An association with premature delivery and increased perinatal mortality rate has been described although this has not been confirmed in all studies. A 10–14 year follow-up, after an episode of bacteriuria in pregnancy, found over a quarter of the women had significant bacteriuria at the time of follow-up and 29% had pyelographic evidence of chronic pyelonephritis[10]. Although a randomized trial of sulphonamide and placebo in the original group of women had reduced the incidence of symptoms during pregnancy, this treatment had no significant effect on the prevalence of bacteriuria at follow-up 10–14 years later. It is not known whether continuous or intermittent treatment with antibiotics would reduce the incidence of renal involvement.

Microscopic examination of the urine is less useful in epidemiological studies. Pyuria (defined as more than 5 polymorphonuclear leucocytes per high power field) is only present in one-third to one-half of the subjects who have significant bacteriuria[4]. Epidemiological studies have shown that *Escherichia coli* is the commonest pathogen producing urinary tract infection. In hospital in-patients the proportion of urinary infections with *E. coli* is less than in the general population (often less than half the cases) and in out-patients and domiciliary patients it is found in about two-thirds of infected patients. In community surveys about 80–90% of organisms are *E. coli*. Other pathogens include *Proteus mirabilis*, *Klebsiella aerogenes*, coliforms, *Streptococcus faecalis*, and uncommonly *Pseudomenas pyocyanea* and *Staphylococcus albus*.

Localization

The clinical importance of urinary tract infection depends mainly on whether or not there is involvement and damage to the kidneys. Infections are almost always ascending from the perineum, although haematogenous infections may occur particularly during the neonatal period. It is, however, often difficult clinically to localize the site of infection. Using a bladder-washout technique in women presenting to their general practitioners with symptoms, a poor correlation was found between symptoms and signs and the site of infection[11]. Loin pain, temperature, rigors and nausea were more likely to occur with renal infection than bladder infection, but some patients with symptoms usually regarded as evidence of bladder infection, such as frequency, burning and suprapubic pain, did have proven renal infection.

In a series of women consulting general practitioners in Australia, half the patients with confirmed infection on catherization had renal infection. The site of infection was renal in most of the Proteus infections, but the study found raised serum antibody titres to the infecting organism to be of no value in assessing the site of infection[11]. However, other studies have suggested a useful correlation between antibody titres and renal infection[12]. Renal tenderness, regarded as prima-facie evidence of kidney inflammation, was found in over half the women with symptoms[13]. Despite the fact that urine is an excellent culture medium, organisms which enter the bladder do not inevitably lead to infection, owing to dilution, voiding and the mucosal defence mechanisms[14].

Prognosis of bacteriuria

There are now several follow-up studies of bacteriuria from both pregnant and non-pregnant groups. These show that bacteriuria may persist, continuously or intermittently, for many years. The controversial question is how often this leads to renal involvement, renal damage and eventual renal failure. Bacteriuria is probably often the result of renal damage rather than its cause. About a fifth of patients with end-stage kidney failure have chronic pyelonephritis. Initially there were high hopes that screening for bacteriuria might be an important service. The screening tests were acceptable, reasonably reproducible and inexpensive. During pregnancy (when the urine is invariably at optimal pH for the growth of *E. coli*), screening for bacteriuria attained widespread acceptance and treatment has been shown to reduce the incidence of symptomatic attacks. Treatment at other times, however, proved difficult because relapse is common and reinfection with a different organism is sometimes associated with the development of symptoms[8].

Mortality

It was hoped and expected that the establishment of the concept of 'significant bacteriuria' and the increased use of antibiotics in the late 1950s and 1960s would reduce mortality from infections of the kidney. In fact, statistics based on death certificates in England and Wales showed a steadily increasing mortality during this period. This is likely to have been an artifact, produced perhaps by an increased attention to urinary tract infection, as deaths from other kidney diseases showed a decline during the same period[15]. More recently the number of deaths from infections of the kidney (ICD 590) in England and Wales has fallen (1179 in 1967, 514 in 1977 amongst men; 1923 in 1967, 1135 in 1977 amongst women). However, the number of deaths from nephritis and nephrosis (ICD 580–584) have increased in both sexes during the same period. Therefore, any trends in death rates from infection of the kidney must be considered with care, and include analysis of trends in deaths from other kidney diseases.

References

1. Office of Population Censuses and Surveys. *Morbidity Statistics from General Practice.* Studies on medical and population subjects. No 26. London: HMSO, 1974.
2. Waters WE. Prevalence of symptoms of urinary tract infection in women. *British Journal of Preventive and Social Medicine* 1969; **23**: 263.
3. Waters WE, Elwood PC, *et al.* Clinical significance of dysuria in women. *British Medical Journal* 1970; **ii**: 754.
4. Kass EH. Asymptomatic infections of the urinary tract. *Transaction of the Association of American Physicians* 1956; **69**: 56.

5. International Committe for Nomenclature and Nosology of Renal Disease. *A handbook of kidney nomenclature and nosology: criteria for diagnosis including laboratory procedures.* Boston: Little Brown, 1975.

6. Kunin CM. *Detection, prevention and management of urinary tract infections.* 2nd ed. Philadelphia: Lea and Febiger, 1974.

7. Buckley RM, McGuckin M, MacGregor RR. Urine bacterial count after sexual intercourse. *New England Journal of Medicine* 1978; **298**: 321.

8. Asscher AW, Sussman M, *et al.* Asymptomatic significant bacteriuria in the non-pregnant woman. *British Medical Journal* 1969; **i**: 804.

9. Kass EH. Bacteriuria and pyelonephritis of pregnancy. *Transactions of the Association of American Physicians* 1959; 72; 257.

10. Zinner SH, Kass EH. Long-term follow-up of bacteriuria of pregnancy. *New England Journal of Medicine* 1971; **285**: 820.

11. Fairley KF, Carson NE, *et al.* Site of infection in acute urinary tract infection in General Practice. *Lancet* 1971; **ii**: 615.

12. Percival A, Brumfitt W, Louvois J. Serum antibody levels as an indication of clinically inapparent pyelonephritis. *Lancet* 1964; **ii**: 1027.

13. Eastwood WB, Bruce RG, Wren WJ. Prevalence of inflammation of the urinary tract. *Journal of the College of General Practitioners* 1963; **10**: 257.

14. Asscher AW. Urinary tract infection in women. In Jones NF, ed. *Recent advances in renal disease.* London: Churchill Livingstone, 1975: 272.

15. Waters WE. Trends in mortality from nephritis and infections of the kidney in England and Wales. *Lancet* 1968; **i**: 241.

Further reading

Brumfitt W. Asscher AW. *Urinary tract infection.* Oxford. Oxford University Press, 1973.

Jones NF. *Recent advances in renal disease.* London: Churchill Livingstone, 1975.

Kass EH, Brumfitt W. *Infections of the urinary tract.* Chicago: University of Chicago Press, 1978.

Kunin CM. *Detection, prevention and management of urinary tract infections.* Philadelphia: Lea and Febiger, 1974.

Stamey TA. *Urinary infections.* Baltimore: Williams and Wilkins, 1972.

Chapter 21 · Prostatic Hypertrophy and Carcinoma

R J BERRY AND D R JONES

Obstruction of the flow of urine is a common problem in elderly men. Usually this is due to benign prostatic hypertrophy; it may also be caused by carcinoma of the prostate.

About 95% of malignant neoplasms of the prostate are adenocarcinomata; most of the remainder are sarcomas. Adenocarcinomas usually arise in the prostatic acini and are frequently multifocal. Once extension beyond the gland occurs the commonest pattern of spread is by both the lymphatic and vascular systems, simultaneously with consequent involvement of the regional lymph nodes and growth of metastases in the bones and lungs.

Patients who present with prostatic cancer frequently have a history of prostatic infection, including venereal infections, or prostatic calculi. In about 20% of patients with adenocarcinomas, benign prostatic hyperplasia is also present. Patients with benign hypertrophy may have an increased risk of the carcinoma[1].

The treatment of carcinoma of the prostate has undergone major changes since supervoltage radiotherapy became widely available. Previously, radical prostatectomy, with its certain consequence of impotence and a relatively high morbidity, was the normal approach. Now supervoltage radiotherapy gives a high rate of local tumour control with relatively few associated symptoms. Survival times vary according to the stage and grade of the tumour[1]. Extensive neoplasms and those with a poor degree of differentiation have a poor overall prognosis. However, the combination of radiotherapy for the primary tumour, and hormonal treatment (orchidectomy, oestrogen therapy) for the metastases, controls the disease in the vast majority of patients for the remainder of their lives.

Sources of data

Mortality data from death registration probably overstate the importance of carcinoma of the prostate as a cause of death. When a patient has carcinoma of the prostate this is likely to be certified or coded as the cause, whereas in many cases it is no more than concomitant with the disease which actually caused death. The death rate may give a good estimate of incidence but a false impression of the impact of the disease on total mortality.

Morbidity data accrue from 2 sources in the United Kingdom, cancer registration and the hospital in-patient enquiry. The usefulness of cancer registry data is limited by variations in the completeness from one National Health Service region to another. There is some suggestion that the proportion of cases registered increased during the 1970s as the awareness of cancer registration schemes increased.

The hospital in-patient enquiry (HIPE) deals with episodes of illness. For epidemiological purposes, the data must be interpreted with caution, because an unknown number of in-patient episodes may result from a single case.

Incidence and prevalence

Variations with age and calendar period

In England and Wales malignant neoplasms of the prostate accounted for about 4600 deaths in 1976 (a crude death rate of 192 per million population). This represents just under 7% of male cancer deaths. Thus prostatic cancer is exceeded by only 2 other sites – lung and stomach – and roughly equals large bowel, in a table of male deaths from cancer by site. Deaths below the age of 50 are very rare indeed, but the death rate increases rapidly with age thereafter. The age-specific death rates in 1976 were: age 55–64, 187 per million; 65–74, 875 per million; 75–84, 2688 per million.

There has been a substantial increase in the death rate over the past 50 years (Fig. 21.1). This was probably due in large part to an increase in the awareness of the diagnosis rather than a true increase in the incidence of the tumour. Death rates increased with each cohort up to that born around 1881, but subsequently decreased slightly.

The pattern of registrations of new cases of prostatic cancer is broadly similar to that of mortality. About 6500 cases were registered in 1973, representing just over 7% of all male cancer registrations. Thus, there were more new cases of prostatic carcinoma reported than there were deaths, and even more episodes of hospital in-patient care for the carcinoma (almost 12 000 episodes in 1976).

Benign prostatic hyperplasia is sometimes reported as a cause of death however unlikely this may seem on basic biological grounds: 1000 such deaths were registered in 1976. The reported death rate from this cause has decreased from about 300 per million in the early 1940s. This is probably due to better quality of diagnosis, with some deaths previously assigned to hypertrophy now being assigned to the carcinoma.

International variations

Very low incidence and death rates for carcinoma of the prostate are reported in Japan, which has an age-adjusted death rate of 30 per million compared with

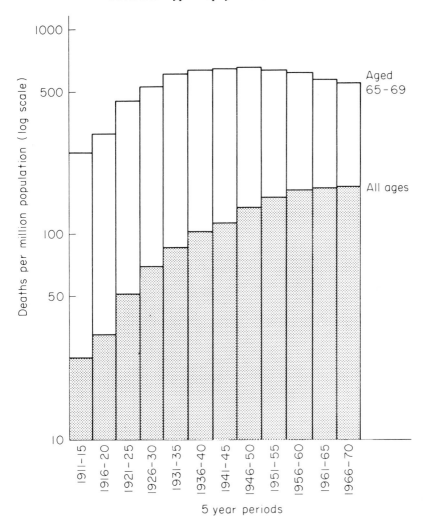

Fig. 21.1. Carcinoma of the prostate: death rate in 5 year periods, England and Wales, 1911–70. (Office of Population Censuses and Surveys. *Cancer mortality, England and Wales, 1911–70. Studies on medical and population subjects.* No 29. London: HMSO, 1975.)

between 150 and 200 per million in most Western countries. The same may be true generally in Mongoloid races, but the data from other relevant countries are less reliable[2,3]. With such a strong disparity between the rates in Japan and in the USA, where prostate is the second most common fatal cancer site, the study of death rates in Japanese immigrants to the United States, and in their offspring, is of special interest. Amongst the Japanese migrants (Issei) there is a substantial increase in the death rate, to a value about midway between the Japanese and

USA national rates[4]. This suggests an aetiology associated with some aspect of their environment or culture which changes on the migration of Japanese to the USA – perhaps a dietary factor. As yet, the data on the offspring of the migrants are insufficiently clear to add much to this picture. There is a similar, although less marked, accommodation to the death rate in the host population among Polish immigrants to the USA.

Clear patterns in the international variations are otherwise hard to find. For example, there is some evidence that rates among Jews in the USA and in Sweden are lower than those in the remainders of the populations of these countries. In contrast, Israeli rates are not unusually low. Steady increases in death rates from carcinoma of the prostate have been seen over the last 20 years in many European countries[5] as well as in the USA.

Variations with other factors

There are no clear patterns of variation in death rates from prostatic cancer with socio-economic groups in either England or Wales or in the USA. However, manual workers have higher standardized mortality ratios (SMR) than non-manual workers in England and Wales[6]; the SMR for Social Class I was about 90 in 1970–72 compared with 115 in Class V. Although enhanced risks in certain occupations were identified in the same study, no confirmation from other more specific studies is available.

Prevalence

A review[3] of autopsy studies has shown that the prevalence of carcinoma of the prostate greatly exceeds the level which the morbidity and mortality would suggest. Prevalence increases with age. For example, of those autopsied between the ages of 50 and 59, 5 % had latent carcinoma, whereas by the age of 70–79, 70 % of patients who came to autopsy had demonstrable carcinoma of the prostate. In another study[7] benign prostatic hyperplasia was found to be present at autopsy in over 80 % of men who died after their 40th birthday.

Relationship between hypertrophy and malignancy

In view of the widespread prevalence of prostatic hypertrophy in elderly men, the presence of hypertrophy in approximately 20 % of all cases of invasive carcinoma of the prostate does not necessarily imply that it is a pre-malignant lesion. There is however some evidence of increased risk of malignant neoplasm in patients with prostatic hypertrophy. The relative risk is between 3 and 5, but it is possible that this merely reflects the increased chances of finding cases of one disease if the other is present and is under investigation or treatment[1]. It appears that the risk of prostatic neoplasm is also increased by prior multiple prostatic infections, including a range of venereal infections, and by the presence of calculi.

Interpretation and conclusions

In his review of prostatic cancer, Franks[8] commented 'We know practically nothing about (its) aetiology and little about (its) epidemiology . . .'. This statement is still true; little new has been added to our information over the past 30 years. It has been suggested that its incidence is related to sexual activity[9]. However its aetiology remains unclear. A second hypothesis is that the incidence of carcinoma of the prostate is related to the intake of dietary fat[10]. This is indirectly supported by evidence from the migrant studies.

Despite its apparent ubiquity, this is a disease largely of old men and only rarely a clinical problem during the active life of the patient.

References

1. Catalona WJ, Scott WW. Carcinoma of the prostate: a review. *Journal of Urology* 1978; **119**: 1–8.
2. Doll R, Muir CS, Waterhouse J. eds. *Cancer incidence in five continents. Vol 2.* Geneva: International Union Against Cancer (UICC), 1970.
3. Wynder EL, Mabuchi K, Whitmore WF. Epidemiology of cancer of the prostate. *Cancer* 1971; **28**: 344–60.
4. Haenszel W, Kurihara M. Studies of Japanese migrants 1. Mortality from cancer and other diseases among Japanese in the United States. *US Journal of the National Cancer Institute* 1968; **40**: 43–68.
5. Campbell H, *et al.* Trends in cancer mortality in Europe. *World Health Statistics Quarterly* 1980.
6. Office of Population Censuses and Surveys. *Occupational Mortality 1970–72.* Series DS1. London: HMSO, 1978.
7. Walsh PC. Benign prostatic hyperplasia: etiological considerations. In: Marberger H, ed. *Progress in clinical and biological research 6.* New York: Liss, 1976: 1–8.
8. Franks LM. Etiology, epidemiology and pathology of prostatic cancer. *Cancer* 1973; **32**: 1092–5.
9. Steele R, *et al.* Sexual factors in epidemiology of cancer of the prostate. *Journal of Chronic Diseases* 1971; **24**: 29–37.
10. Armstrong B, Doll R. Environmental factors and cancer incidence and mortality in different countries with special reference to dietary practices. *International Journal of Cancer* 1975; **15**: 617–31.

Further reading

King H, Diamond E, Lilienfeld AM. Some epidemiological reports of cancer of the prostate. *Journal of Chronic Diseases* 1963; **16**: 117–53.
Higgins ITT. Epidemiology of cancer of the prostate. *Journal of Chronic Diseases* 1975; **28**: 343–8.
Klein LA. Prostatic carcinoma. *New England Journal of Medicine* 1979; **300**: 824–33.

Chapter 22 · Carcinoma of the Bladder

R J BERRY

Carcinoma of the bladder is a disease of high potential mortality, resulting in 4 % of cancer deaths in men and 2 % in women. It is the sixth commonest cause of cancer mortality in men in the United Kingdom. The usual clinical presentation is painless haematuria, the diagnosis is made by cystoscopic examination with histological confirmation. Staging is based on the depth of penetration of the tumour into the wall of the bladder. The disease commonly has a long natural history with control being attained by repeated cystodiathermy until deep invasion (more than half the thickness of the muscular wall) occurs. At this stage radical radiotherapy and/or total cystectomy becomes the only potentially curative treatment. The development of malignant bladder tumours is often preceded by pre-malignant papillomata or carcinoma *in situ* in the bladder. These also produce haematuria and, if not completely controlled by cystodiathermy, progress to papillary carcinoma. The majority of invasive bladder neoplasms are of the transitional cell type, varying in differentiation between a well-differentiated papillary tumour to undifferentiated carcinoma. Less commonly, squamous carcinomata can be found, often in conjunction with areas of squamous metaplasia. Adenocarcinoma may be found particularly in the bladder diverticulum or the remains of a patent urachus.

Known causal agents

Benzidine was one of the first bladder carcinogens to be described. Exposure to a number of aromatic amines has been shown to cause malignant change in the bladder. These include β-naphthylamine, the nitro, primary amino, and halogen substituted derivatives of diphenyl, and dyes such as magenta. Several retrospective studies in England, Scandinavia and America have established cigarette smoking[1,2,3] as a major cause of bladder cancer in the Western world. Prior irradiation of the pelvis, and the administration of some cytotoxic drugs such as cyclophosphamide for the treatment of other malignant conditions, are correlated with increased risks of bladder cancer.

Nitrosamines, whether metabolized from food or produced *in situ* by bacterial action in infected bladders, are known to induce bladder cancer in experimental animals. There is equivocal epidemiological evidence as to whether the excessive use of the cyclamates affects bladder cancer incidence. A weak association between the risk of bladder cancer and excessive coffee drinking[4],

266

and a possible association with the use of opium has also been found. Finally, in some areas of Africa and the Middle East, where bilharzia is endemic, the incidence of bladder cancer is elevated, and is correlated with persistent infection with *Schistosoma haematobium*.

Sources of data in England and Wales

Mortality data for carcinoma of the bladder can be obtained from registered causes of death. The data are classified by age, sex, and time period and by social class. Morbidity data can be obtained from cancer registries.

During the 1970s the proportion of new cases registered has tended to increase. Registry data usually only includes malignant tumours but in the case of bladder tumours, benign (and unspecified) neoplasms are also registered.

A further source of information is provided from claims for industrial disablement and death benefits, made in respect of cases of primary neoplasms of the epithelium of the bladder which is a prescribed disease under the Social Security Act 1975. However, as the numbers of new, successful claims each year is generally less than 25, they are of limited value to the epidemiologist.

Mortality

Available data are largely confined to incidence. In the United Kingdom carcinoma of the bladder is the sixth commonest cause of cancer deaths in men (1976) after lung, stomach, prostate, colon and rectum. In that year, 4.3 % of all cancer deaths in men (a total of 2951 deaths) were due to bladder cancer (an overall rate of 123 per million). Although its incidence is far lower in women, it caused 2.2 % of cancer deaths (1291 deaths) in 1976, a rate of 51 per million per annum.

Bladder tumours are exceedingly rare in the young. The age-specific death rates rise dramatically above 45 years, so that by age 75–84 years the rate is 1278 per million in men and 327 per million in women (Fig. 22.1). Very occasionally, death is recorded from benign or unspecified tumours of the bladder. These account for only about 1 % of all deaths from bladder neoplasms.

In evaluating trends in the incidence of bladder cancer, there are difficulties in the comparability of data in the United Kingdom before 1951 with later years. However, since then age-standardized incidence rates have increased little in men, from 88 to 105 per million. They have remained steady in women. Mortality increases with each male cohort (segment of the population born around the same time period) until the 1901 Cohort, but it is steady in women. Similar changes have been noted in the USA.

Bladder cancer incidence is related to social class, ranging from a standardized mortality ratio (SMR) of 79 for Social Class I to 115 for Class V. The

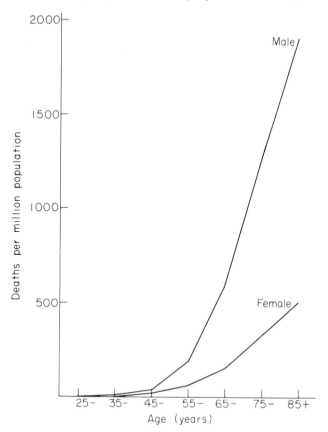

Fig. 22.1. Age-specific death rates from carcinoma of the bladder, England and Wales, 1978.

gradient is consistent, except that Group III M has an SMR around 120 (this may have some correlation with occupation) and correspondingly the socio-economic group of skilled manual workers has an SMR of 125. However, the variation in incidence with social class for women (classified by their husbands' occupation) is more marked, ranging from 54 in Social Class I to 123 in Social Class V. The wives of Social Class III M men have a higher SMR (131). The overall pattern of variation in incidence is similar for benign neoplasms.

Bladder cancer has been recognized as associated with occupational risks since Rehn in 1895 noticed an unexpectedly high incidence amongst patients who were workers with aniline dyestuffs. Clear risks with identified carcinogenic chemical aetiology have been demonstrated following exposure to aromatic amines amongst dyestuffs workers, where the relative risk can be as high as 30. Similar risks has been found in workers in the rubber industry and in those involved in the production and insulation of electrical cables. Bladder tumours occur after a long latent period, often of more than 20 years. Therefore, despite the safety measures taken by these industries, a number of further cases of occupational bladder cancer are likely to appear. The monomer of polyvinyl chloride that has been identified as a risk factor in industry may have wider connotations because of the widespread use of PVC films for the packaging of food. Other occupational risk groups include the printing, plastics, textile, coal and leather industries, and ladies' hairdressing, where the carcinogen has not been clearly identified.

There are specific occupational groups where high SMRs for bladder cancer occur for no apparent reason. These include the Armed Forces (285), transport and communication workers, painters and decorators (152) and woodworkers. In these groups bladder cancer incidence is low amongst the wives, except in the case of members of the Armed Forces and in managers. In the United Kingdom carcinoma of the bladder has a higher incidence in urban than in rural areas. Mortality rates from carcinoma of the bladder correlate internationally with the intake of oils and fats.

Registration

Since 1970 when registration of benign and unspecified tumours of the bladder, in addition to malignant tumours, was recommended, the reported rates of these lesions have increased markedly. Previously benign bladder tumours (well differentiated papillomata) were often included with transitional cell neoplasms if registered at all. This compounds the usual problems of determining the completeness of cancer registration data and interpreting it. In one cancer registry in the United Kingdom (Wessex) there is now an ominously high rate of registration of so-called benign bladder tumours ($2\frac{1}{2}$ times the national rate) and unspecified bladder lesions (10 times the national rate).

In 1973 the bladder was the fifth commonest site for registration of new neoplasms in men. It comprised 6.6 % of all registrations of new cancers, a total of about 5500 giving a rate of 233 per million per year. In women the rate was 78 per million per year. The number of bladder cancers registered increases markedly with increasing age, but at all ages the rate in men is about 3 to 4 times that in women. The rates for benign tumours were 41 and 13 per million in men and women respectively in 1973, with rates of 4 and 1 per million for unspecified neoplasms.

Internationally age-standardized rates in the majority of Western European countries, Israel, Canada and USA Whites are similar at around 100 per million per year, although the incidence in the USA non-White population is half that in Whites. Incidences in most Eastern European countries are somewhat lower, with Hungary at 30 per million, Yugoslavia at 50 per million and Poland at 60 per million per year. The reported incidence is lower in Asian countries than it is in

Europe, 50 per million in Japan and 20 per million in India. Further suggestion that race may play a part in the incidence of bladder cancer comes from the low incidence in the Phillipines and in Hawaii (15 per million) and in the Australian and New Zealand Maori populations (9 per million)[5]. However, the rate for bladder cancer of New Zealanders of European origin is also low, 12 per million.

Special features

Bladder cancer is unusual in having been recognized early as a lesion caused by identifiable carcinogens, particularly those present in specific industrial environments, although perhaps only 1 % of all cases are clearly attributable to exposure to industrial carcinogens. It has been used as a model for developing and understanding both the mechanisms of carcinogenesis and of the evaluation of potential carcinogenic hazards in other environments where risks are less easily defined. The study of bladder cancer[6] using the cohort method was the earliest satisfactory model for the investigation of a potential industrial hazard.

Interpretation of data

Natural history

Bladder tumours commonly present as multiple lesions but the disease often has a long natural history. There is evidence that carcinogenesis is a multi-stage process involving tumour initiation and promotion. The length of the latent period before symptoms develop is affected by the exposure of the promoting agents. Whilst many tumours grow to great size and produce symptoms by mechanical effects on micturition before the disease is disseminated, others metastasize rapidly. Distant metastasis is common only in the deeply invasive tumours, particularly from those which have arisen from areas of carcinoma *in situ*. Often these are tumours of relatively undifferentiated histology and the metastases may be to lungs or liver, but commonly to bone where they cause painful symptoms.

The overall efficiency of treatment is related to the long natural history of the disease, 60 % of all patients survive 3 years after diagnosis, over 50 % survive 5 years after initial diagnosis. However, as the majority of bladder cancers develop in the sixth decade of life, the statistics are complicated by the concomitance of other life-threatening diseases.

Cause and determinants

Among the known causative agents, aromatic amines, carcinogenic in themselves, are present in the urine. The bladder mucosa is thus exposed over extended periods of time and the latent period for the development of frank malignancy is long. As noted above there is evidence for a multi-stage process, involving initiation and promotion, but some agents can act as complete carcinogens. Mutagenic cytotoxic drugs may be among these although cyclophosphamide, which is widely used in the treatment of other malignancies, is known to be toxic to the bladder but appears to act solely as a promoter in the development of bladder cancer. The retention of urine, a common feature of urinary outflow obstruction, experienced by many middle-aged and older men, probably enhances the chance that carcinogens in the urine will act to produce bladder tumours.

The use of tobacco carries a 2- to 4-fold increased risk of bladder cancer, especially in cigarette smokers, and it appears that there may be a dose – response relationship[7]. However, as the total number of bladder cancers in men is far smaller than the number of lung cancers, it may be that the long latent period for the development of bladder cancer exceeds that for the development of lung cancer amongst smokers, whilst the high mortality rate from lung cancer prevents patients from living long enough to develop their bladder lesions. Studies of national death rates show that the mortality for bladder cancer correlates well with the mortality for lung cancer in different countries. In the USA, at county level, mortality from bladder cancer correlates with *per capita* cigarette consumption[8]. The aetiology of the induction of bladder cancer by tobacco smoking may be direct through β-naphthylamine and/or other aromatic amines or nitrosamines in the smoke. These may be present in just sufficient concentration to be carcinogenic or may only be indicators of the presence of other carcinogens. There may also be indirect carcinogenesis through aberrant tryptophan metabolism in smokers. Other potential ingestion hazards have been suggested including coffee, but coffee consumption is strongly correlated with cigarette smoking[9].

The mechanism for the development of bladder cancer in patients infected with *Schitosoma haematobium* is not known, but is presumably related to the increased rate of epithelial cell turnover which this infestation demands. A higher proportion of these cancers are of the squamous type, which would be expected if the changes were occurring in metaplastic squamous epithelium. The relationship between incidence of bladder cancer and Bilharzia bladder is firmly established in Egypt[10].

Prevention

With the recognition of potential industrial hazards the surveillance of workers at risk using urine cytology has been widely practiced. Benzidine is no longer used as a laboratory reagent in the United Kingdom and there are restrictions on the manufacture, import and handling of most known bladder carcinogens[11].

The attempt to reduce cigarette consumption in Western society has been neither whole-hearted nor as yet successful.

References

1. Stevens RG, Moolgarkar SH. Estimations of relative risk from valid data: smoking and cancers of the lung and bladder. *US Journal of the National Cancer Institute* 1979; **63** (6): 1351–7.
2. Armstrong B, Doll R. Bladder cancer mortality in England and Wales in relation to cigarette smoking and saccharine consumption. *British Journal of Preventive Medicine* 1974; **28**: 233–40.
3. Howe GR, Burch JD, *et al.* Tobacco use, occupation, coffee, various nutrients and bladder cancer. *US Journal of the National Cancer Institute* **64**: 701–13.
4. Cole P. Coffee drinking and cancer of the lower urinary tract. *Lancet* **i**: 1335–7.
5. Segi M, Kurihara M. *Cancer morbidity for selected sites in 24 countries.* Japan Cancer Society. Report No 6. 1972.
6. Case RAM, Hosker MG. *et al.* Tumours of the urinary bladder. *British Journal of Industrial Medicine* 1954; **11**: 75–104.
7. Miller AB. The etiology of bladder cancer from the epidemiological viewpoint. *Cancer Research* 1977; **37**: 2939–42.
8. Fraumeni JF. Cigarette smoking and cancer of the urinary tract – geographical variations in the US. *US Journal of the National Cancer Institute* 1968; **41**: 1205–11.
9. Wynder EL, Goldsmith R. The epidemiology of bladder cancer: a second look. *Cancer* 1977; **40**: 1246–68.
10. Makhyoun NA, El-Kashlan KM, *et al.* Aetiological factors in bilharzial bladder cancer. *Journal of Tropical Medicine and Hygiene* 1971; **74**: 73–78.
11. Waldron HA. *Lecture notes on occupational medicine.* Oxford: Blackwell Scientific Publications, 1976.

Chapter 23 · Gynaecological Cancers

J. CHAMBERLAIN

The three principal cancers of the female genital tract are those of the uterine cervix, the endometrium and the ovary. Cancers of the vulva, vagina and Fallopian tube also occur, as do other rare malignant neoplasms such as myosarcoma and chorionepithelioma but these are not considered here. The 3 major cancers occur with approximately equal frequency in Britain today, but their mortality rates differ, carcinoma of the ovary having a poor prognosis, carcinoma of the cervix intermediate, and carcinoma of the endometrium a favourable prognosis. Table 23.1 derived from routinely collected statistics on cancer registration and mortality, shows the number of women in England and Wales newly diagnosed as having cancer of one of these sites in 1973, and the numbers of deaths in 1977 from these cancers.

Table 23.1. Registrations, 1973, and deaths, 1977, from principal gynaecological cancers in England and Wales.

Type of cancer	Number of Registrations	Number of Deaths
Ovary	3819	3670
Body of the uterus	3681	1512
Cervix	4065	2145

Although there are some similarities in the types of women who develop carcinoma of the ovary and endometrium, carcinoma of the cervix is very different in its epidemiology. Moreover, all 3 cancers differ in their natural history and hence in the organization of health services most appropriate to their control. Therefore, each is considered separately.

Carcinoma of the uterine cervix

The term 'carcinoma of the cervix' includes both squamous carcinoma and the relatively uncommon adenocarcinoma. For a malignant neoplasm of epithelial origin the disease affects relatively young women, with incidence increasing rapidly from the age of 25 to 45, then levelling off and finally falling again after the age of 60.

273

Secular trends

During the past 20 years there has been a decline in frequency of the disease shown both in mortality data and in registration data. The standardized mortality ratio (SMR) in England and Wales fell from 103 in 1966 to 89 in 1976 (base year 1968 = 100) and the standardized registration ratio fell from 106 in 1964 to 94 in 1973 (base year 1968 = 100). This decline is almost certainly a continuation of a trend extending back for several decades but, prior to 1951, the International Classification of Diseases (ICD) did not distinguish carcinoma of the cervix from other cancers of the uterus.

Within this general decline however, it is possible to discriminate some cohorts (segments of the population born around the same time period) of women, who have had a greater than average mortality from cervical cancer. Beral[1] examined mortality rates in successive generations of women born between 1902 and 1947 and found that 5 year cohorts of women born around 1917, 1942 and 1947 each stood out as having a reversal of the general downward mortality trend, this reversal being maintained even as they grew older (Fig. 23.1). Moreover the most recently available data suggest that the next

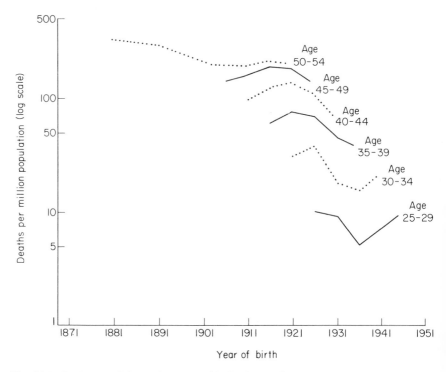

Fig. 23.1. Carcinoma of the cervix: age-specific death rates for successive birth cohorts, showing increasing death rates in the most recent cohorts[2].

cohort (born in 1950–54) is likely to experience an even higher mortality than its predecessor. The mortality rate below the age of 35, although still very small at less than 3 deaths per 100 000 women, has doubled in the past decade; if this trend is continued as these women grow older, an increase in mortality rates at older ages can be predicted.

Geographical variation

As well as temporal variations, there are also interesting variations between countries in the frequency of cervical carcinoma. These need to be interpreted with caution because of differences in the extent to which cervical carcinoma is classified as such, or is included under the general heading of 'malignant neoplasm of the uterus, unspecified'. Also, for the incidence data, there is considerable variation between registries in their classification of *in situ* carcinoma of the cervix. It is now recommended that this should be treated as a separate entity, but many registries have in the past included it with invasive cervical cancer.

Despite these reservations, there is, in general, consistency between incidence and mortality rates, in that registries reporting high incidence are in countries with high mortality, suggesting that the differences in frequencies of the disease are real (Table 23.2). Highest rates are reported in Central and South America with a decreasing gradient across Europe into Asia, the Far East and Australasia. There is also a suggestion that the disease is more common in developing countries. However, there are many exceptions to these trends, and some puzzling anomalies where adjacent countries sharing a common culture differ markedly from one another. For example, Spain has a registry reporting the lowest incidence in the world[3] and is also among the countries with a low

Table 23.2. Some geographical comparisons of mortality[2] and incidence[3] of carcinoma of the cervix, age-standardized per 100 000 women aged 35–64.*

Country	Mortality	Cancer Registry	Incidence
Colombia	—	Cali 1967–71	148.8
Venezuela	29.0		—
USA 1965–69	13.5	Connecticut 1968–72	20.7
Canada 1971	11.6	Quebec 1969–72	33.4
Denmark 1871	23.6	Denmark 1963–67	80.0
Romania 1971	23.5	Timis 1970–72	64.4
United Kingdom 1971	14.3	South London 1967–71	34.0
Spain 1970	1.8	Zaragoza 1968–72	10.2
Japan 1971	5.4	Osaka 1970–71	39.8

* There may be differences between countries in the extent to which carcinoma of the cervix is coded separately from other uterine carcinomas, and, in the incidence figures, in the extent to which carcinoma *in situ* is excluded.

mortality[4], whereas Portugal has a relatively high mortality; similarly the rates in Romania are high whereas those in Bulgaria are low, Denmark and the Federal Republic of Germany are high but other countries in north western Europe, including Britain, are relatively low.

Aetiological factors

The variations in frequency of carcinoma of the cervix in time and space do not provide any immediately obvious clues to its aetiology. However, clinical observations of the kind of women who develop carcinoma of the cervix have made large contribution to understanding its aetiology. Subsequent case control studies and other epidemiological studies have enabled relevant factors to be more clearly defined[5] and various hypotheses about causative agents suggested.

Demographic characteristics

When compared with age-matched controls, patients with carcinoma of the cervix are less likely to be single; more likely to be widowed, divorced or separated, to have married early, to have had more pregnancies, and to have started child bearing at a young age. In the USA there are racial differences, with a higher proportion of Black women among the cases than controls, and a lower proportion of Jews. Cases tend to be of lower social class and within each class (which is based on husband's occupation) their husbands tend to be employed in jobs which entail periods away from home.

Sexual experience

Leading from the general points above, various specific aspects of sexual and reproductive activity have been investigated in case–control studies and it has been found that cervical cancer patients tend to have started sexual activity at an earlier age and to have had a greater number of sexual partners. They are also more likely to have had venereal disease and it has been shown that cohorts of women experiencing high mortality from cancer of the cervix have also experienced high rates of gonorrhoea in their early adult life[1]. In addition an association has also been shown between carcinoma of the penis and carcinoma of the cervix occurring in husband and wife. Cases are less likely to have used occlusive methods of contraception than controls.

Causal hypotheses

The link between the disease and early and promiscuous sexual activity has generated 2 principal hypotheses about its causation. Both of these emphasize that in adolescence and during a first pregnancy the cervical epithelium is particularly metaplastic. It is thought that the nucleic acid of actively dividing cervical epithelial cells at this time is susceptible to potential mutagens, thus accounting for the risk factor of early sexual experience.

1   One hypothesis implicates herpes simplex virus (HSV) – type 2 – (see Chapters 3 and 5) which is known to be oncogenic. It has been shown that herpes infection and HSV2 antibodies occur more often in cases than controls but this merely shows an association between the infection and the cancer similar to that already known for venereal disease in general. Antibodies have not been found in all cases of cervical cancer as might be expected if HSV2 (with or without other factors) were causative; but a negative conclusion cannot be drawn because of the interchangeability of HSV1 and HSV2 antibodies and variation in strains and in test methods. Attempts have been made to identify HSV antigens in tumour cells, and current work is focussing on identification of viral nucleic acids in cancer cells. At present the viral hypothesis remains unproven[6].

2   Another hypothesis implicates basic proteins from the sperm head as carcinogenic agents. It suggests that there are some men with a particular histone/protamine ratio in their sperm who are more likely than others to initiate neoplasm in the cervical epithelium of their partners, particularly if the epithelium is in a metaplastic phase. This theory too is unproven and it is clear that much work remains to be done to disentangle the particular factors associated with early coitus which contribute to the causation of cancer.

Future prospects

Until the causative factor is more clearly understood there is no prospect of primary prevention of this disease. Social changes in Western societies in the past 20 years, towards more permissive sexual behaviour, suggest that the disease is likely to become more common in the future. This is borne out by the cohort analysis of mortality which shows that women now in their 20s and 30s are already experiencing higher mortality than their predecessors. There is, therefore, a need to look for other methods of controlling cervical cancer.

Natural history and prognosis

Cytological examination of exfoliated cervical cells stained by the Papanicolaou technique has enabled a picture to be built up of the early stages of cervical neoplasia. It seems to follow a progressive course from epithelial dysplasia to carcinoma *in situ* to invasive cancer (Fig. 23.2). This picture though, is necessarily incomplete because a biopsy is needed to confirm the cytological diagnosis and the biopsy may itself remove the whole lesion (thus preventing further observation of natural history). Alternatively it may be incomplete and leave behind some areas which were already invasive. In selected series of patients with carcinoma *in situ* treated only by limited (punch) biopsy, the proportion of cases progressing to invasive carcinoma has ranged from 8.5% over 8 years to 35% over 15 years[7]. On screening many more women are found to have pre-neoplastic and pre-invasive disease than would be expected on the basis of past experience to develop invasive cancer, which suggests that most of these lesions do not progress to invasion. However, the age-specific incidence of the earlier stages reaches its maximum 15–20 years before that of invasive cancer, and the cohort effect already mentioned may be contributing to the higher incidence of pre-malignant disease in younger women. It is thus not possible to predict with certainty what proportion of pre-malignant disease will progress to invasion, much less to identify which cases are likely to do so. Nor is it possible to say how many cases of invasive disease go through a recognizable pre-invasive phase.

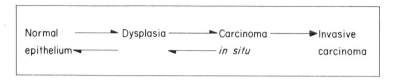

Fig. 23.2. Hypothetical model of the natural history of carcinoma of the cervix.

Once an invasive carcinoma of the cervix has become established it spreads by direct extension into the surrounding pelvic organs, and involves the pelvic lymph nodes, but extra-lymphatic distant metastases are uncommon. Treatment is therefore, directed at control of the local disease. The early stages may be treated by radical surgery but this carries substantial morbidity. Radiotherapy is therefore more often used as the primary treatment, this being facilitated by the ability to place a source of high radiation dose such as radium or caesium in the endocervical canal and vaginal fornices, which gives a tumourcidal dose in the immediate vicinity but falls off very rapidly after only a few centimetres. If the pelvic lymph nodes are involved the centrally placed intracavitary source of radiation needs to be supplemented by external beam irradiation.

Age-corrected survival rates from cancer of the cervix, based on national cancer registration[8] have shown an improvement over the past 30 years, the 5-year survival rate being 39% for cases diagnosed in 1959 rising to 54% for those diagnosed in 1971–73. Deaths from the disease continue to occur up to 10 years following diagnosis but thereafter level off, the 15 year survival rates of about 32% (for cases diagnosed in 1959) approximating to the proportion of patients who are cured. The extent to which the recent improvement in survival is due to improved radiotherapy treatment methods, or to an increasing proportion of cases diagnosed at an earlier stage is not known.

The role of screening

In theory regular cytological screening of all women who have had sexual experience would appear to be the most likely means of diminishing mortality from cervical cancer, and keeping at bay the predicted increase in incidence of the disease. However, the initial optimism with which population screening was introduced has not been justified in practice and considerable scepticism now exists about its effectiveness. Unfortunately, a randomized controlled trial was not done when the technique was being introduced for population screening about 25 years ago. It has become accepted as clinical practice and a trial in which some women were offered screening and others not would now be regarded as unethical in most societies. Consequently the evidence for its effectiveness rests on comparisons of incidence and mortality before and after screening was introduced, or geographical comparisons between populations in which it is practised with greater or lesser intensity.

The crux of the matter is uncertainty about the natural history of the disease itself. The proportion of cases of invasive cervical cancer which go through a pre-invasive phase, and their duration in that phase are still not known, although attempts to estimate the latter by comparisons of age-specific incidence of pre-invasive and invasive cancers suggest that it may average about 15–20 years, or in one recent estimate as long as 35 years[9]. This implies that a follow-up of that duration is required before the impact of screening on reducing incidence of invasive cancer can be assessed, and even longer for assessing the impact on mortality. These estimates assume that the average case of pre-invasive cancer does eventually progress to invasion, but this too is unknown and there is evidence to suggest that some of them do not. The argument centres not so much on whether indentification and extirpation of pre-invasive lesions does ever prevent invasive cancer (most agree that it almost certainly does in some cases) as on how much good a screening programme could achieve in reducing mortality in the population, and at what cost in terms of unnecessary treatment of women with lesions which would not have become invasive, as well as in use of health service resources.

The difficulty of answering these questions by temporal or geographical comparisons of different populations is compounded by the practical difficulties of mounting and maintaining an efficient screening service. Two particular aspects which influence the potential benefit of screening are the response rate and the sensitivity of the test. Numerous studies have shown that response to an initial invitation to be screened is of the order of 50–60 %, but that response drops off with increasing age and with socio-economic group, the poorest, least educated women coming least readily. Thus response is lowest in those women previously thought to be most at risk, although recent changes in attitude towards sexual relationships may lessen the risk differential between different social groups of women. These studies of response have been based on invitations to be screened, but, as practised in most places, screening is merely provided as a service which women may seek out themselves if they are sufficiently aware, or which is provided automatically (often without their knowledge) when they are having a gynaecological examination for other reasons. Such a system accentuates the inverse take-up between those least and those most at risk.

The second factor influencing benefit is the sensitivity of the test in detecting neoplastic changes. There is no way in which this can be assessed directly but studies have been done in which women with negative cytology have been retested after a short interval, (such as 3 months). On the assumption that lesions detected at this second test were present but were missed at the first test, it has been estimated that the false negative rate is of the order of 20 % (sensitivity 80 %). The false negatives are thought to be more or less equally divided between laboratory error, faulty technique in taking the smear, and variation in the rate of exfoliation within the subject. The implications of this poor sensitivity are that a first negative test should be followed after a relatively short interval by a second test and possibly a third, before settling into a routine pattern of testing at set intervals. Current policy in Great Britain suggests that routine screening should be repeated every 3–5 years although this is an arbitrary interval which is probably not observed to any extent. Although in England and Wales over 2 million smears are taken annually, it seems likely that some of these are unnecessarily frequent tests in women who need them least (e.g. annual tests in young educated women attending family planning clinics) with little attempt on the part of the health services to follow a planned screening policy. It is small wonder that the cytology service which has been in existence for about 20 years has not yet been seen to have any great effect.

However, there are some places in which particular populations have been subjected to more positive screening policies and in which a falling incidence of invasive cancer has been shown to be related to the intensity of screening. These include parts of Canada[8], Finland, Iceland and, within Great Britain, Aberdeen. There is a suggestion too that mortality from cervical cancer is also falling, but interpretation is still bedevilled by the relatively small populations on which these data are based, by the probably long duration of pre-invasive lesions, by confounding variables such as the number of hysterectomies for unconnected diseases, by possible improvements in results of treated invasive disease, and by secular changes in the frequency of carcinoma of the cervix.

Carcinoma of the endometrium

Carcinoma of the endometrium (or *corpus uteri*) is a clearly defined disease occurring principally in postmenopausal women. It is extremely rare in women under the age of 40 but rises steeply thereafter to reach its peak incidence around 70 years of age, falling off slightly thereafter.

Secular trends and geographical variation

The World Health Organization's International Classification of Diseases (ICD) did not distinguish between carcinomas of the corpus and cervix until 1951, and there still remain some cases coded as 'Uterus unspecified'. During this century there has been a marked decline in carcinoma of the uterus as a whole. If it is assumed that this is accounted for by the same downward trend in cervical cancer that has occurred subsequent to 1951, there seems to have been little change in the frequency of endometrial cancer. Taking 1968 as the base-year ($= 100$) the standardized mortality ratio has fluctuated around this point between 1966 and 1976, never falling below 90 nor rising above 102. Similarly the standardized registration ratio has been ranged between 98 and 108; in the latest year (1973) for which registration data are available there appears to have been a slight increase, caused by an increase in registrations among women aged over 65. It is not possible to predict whether this will be maintained. No marked cohort effects have been observed. Geographically, carcinoma of the endometrium is commoner in the West than the East, with North America reporting the highest incidence. Within North America, which up until 1970 had steady rates, there appears to have been an increase in incidence in the past decade.

Intrinsic aetiological factors

It has been recognized for many years that endometrial cancer occurs more commonly in nulliparous women. Case–control studies[10] have established a firm inverse association with parity*, increasing parity conferring increasing protection against the disease. There appears to be no association between endometrial cancer and age at first birth, or number of spontaneous abortions. Early menarche and late menopause are associated with increased risk. Risk is greater for married nulliparous women than for unmarried women which suggests that the risk factor may be related to infertility rather than to nulliparity *per se*, for infertility probably characterizes married nulliparae to a greater extent than unmarried nulliparae.

Very obese women are at significantly greater risk than those of normal build. There appears to be no association with height. Primary cancers of the breast and of the ovary occur with above average frequency in women with endometrial cancer. Each of these cancers indicates greater risk of developing the other two. Diabetes, hypertension, and in one study arthritis, have all been found more frequently among cases than controls.

Hypothesis

One factor common to infertility, early menarche and late menopause, is the occurrence of anovular cycles, during which the main source of oestrogens is

---

* In the context of this analysis 'parity' refers to the number of previous births.

adrenal androstenedione which is converted to oestrone by adipose tissue. This is also the main source of oestrogen in postmenopausal women. Therefore, it has been suggested that a high ratio of oestrone to other oestrogen compounds is a cause of endometrial cancer.

External factors: oestrogen replacement therapy

Oestrogen compounds have been increasingly used for the relief of menopausal symptoms and the prevention of osteoporosis, particularly in the USA, during the past 10–15 years. A number of recent case–control studies of women with endometrial cancer have consistently shown considerable increase in risk in women who have used these drugs[11]. The risk increases with increasing dose and duration of therapy and decreases after stopping therapy. Hyperplasia of the endometrium is a well recognized complication of oestrogen therapy and is a precursor of malignant change. It was postulated that the risk of cancer could be reduced by cyclical rather than continuous therapy but this proved to be unfounded. More recently the addition of progestagens to the hormone therapy has been shown to reduce the incidence of hyperplasia, but there is no direct evidence that this applies to endometrial cancer and at least one study has implicated it as well. In the light of this convincing evidence of an association between hormone replacement therapy and endometrial cancer and the continued use of these drugs, it is remarkable that evidence of their benefit is not more clearly established.

Natural history of prognosis

Adenomatous hyperplasia of the endometrium appears to be a precursor of malignant change, particularly if associated with failure of ovulation and dysfunctional uterine bleeding. It is not at all clear however, how many endometrial cancers go through this premalignant phase nor how long is its duration, since the typical patient with endometrial cancer presents with postmenopausal bleeding. It is possible that the clarity of this unexpected sign of disease leads to early presentation, which, combined with the thickness of myometrium surrounding the endometrium, means that the carcinoma is still localized to the uterus in the majority of cases. Treatment by hysterectomy results in age-corrected 5-year survival of about two-thirds of cases, and there is only a small drop-off in the survival thereafter, so that well over half the patients with endometrial cancer are cured.

Cancer of the ovary

Some confusion may be expected in examining the epidemiology of ovarian cancer because no fewer than 12 different categories of malignant neoplasm may be recognized histologically in this organ. Moreover in routine statistics of cancer registration and mortality, cancers of the Fallopian tubes and broad ligament are also included with those of the ovary. However, about 90 % of ovarian tumours arise from the germinal epithelium. Most of these are various forms of cystadenocarcinoma,[12] (the exceptions being those of apparently endometrial origin) and it has been shown that the principal epidemiological characteristics are common to all epithelial tumour types. Therefore, they are all included as one disease in this section. The age-specific incidence of ovarian cancer rises very steeply from the age of 30 levelling off slightly at about 50, but continuing upwards to reach its peak at the age of 70, whereafter it falls off slightly.

Secular trends

The mortality rate from ovarian cancer in England and Wales has been rising steadily throughout this century, although in recent years it has levelled off in all but the oldest women. A closer analysis of mortality trends[13] has shown that each successive 5 year birth cohort of women between 1861 and 1901 experienced greater mortality from ovarian cancer at all ages than the previous cohort. Subsequently, for each 5 year birth cohort between 1906 and 1931, ovarian cancer mortality at all ages has been less than in the previous cohort. Because survival of patients with ovarian cancer is poor and there is no reason to suppose that it has changed over time for women of different age groups, the patterns of mortality may be taken to reflect those of incidence. Therefore, it can be concluded that ovarian cancer became increasingly common in women born up to the 1901 birth cohort but that it has subsequently declined (Fig. 23.3).

Geographical variation

Comparison of age-standardized incidence rates of ovarian cancer in different countries[3] shows that it is relatively stable at around 10–15 cases per 10 000 women per annum in most of Europe and North America but incidence rates are lower in South America, Africa and India. The lowest incidence in the world is reported from Japan (2.8 per 10 000) but, like breast cancer, it has been shown to increase in Japanese imigrants to the USA. This suggests that the geographical and racial differences are more likely to be due to some environmental and/or behavioural influence than to genetic susceptibility.

Intrinsic aetiological factors

Parity

Retrospective case–control studies[12] have shown an inverse relationship between parity and risk of ovarian cancer, increasing parity being associated with decreasing

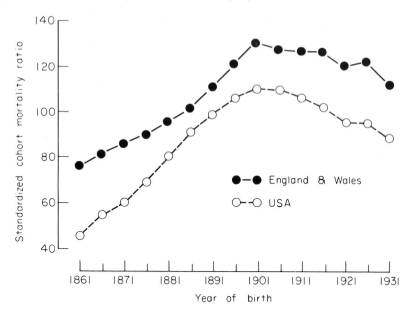

Fig. 23.3. Ovarian cancer: age-standardized mortality ratios, England and Wales and the USA, for generations of women born at 5 year intervals between 1861 and 1931. (Reproduced, with kind permission of the authors and publishers, from Beral V, Fraser P, Chilvers C. Does pregnancy protect against ovarian cancer? *Lancet* 1978; **1**; 1083–7.)

risk. In order to determine whether this association is due to a protective effect of pregnancy or to some endocrine abnormality affecting both fertility and ovarian cancer, Beral *et al.*[13] related the standardized cohort mortality ratio to the average completed family size for different cohorts of women. A striking negative correlation was found between ovarian cancer mortality and cohort fertility, which showed an identical pattern both for the USA and for England and Wales, and held up in every birth cohort (Fig. 23.4). A similar analysis of different countries showed an inverse relationship between mortality from ovarian cancer and average completed family size, and this association also explains the difference in ovarian cancer rates between single and married women and between different ethnic groups within the general environment. Variations in completed family size are largely the result of intentional control of fertility rather than the result of hormonal changes, so that it can be concluded that pregnancy affords protection. Since family size has decreased in the past 3 or 4 decades, an increase in incidence of ovarian cancer seems likely.

Mumps

Patients with ovarian cancer are less likely to report having had mumps than control women. This could be explained by mumps oophorities (see Chapter 3) causing permanent impairment of ovarian function, but other infectious diseases, not associated with oophoritis, have also been reported less frequently by cases than controls, possibly suggesting that patient's exposure to infection may have been less, for instance because of a smaller number of siblings.

Hypothesis

Fathalla[14] put forward the hypothesis of 'incessant ovulation' to explain the relationship between parity and ovarian cancer, suggesting that the germinal epthelium suffers minor trauma at ovulation during which it is exposed to oestrogen-rich follicular fluid. If this continues without any rest period such as that afforded by pregnancy, malignant change may ensue. This hypothesis is supported by comparative animal physiology, since ovarian tumours are rare in mammals with infrequent oestrous, and are of histological types which are also rare in man; whereas epithelial adenocarcinomas (the usual human variety) are extremely common in birds, particularly domestic fowl in which egg production is enhanced. If rest periods from ovulation have a protective effect, oral contraceptive agents, which mimic pregnancy by suppressing ovulation, may

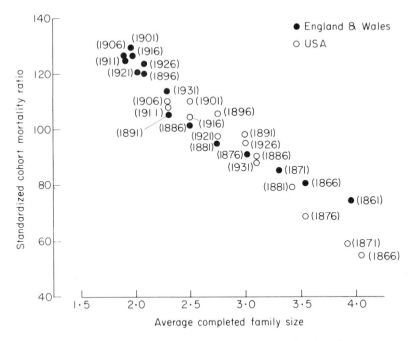

Fig. 23.4. Ovarian cancer: age-standardized mortality ratios plotted against the average completed family size for different generations of women, England and Wales and the USA. The mid-year of birth of each generation is shown in brackets. (Reproduced, with kind permission of the authors and publishers, from Beral V, Fraser P, Chilvers C. Does pregnancy protect against ovarian cancer? *Lancet* 1978; 1; 1083–7.)

afford protection against ovarian cancer. In a case–control study of women under the age of 50,[15] relative risk decreased with increasing numbers of live births, increasing numbers of incomplete pregnancies and increasing duration of oral contraceptive use; none of these factors on its own was statistically significant but when combined into an index of 'protected time' there was a significant decrease in risk.

The implication of this hypothesis for the trend in ovarian cancer in the immediate future is that an expected rise in incidence due to decreasing family size among women born after 1931 may be at least partly offset by increasing use of oral contraception.

External factors: talc

The case against talc as a carcinogen arises because of its chemical similarity to asbestos which promotes mesotheliomatous tumours. Talc particles have been found embedded in ovarian cancers, but also in normal tissues of the pelvis. In one study of female asbestos workers an excess risk of ovarian cancer amongst those with long and severe exposure has been found but reproductive factors cannot be ruled out as a possible explanation for this[16]. There is at present no real evidence to support the contention that talc is carcinogenic to the ovary.

Natural history treatment and prognosis

The early stages of development of epithelial adenocarcinomas which make up the great majority of ovarian cancers are inaccessible to investigation. Once these tumours have been diagnosed they grow rapidly and spread, not locally, but by intraperitoneal routes to other abdominal organs including omentum and liver. Initial treatment is by surgical removal, usually followed by chemotherapy to attack occult metastases. Ovarian tumours respond to alkylating agents, and the addition of cis-platinum has improved response greatly. In advanced disease many clinicians now advocate 'second look' laparoscopies, performed to assess response to courses of chemotherapy and to remove any overt residual disease. Nevertheless the disease is likely to recur repeatedly, and the quality of some extra months of survival punctuated with repeated surgery and courses of chemotherapy may be questionable for some patients. The age-corrected 5 year survival rate is of the order of 20–25%, probably fewer than a fifth of patients being cured of their disease.

Implications for control of gynaecological cancers

It seems likely that these three cancers are going to pose an increasing threat to women in the foreseeable future. Current hypotheses about their underlying causes suggest that the principal factors are early and promiscuous sexual activity in the case of cancer of the cervix, infertility in the case of cancer of the endometrium, and limitation of family size in the case of cancer of the ovary. Although the first and third of these are to some extent under the control of the individual woman, they are in reality determined by the attitudes and behaviour of our society as a whole, and any attempt to control these cancers by health education would need to be offset against society's views of the benefits of present trends in reproductive practices. It is possible however, that oral contraception may be protective against ovarian cancer and so the predicted rise due to limitation of family size may be averted.

A much more remote possibility for controlling cervical cancer might be feasible if the causative agent were definitely identified as a virus and anti-viral treatment or immunization were developed. At present, though, screening in order to detect and treat the disease at a pre-invasive stage seems to offer the best hope. Endometrial cancer, by virtue of its association with primary infertility, is unlikely to change from its background level unless some breakthrough in endocrine therapy occurs. However, the predicted rise in incidence already being seen in North America is most probably associated with increasing use of oestrogen replacement therapy, which puts the means for its limitation in the hands of the same professional group responsible for its treatment – the gynaecologists. Further consideration of the benefits of hormone replacement therapy, including dose and duration, is urgently required.

The organization of health services for management of these three cancers requires provision of adequate gynaecological and histopathology expertise in diagnosis as the first essential. For treatment, collaboration between gynaecology and radiotherapy is necessary in the case of cervical cancer, and collaboration between gynaecology and medical oncology for cancer of the ovary.

Undoubtedly the principal challenge to efficient organization of services concerns screening for detection of pre-invasive cervical cancer. The present policy of merely making it available to those women and doctors who wish to use it needs to be altered to a more positive approach aimed at bringing in high risk women, early re-screening to diminish the false negative problem, and thereafter re-screening at deliberately chosen rather than *ad hoc* intervals. Such a policy would result in a greater yield of cases and avoid the present wasteful use of cytology resources in unnecessary frequent testing of those women who need it least.

References

1. Beral V. Cancer of the cervix: a sexually transmitted infection?, *Lancet* 1974; i: 1037–40.
2. Office of Population Censuses and Surveys. *Trends in mortality 1951–75*. Series DH1.3. London: HMSO, 1978.

3. Waterhouse J, Muir C, *et al. Cancer incidence in five continents. Vol 3.* Lyon: IARC Scientific Publications, 1976.

4. Hill GB. Mortality from malignant neoplasm of the uterus since 1950. *World Health Statistics Quarterly* 1975; **28**: 323.

5. Rotkin ID. A comparison review of key epidemiological studies in cervical cancer related to current searches for transmissible agents, *Cancer Research* 1973; **33**: 1353–67.

6. Roizman B, Frenkel N. Does genital herpes cause cancer? A midway assessment. In: Caterall RD, Nicol CS, eds. *Sexually transmitted diseases.* London: Academic Press, 1976, 151–70.

7. Green GH. The Progression of pre-invasive lesions of the cervix to invasion, *New Zealand Medical Journal* 1974; **80**: 279–87.

8. Office of Population, Censuses and Surveys. *Cancer statistics, survival.* Series MBI. 3. London: HMSO, 1980.

9. Task force appointed by the conference of the Deputy Minister of Health. Cervical cancer screening programmes, the Walton report, *Canadian Medical Association Journal* 1976; **114**: 2–32.

10. Elwood JM, Cole P, *et al.* Epidemiology of endometrial cancer. *US Journal of the National Cancer Institute* 1977; **59**: 1055–60.

11. Editorial. Oestrogen therapy and endometrial cancer. *Lancet* 1979; **i**: 1121–2.

12. Newhouse ML, Pearson RM, *et al.* A case control study of carcinoma of the ovary. *British Journal of Preventive and Social Medicine* 1977; **31**: 148–53.

13. Beral V, Fraser P, Chilvers C. Does pregnancy protect against ovarian cancer? *Lancet* 1978; **i**: 1083–7.

14. Fathalla MF. Factors in the causation and incidence of ovarian cancer. *Obstetrical and Gynecological Survey* 1972; **27**: 751–68.

15. Casagrande JT, Pike MC, *et al.* 'Incessant ovulation' and ovarian cancer. *Lancet* 1979; **ii**: 170–3.

16. Newhouse ML. Cosmetic talc and ovarian cancer. *Lancet* 1979; **ii**: 528.

Chapter 24 · Carcinoma of the Female Breast

J CHAMBERLAIN

In British women, carcinoma of the breast is the most common type of cancer, cause of cancer death (although likely soon to be overtaken by cancer of the lung) and single cause of death between the ages of 30 and 59. It is justifiably a disease which causes much public concern, not only because of its high toll of deaths of women at the peak of their family and occupational responsibilities, but also because of the mutilating nature of the standard form of treatment, mastectomy.

Information on its frequency in Great Britain is available from routinely collected statistics derived from cancer registrations and death certificates. Mortality statistics are thought to be accurate although there may be some undercertification of breast cancer as the cause of death, particularly in very elderly women. The cancer registration scheme is based on regional cancer registries which receive notification of newly diagnosed cancers from all hospitals in their region. There is known to be variation in completeness of recording between different regions and even the best of them are likely to miss cases not admitted for hospital treatment. Thus national registrations give an underestimate of the true incidence. In spite of these reservations about their accuracy, however, routine incidence and mortality data are still of value in examining trends over time and in making geographical or other comparisons between different populations. In 1973, 20 112 newly diagnosed cases of breast cancer were registered, an incidence rate of 80 per 100 000 women of all ages[1]. In 1977, 11 820 women died from breast cancer, a mortality rate of 47 per 100 000 females of all ages[2].

Secular trends

Mortality from breast cancer has been increasing steadily throughout this century, the crude death rate per 100 000 women has more than doubled from 20 in 1915 to 47, its present level[3]. Some of this increase is, of course, due to the increasing proportion of elderly women in the population. However, an increase of 15–20 % has occurred within each 5 year age group between 25 and 70 (Fig. 24.1). Within the last decade, the standardized mortality ratio (SMR) (1968 = 100) has risen from 98 in 1966 to 111 in 1976. An analysis by age group shows an increase in mortality in all ages above 44.

National information on incidence has only been available since the cancer registration scheme was started in the early 1960s. During the decade ending in

1973, the incidence of breast cancer showed a steady increase (Fig. 24.2). It was most marked in the later years and in women aged over 45 years of age. Again taking 1968 as the standard, the standardized registration ratio for breast cancer has increased from 95 in 1964 to 114 in 1973[1]. Some of this apparent increasing incidence is undoubtedly due to more complete registration in recent years, nevertheless there is almost certainly an underlying real increase. This is borne out by the increasing mortality which is more likely to be due to increasing incidence than to poorer survival rates; and by the fact that longer established comprehensive registries in similar countries, such as those in Connecticut (USA) and Denmark, have also shown the same trend. The increasing mortality and incidence within each age group indicates that each successive cohort of women suffers a higher rate. This suggests that there has been an increase in exposure to a carcinogenic agent, rather than exposure being limited to a specific time period. However, the rates below age 45, based on relatively small numbers, do not show a clear trend in recent years.

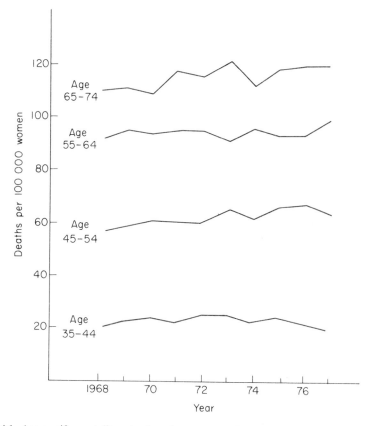

Fig. 24.1. Age-specific mortality rates from breast cancer, England and Wales, 1968–77.

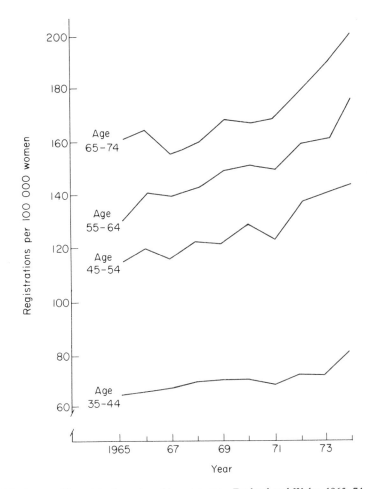

Fig. 24.2. Age-specific registration rates of breast cancer, England and Wales, 1965–74.

Geographical variations[4]

There is marked international variation in the frequency of breast cancer. The incidence is much higher in Western countries than it is in the East and the lowest rates occur in Asia. Studies of Japanese migrants to the USA have shown that their incidence of breast cancer gradually increases, approaching the level of American women after 2–3 generations. A sharp increase in breast cancer has occurred during the past half-century in Iceland, concomitant with the social change to a Western life-style. Within Britain, there is little geographical variation in either incidence or mortality rates.

Demographic variations[4]

Age

In England and Wales breast cancer is very rare under the age of 30. Thereafter age-specific incidence rates increase rapidly until the 45–49 age group when they level off for about 5 years before increasing at a slightly less steep gradient (Fig. 24.3). This is typical of age-specific curves in Western high incidence areas, all of which show a levelling or even dip in incidence at the time of the menopause (sometimes known as 'Clemmeson's Hook'). By contrast, age-specific curves in low incidence areas tend to plateau at age 50 (e.g. in Eastern Europe) or to fall (e.g. Asia) (Fig. 24.3). The difference in incidence between Eastern and Western populations is thus concentrated in postmenopausal women.

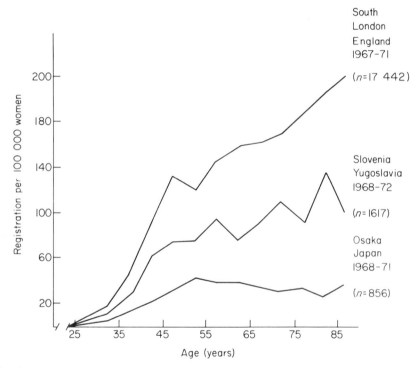

Fig. 24.3. Geographical differences in age-specific incidence rates of breast cancer[5]. *n* Total number of cases observed.

Parity

Nulliparous women are at greater risk than parous women, and increasing parity (number of previous children) is associated with a decreasing risk of breast cancer. Women with many children are likely to have started their families at a young age and much, but not all, of the association with parity is explained by the fact that early age at first birth seems to have a protective effect. Parous women who have had their first full-term pregnancy aged 30 or over are at even higher risk than nulliparous women.

Marital status

One of the earliest recorded epidemiological observations about breast cancer was that by Rammazzini in Italy in the 18th century, who noted its frequency in nuns. Since then it has been substantiated that single women are more likely to develop breast cancer than married or divorced women or widows. This difference is explained by the inverse association of the disease with parity.

Socio-economic status

Breast cancer is one of the few diseases which is more common among professional and managerial classes than among semi-skilled or unskilled working classes. The association is not very marked and may be explained by the risk factor of age at first birth.

Reproductive variations[4]

The association with parity and age at first full-term pregnancy has already been noted. There is also a suggestion that women who have had spontaneous abortions are at greater risk.

Menstruation

Both early menarche and late menopause are associated with increased risk. Premenopausal oophorectomy reduces risk, this latter finding also being evident in dogs which have been spayed at a young age.

Breast feeding

Breast feeding was long thought to have a protective effect, but when parity and age at first full-term pregnancy are taken into account there appears to be no association.

Oral contraceptive hormones

These have not so far shown any association with subsequent breast cancer although they have been shown to have a protective effect against benign breast disease. A latent interval of at least 10–15 years between exposure and development of cancer would be expected and prospective follow-up of oral contraceptive users is still continuing. Similarly, administration of oestrogen replacement therapy to alleviate menopausal symptoms may be of relevance to subsequent risk of breast cancer and a longer follow-up of women receiving this treatment than is yet available is required.

Other risk factors[4]

Family history

Women with an affected relative on either the maternal or paternal side of the family are more likely to develop breast cancer than others. In general, this is a rather weak association, but in some families there seems to be a strong genetic susceptibility. In these families the disease is usually diagnosed premenopausally and is often bilateral.

Previous breast disease

Women who have had previous biopsies for benign breast disease are at increased risk of breast cancer. However, the diverse histopathology of benign disease makes retrospective study of the association difficult. It is possible that some particular types of epithelial hyperplasia are pre-malignant, or at least are provoked by the same factors as breast cancer. Women who have cancer in one breast are at high risk of developing a second primary cancer in the other breast.

Other primary cancers

There is an association between carcinoma of the breast and carcinomas of the ovary and the endometrium.

Height and weight

An association between body build and breast cancer has been noted, with large women being at greater risk than thin women; this association seems to be limited to postmenopausal breast cancer.

External factors

An increased incidence of breast cancer has been observed in women exposed to radiation. This has been shown both in atom bomb survivors in Japan, and in various follow-up studies of women who received large doses of radiation to the chest for medical reasons. A dose of 1 rad to the breast is estimated to induce around 5 cancers per million women-years, starting after a latent interval of 10–20 years.[6]

Hair dyes

Known to contain mutagenic chemicals, hair dyes have been studied in relation to breast cancer. The evidence of an association, derived from a number of case–control studies, is conflicting, with a majority finding no connection.

Reserpine

A suggestion that reserpine, used in the treatment of hypertension, was associated with subsequent breast cancer has also been the subject of various case–control studies. In general, they show only a very slight increase in risk which could be attributed to the drug, and there is no consistent dose–response effect.

Aetiological hypotheses[7]

Endocrine factors

Apart from family history and external risk factors, all the evidence points to endogenous endocrine steroids as being implicated in the development of breast cancer. One hypothesis is that the ratio of oestriol to oestrone and oestradiol in young adult life is important. A high oestriol ratio seems to confer protection whereas a low ratio initiates or promotes breast cancer. Oestriol competes with the other two hormones for oestrogen receptor binding sites and thus a high oestriol level would indicate that oestrone, which is carcinogenic in animals, would have less opportunity to affect the breast. Although there is circumstantial evidence to support this hypothesis, the carcinogenic effect of oestrone and the protective effect of oestriol have not been proved in humans. Progesterone may also have a protective effect and it is thought that anovulatory cycles in which oestrogens are unopposed by progesterone may increase risk. Subnormal production of androgen metabolites by the adrenal glands has been shown to be associated with breast cancer risk, but the mechanism involved is not clear. Prolactin, produced by the pituitary gland, has also been studied and there is a suggestion that an elevated level of prolactin at night is an indicator of increased risk.

Diet

The international variation in incidence of postmenopausal breast cancer has led to the suggestion that diet may have a role in its aetiology. In particular, a high calorie, high fat diet, such as is found in Western societies, may influence hormonal production. This could occur directly, by promoting nocturnal prolactin synthesis, or indirectly by promoting obesity and thereby increasing conversion of androstenedione to oestrone (adipose tissue is the principal source of postmenopausal oestrone). Another hypothesis is that the diet may stimulate production of bile acids which may then be converted by certain gut bacteria into oestrogen-like compounds.

Although these possible interrelationships between diet, obesity and endocrine steroids provide plausible hypotheses to explain the known risk factors, attempts to test them by endocrine measurements and dietary measurements in cases and controls have, in general, led to inconclusive results. One difficulty is that measurements in women who already have breast cancer (the cases) may be influenced by the disease itself and, in any case may be quite different from measurements made at the time of initiation of the tumour, which is likely to be many years earlier.

Viruses

A quite separate aetiological hypothesis concerns the possible role of viruses. There is no doubt that viruses can be carcinogenic and discovery of the mouse mammary tumour virus led to speculation that a similar organism might cause human breast cancer. However, there is at present no evidence to support this hypothesis. Even if a virus is involved, endocrine factors are also likely to be important in promoting the tumour.

Primary prevention

Current knowledge of the aetiology of breast cancer is of possible value in enabling a high risk group to be identified but as yet it offers little prospect for primary prevention. It is conceivable that administration of hormones such as oral contraceptives may, in future, be shown to be protective, and topical application of progesterone has also been suggested as a prophylactic measure, but these are still of unproven value.

Natural history and results of treatment

Breast cancer has a variable natural history, some cases progressing very rapidly while others, even if untreated, may persist in a localized form for many years[8]. Follow-up studies of treated patients show that it is 20 years or more before their life expectancy runs parallel to that of the general population, and even after this time they may still die of recurrent metastatic disease[9]. Some data on survival are available from cancer registries which show that nearly half the patients die within 5 years of diagnosis and two-thirds within 10 years. In one region it was estimated that the 'cure' rate (i.e. those with normal life expectancy) for cases diagnosed in 1947–50 was only 20 % but that this had increased to 29 % for cases diagnosed in 1960–71, suggesting a trend towards improved survival[10].

The standard treatment in the first half of this century was radical mastectomy with radiotherapy to the supraclavicular and internal mammary nodes. The results of this were often unsatisfactory both in morbidity and cosmetic appearance. Realization that this radical and unpleasant treatment by no means guaranteed cure gradually led to trials of more conservative methods, involving only simple mastectomy or even tylectomy (local removal of the tumour) with radiotherapy. By and large, these trials showed that radical treatment had no advantage over the more conservative approach, although patients treated by tylectomy had a greater tendency to local recurrence. Simple mastectomy with axillary node sampling or clearance and with adjuvant radiotherapy if the nodes are involved is widely regarded as the treatment of choice for early breast cancer[11]. In some cases the skin is preserved (subcutaneous mastectomy) and the breast reconstructed at a later date. The introduction of tests such as radioactive scans has enabled patients to be thoroughly investigated before surgery for evidence of occult distant metastases and, if these are present, the patient may be treated by endocrine therapy, chemotherapy or radiotherapy without mastectomy. Trials of chemotherapy adjuvant to primary surgical treatment for cases where the axillary nodes are involved are now under way and early results indicate that, in premenopausal women, there is an improvement in relapse-free survival rate[12].

There is a marked difference in survival between cases diagnosed at different stages. Small tumours of less than 2 cm, with no nodal involvement do very well, having 20 year survival rates of 80 % or more, but there is a progressive decline in survival with increasing size of tumour, skin or muscle involvement, nodal involvement and distant metastases. Measurement of oestrogen receptor status in the tumour is an additional investigation of prognostic importance. Cancers which are receptor-positive do better than those that are receptor-negative within each stage.

If there is a time trend towards improved survival in more recent years, it is pertinent to ask if this is due to better treatment methods or to a different case-mix, with more cases now presenting at an earlier stage. In one study, the proportion of cancers in stages I and II increased from 51.2 % in 1947–50 to 56.7 % in 1960–71[10]. Similarly, in North America, where incidence rates are rising but mortality rates staying steady (implying an improvement in survival), the proportion of 'early' cases is increasing[4]. With the possible exception of adjuvant chemotherapy, which is still under trial, modern methods of treatment within each stage do not give any better results in terms of survival than in previous years, although they may well improve the quality of life, particularly for women with advanced disease. Thus the trend towards improved survival is more likely to be due to earlier diagnosis than to improved treatments.

It is also possible that a small part of the increased incidence and improved survival may be caused by a change in diagnostic practice, with some cases which would previously have been called benign epithelial proliferation now being classified as carcinoma. There is an interesting category of pre-invasive carcinoma, classified histologically either as lobular carcinoma *in situ* or as intraduct carcinoma with no evidence of invasion. These lesions are identified by excision biopsy which makes study of their natural history difficult because the biopsy itself may have excised the affected area completely, or, alternatively, it may have left behind some tumour in which invasion had already begun. Lobular carcinoma *in situ*, which makes up somewhat less than 5 % of the average case-mix of breast cancers, is liable to be multifocal and bilateral. A 20 year follow-up of cases treated by diagnostic biopsy found that the cumulative risk over 20 years of developing invasive cancer in the same breast was 35 % and in the opposite breast was 25 % (some being bilateral)[13].

Screening

Since the best hope of reducing mortality from breast cancer seems to lie in early treatment, there is considerable interest in screening women to detect the disease at a pre-symptomatic stage. However, because the natural history is known to vary from very fast growing to very slow growing tumours, it cannot necessarily be assumed that all cases detected early by screening will behave in the same way as stage I cancers presenting symptomatically; the latter, although called 'early' may, in fact, be slow growing tumours which have been present for some time. There is therefore a need to determine whether pre-symptomatic detection and treatment does improve survival; moreover, since screening is a preventive measure offered to the public at large, there is an ethical responsibility for the health authorities to balance the benefits it can achieve against the costs, in terms both of unnecessary morbidity and use of resources.

The principal methods of early detection now available are clinical examination of the breasts, mammography and thermography[14]. Clinical examination can be performed by medical or paramedical staff, or by the woman herself. Breast self-examination has obvious advantages in convenience, cost, and the frequency with which it can be repeated, but its sensitivity (ability to detect cancers) and specificity (ability to classify breasts without cancer as normal) have not been tested. Moreover, little is known about women's reactions to it and their compliance, nor about possible anxieties it may engender. Clinical examination by a health professional is widely practised but is not a very efficient test. Its sensitivity is only about 50 % and its specificity is about 95 %, implying that 5 % of women without cancer will have a positive test necessitating referral to a surgeon and, possibly, biopsy. In spite of these drawbacks, clinical examination is still used because it detects a small proportion of cancers that are missed by other methods.

Thermography, a technique which records heat patterns emitted from the breast, has an even lower sensitivity and specificity than clinical examination and has fallen out of favour, although its role as an indicator of high risk women is still being evaluated.

The remaining test, mammography, is at present the most efficient. Its sensitivity has been variously reported as between 75 % and 90 % and its specificity about 98 %. However, it has one serious drawback, a possible radiation hazard, which might actually induce some new breast cancers at a later date. Much has been done in recent years to reduce the dose, and the technique has been changed from 2 views of each breast to a single oblique view, so that present dosage levels are below 0.5 rad. For every 350 000 women screened this implies a risk of inducing 1 cancer per annum after a latent interval of 10–15 years. Thus the risk of cancer induction is very small but nevertheless mammography cannot be advocated for screening without clear evidence that it is of benefit.

The only firm evidence on the benefits of screening comes from a large trial conducted in New York in the 1960s, in which 62 000 women aged 40–65 were randomly allocated to a study group or a control group[15]. The 31 000 women in the study group were offered annual screening by clinical examination and mammography for 4 years. 10 years from the start of the trial there had been 97 deaths from breast cancer in the study group and 137 in the control group. The difference was concentrated in women aged 50–59, with a lesser difference in those over 60 and no difference in those under 50. Despite the fact that only 65 % of the study group accepted the initial invitation to screening and less than half had all 4 screens, and despite the fact that the sensitivity of the combined tests was no more than 75 %, a one-third reduction of mortality in the whole study group (including cancers not detected by screening) indicates that a screening service could make a major contribution. The 8 year survival rate of cases detected at screening was 72 % compared with 50 % in the control group, also suggesting considerable benefit from early detection. However, as with screening for other conditions, survival comparisons are biased by 'lead time'–the time gained by pre-symptomatic diagnosis over the time when the case would have otherwise presented–and by the fact that screening is likely to detect cases with a long pre-symptomatic phase which are probably slow growing.

Although an excellent example of the type of trial required to evaluate health services, the New York study is now outdated in its mammography technique and provided very little information on either human or resource costs. Further evaluation studies have now been launched in Sweden and in Great Britain, the latter comprizing a comparison between 2 groups of women offered screening, 2 offered education in breast self-examination, and 4 only receiving conventional diagnostic services.

Implications for provision of health services

Until the results of the current trials of early detection are known, additional services for screening or self-examination are not justified. Nevertheless, it is likely that some improvement in existing diagnostic and treatment services is possible. Considerable delays are known to occur, attributable in part to the patients themselves but also to their general practitioners and hospital staff, particularly those concerned with scheduling out-patient appointments and in-patient admissions. Education of all concerned about the significance of breast symptoms in women aged over 40 could do much to reduce delay.

A recent study of services in the West Midlands[16] has shown little concentration of facilities and expertise, many patients being treated by surgeons who see very few cases of breast cancer. While there is no evidence that patients treated in specialized breast units do any better in terms of survival than those treated elsewhere, it is possible that they receive better care if not cure. These units are likely to be the forerunners in modern trends towards more conservative local treatment, more awareness of the psychological effects of the disease and better palliative care for late diseases. Moreover, they are frequently active in research into aspects of breast cancer and trials of alternative treatments. Hence concentration of cases may have additional spin-off benefits for the future management of this increasingly common disease unless or until methods of primary or secondary prevention are shown to be of value.

References

1. Office of Population Censuses & Surveys. *Cancer Statistics 1972–73.* Series MB1. No 2. London: HMSO, 1979.
2. Office of Population Censuses & Surveys. *Mortality Statistics 1977.* Series DH2. No 4. London: HMSO, 1979.
3. Office of Population Censuses & Surveys. *Cancer mortality, England & Wales, 1911–1970.* Studies on medical & population subjects. No 29. London: HMSO, 1975.
4. Kelsey JL. A review of the epidemiology of human breast cancer. *Epidemiologic Reviews* 1979; **1**: 74–109.
5. Waterhouse J, Muir C, *et al. Cancer incidence in five continents. Vol 3.* Lyon: IARC Scientific Publications, 1976.
6. Upton AC, Beebe GW, *et al.* Report of National Cancer Institute ad hoc working group on the risks associated with mammography in mass screening for the detection of breast cancer. *US Journal of the National Cancer Institute* 1977: **59** (2): 480.
7. MacMahon B, Cole P, Brown J. Etiology of human breast cancer: a review. *US Journal of the National Cancer Institute* 1973; **50**; 21.
8. Bloom HJG, Richardson WW, Harries EJ. *British Medical Journal* 1962; **ii**: 213.
9. Brinkley D, Haybittle JL. The curability of breast cancer. *Lancet* 1975; **ii**: 95.

10. Haybittle JL. Results of treatment of female breast cancer in the Cambridge area 1960–71. *British Journal of Cancer* 1979; **40**: 56–61.
11. Duncan W, Kerr GR. The curability of breast cancer. *British Medical Journal* 1976; October **ii**: 781.
12. Bonadonna G. Adjuvant chemotherapy of breast cancer. *British Journal of Hospital Medicine* 1980; **23**: 40–53.
13. McDivitt RW, Hutter RVP, *et al. In situ* lobular carcinoma: a prospective follow-up study indicating cumulative patient risks. *JAMA* 1967; **201**: 96–100.
14. Chamberlain J. Problems encountered in screening for breast cancer. *Technical Report Series* 1978; **40**: 158–82. International Union Against Cancer (UICC).
15. Shapiro S. Efficacy of breast cancer screening. *Technical Report Series* 1978; **40**: 133–57. International Union Against Cancer (UICC).
16. Bywaters JL, Knox EG. The organization of breast cancer services. *Lancet* 1976; **i**: 849.

SECTION 6 · ENDOCRINE DISEASES

Chapter 25 · Diabetes Mellitus

C ᴅᴜ V FLOREY

The existence of diabetes mellitus was recorded as long ago as the 6th century BC in a Hindu manuscript which referred to the sweetness of the urine of patients who presumably had the disease. Despite centuries of observation and interest in diabetes, only about 5 % of patients have diabetes secondary to known causes. In the absence of a definite aetiology, a number of classifications and a wide variety of definitions of diabetes based on the glucose tolerance test (GTT) have been used. Because of this lack of uniformity, prevalence and incidence rates for diabetes derived from different studies are not comparable since a diabetic by one set of criteria may be non-diabetic by another. To overcome this problem, a new classification and revised criteria have been proposed by the National Diabetes Data Group in the USA[1]. As the revisions are based principally on epidemiological investigations, the rationale behind them will be described here as well as the general epidemiology of diabetes.

Diagnosis

Diabetes mellitus is defined as a metabolic abnormality which gives rise to abnormally high levels of glucose in the blood. To diagnose a patient in a clinical setting, the blood–glucose of the patient is measured to determine whether it is above or below a predetermined level which divides 'abnormal' from 'normal'. Casual or postprandial levels of glycaemia, if sufficiently high, may be adequate for clinical diagnosis, though they are not definitive. High fasting levels on more than one occasion are diagnostic, but in many cases a GTT may be required. The interpretation of the GTT has been hampered because until recently there was no evidence that the distribution of blood–glucose in diabetics was distinct from that of normal individuals; diabetic glucose levels merged with normal levels to produce a unimodal distribution curve.

In 2 unusual populations the distribution of plasma glucose has been found to be bimodal. The first consists of the Pima Indians in Arizona[2]. At the turn of the century diabetes was almost unknown in this tribe, but with increasing affluence and a tendency to obesity, diabetes now occurs in about 35 % of the adult population. The venous plasma–glucose distributions 2 hours after a 75g oral glucose challenge show bimodality which becomes increasingly obvious with advancing age. The intersection between the subgroups is between 11.1 and 13.9

mmol/1 (200–250 mg/dl). Retinopathy and proteinuria are found almost exclusively in the hyperglycaemic groups.

The second population is from Nauru[3], an island in the Central Pacific which has rapidly increased in prosperity due principally to phosphate mining. Using the same test procedure and diagnostic criteria as in the Pima study, the investigators found 34.4 % of a sample of people over the age of 15 years to be diabetic. The plasma glucose distribution at 2 hours post-challenge has the same point of intersection between its 2 modes as that for the Pima Indians. In both populations bimodality is also found in the distributions of fasting plasma–glucose with an intersection at about 7.8 mmol/1 (140 mg/dl).

In a cross-sectional study in Bedford (United Kingdom) carried out in 1962, 3 classes of glycaemia were defined – normal, borderline diabetic and definite diabetic. Borderline diabetic levels were defined as capillary blood sugars 2 hours after a 50g oral glucose challenge between 6.7 and 11.1 mmol/1 (120–199 mg/dl), and definite diabetic levels those above this range. 364 borderline and definite diabetics were followed up 5 years after the initial survey. There was an increase in diabetic retinopathy of 2 % in the borderline diabetics compared with increases from 11.8 to 25.3 % according to the initial level of blood sugar in the definite diabetics. After $8\frac{1}{2}$ years follow-up, only 8.5 % of the borderline diabetics became definitely diabetic (a rate of approximately 1 % per annum). In another study carried out by the same group, 204 male civil servants were found to have borderline diabetes using the same criteria. All were subjected to regular ophthalmoscopy. After follow-up for 6–8 years, none had been found to develop diabetic retinopathy.

Since capillary blood glucose levels after a 50g load are approximately the same as venous plasma–glucose levels after a 75g glucose load, the results from the United Kingdom support those for the Pima and Nauruans, suggesting a division at about 11.1 mmol/1 (200 mg/dl) between levels of glycaemia with and without associated risk of complications.

The bimodal distributions of fasting plasma glucose for the Pima and Nauruans indicated that diabetics usually had levels in excess of 7.8 mmol/1 (140 mg/dl). This cutting point is supported by data from a study in Jamaica[4] where venous whole blood was used. A venous whole blood glucose value of 6.7 mmol/1 (120 mg/dl) is approximately equal to 7.8 mmol/1 of plasma–glucose. 92.4 % of the known diabetics in a defined geographical area had fasting levels above 6.7 mmol/1 when not receiving treatment, whereas only 1.5 % of the rest of the population had levels as high as this; a quarter of these (2 out of 8) were later found to have diabetes by the new criteria.

The new criteria for non-pregnant adults are given in Table 25.1. Other criteria are used for children and pregnant women[1].

The test for glucose in the urine, although commonly used in medical practice, is very unsatisfactory for screening for diabetes. In the Bedford study

Table 25.1. Diagnostic criteria for diabetes mellitus in non-pregnant adults[1].*

Diagnosis		Venous plasma glucose levels (mmol/l) at			Comment
		Fasting	Intermediate	2 hours	
Diabetes mellitus	A	Gross elevation			With classical symptoms of diabetes
	B	≥ 7.8			GTT not required
	C	—	≥ 11.1	≥ 11.1	On 2 occasions
Impaired glucose tolerance (IGT)		< 7.8	≥ 11.1	7.8–11.1	
Normal		< 6.4	< 11.1	< 7.8	Glucose values above these concentrations but below criteria for diabetes or IGT are not considered diagnostic for these conditions

* An oral load of 75g glucose is given for the glucose tolerance test (GTT). Other criteria are given for venous whole blood and capillary whose blood, and for children and pregnant women[1].

the sensitivity of the test (proportion of people with disease who have a positive test) after a glucose load was only 10 %. In studies in South Africa the tests for glycosuria after a meal had sensitivities which never exceeded 50 %. Although the specificity of the test was uniformly high – over 90 % – the lack of sensitivity meant that many diabetics would have been missed if this had been the only test. With the new criteria the sensitivity would be much improved but this advantage for screening would be counterbalaneed by a loss in specificity.

Classification

Diabetes may be broadly classified as primary, aetiology unknown, and secondary, when it is due to known processes which exhaust or destroy the insulin-secreting cells of the pancreas or inhibit insulin secretion. Exhaustion of the cells may occur because of increased levels of other hormones antagonistic to the hypoglycaemic action of insulin as occurs in acromegaly, Cushing's syndrome, oral contraceptive therapy and steroid therapy. Destruction of the cells may occur in carcinoma of the pancreas, pancreatectomy, pancreatitis and after some viral infections as well as from certain drugs. Inhibition of insulin secretion occurs in the presence of excess catecholamine activity and in association with potassium depletion as occurs with aldosterone producing tumours and the use of some diuretics. The great majority of patients, however, have primary diabetes.

For many years primary diabetes was divided into 2 groups, juvenile and maturity onset diabetes, to distinguish the disease frequently seen in children and young adults, with the classical symptoms of polyuria, polydypsia and loss of weight and early mortality, from the disease in older adults which tended to occur in the obese, ran a benign course and could be controlled by attention to diet or the use of oral hypoglycaemic agents. Since this classification was created it has become clear that a substantial proportion of young diabetics – possibly 50 % – does not require insulin. The patients have been described as having maturity onset diabetes of the young (MODY). The classification even with this modification remains unsatisfactory as it is internally inconsistent and it relies on a risk factor (age) which is insufficient. A more accurate pathological description is favoured in which diabetes is described as insulin dependent (IDD or type I) and non-insulin dependent (NIDD or type II)[1]. Both are associated with micro and macrovascular changes which may eventually cause death by renal failure, ischaemic heart disease or stroke.

Another type of diabetes has been described in tropical countries in which patients were resistant to ketosis. Known as J-type diabetes because of a report of Jamaican patients, it was characterized by young age, leanness, and the need for high doses of insulin to control blood glucose levels. However, follow-up of the cases in Jamaica and observations on other groups has shown that these patients lose their resistance to ketoacidosis and their high insulin requirements are reduced by dietary change.

Diabetes has also been classified under the 4 headings of severity: potential, latent, asymptomatic and clinical, as shown in Table 25.2[5]. The terminology is that accepted currently in the United Kingdom and Europe but there are some differences with that used in the USA. A new classification has been proposed[1] principally to remove the stigma of the diagnosis of diabetes from those who have only an abnormality of glucose tolerance.

Mortality

The total number of deaths due to diabetes (World Health Organization International Classification of Diseases(ICD) number 250) in England and Wales in 1978 was 4896, small in comparison with the major causes of mortality and similar, for example, to the number of deaths from neoplasms of the rectum (ICD 154) and rectosigmoid junction, neoplasms of lymphatic and haemat-opoietic tissue (ICD 200–209), chronic rheumatic heart disease (ICD 393–398), or hypertensive heart disease (ICD 402). Diabetes accounted for 73.1 % of all deaths from endocrine, nutritional and metabolic diseases (ICD 240–279) in 1978.

Table 25.3 shows the number of deaths and the death rates from diabetes in England and Wales in 1978. The crude death rate for men was only about two-thirds that of women; a ratio reflected in the total number of deaths. However, the age-specific death rates show that men had similar or higher rates at almost all ages and that the sex difference in crude mortality must be due solely to the larger

Table 25.2. The diagnostic classification of diabetes[5].

Potential

People with a normal glucose–tolerance test but with a potential risk of developing diabetes:

1   An identical twin, the other twin being diabetic.

2   A person with both parents diabetic.

3   A person with one diabetic parent whose other non-diabetic parent has, or had, either a diabetic parent, sibling, or offspring, or a sibling having a diabetic child.

4   A woman who has given birth to a live or stillborn child weighing 10 lb (4.5 kg) or more at birth, or a stillborn child showing hyperplasia of the pancreatic islets not due to rhesus incompatibility.

Latent

1   A person with a normal glucose–tolerance test who is known to have had a diabetic glucose–tolerance test at some time during pregnancy, infection, or other stress or when obese.

2   A person who has abnormal blood–glucose responses (similar to those found in diabetes mellitus) to provocative tests such as the cortisone augmented GTT of the intravenous sodium tolbutamide test.

Asymptomatic (sometimes referred to as subclinical or chemical):

1   A person with a diabetic response to the GTT whose fasting blood sugar is below 130 mg per 100 ml (capillary) or 125 mg per 100 ml (venous).

2   As above, but with fasting blood sugars above the stated values.

Clinical

1   A person with an abnormal glucose–tolerance test with the symptoms or complications of diabetes.

2   The term 'pre-diabetic' is reserved for the period in the life of a diabetic before the diagnosis is made.

Table 25.3. Age-specific deaths and death rates from diabetes mellitus, England and Wales, 1978.

	Age (Years)								
	< 1	1–4	5–14	15–24	25–44	45–64	65–74	75+	Total
Men									
Actual deaths	0	1	4	12	97	421	743	730	2008
Deaths per 100 000	0	0.1	0.1	0.3	1.5	7.7	37.5	85.9	8.4
Women									
Actual deaths	1	2	5	13	53	383	879	1552	2888
Deaths per 100 000	0.4	0.2	0.1	0.4	0.8	6.6	34.0	85.2	11.5

number of women than of men in the old age groups, where mortality from diabetes is greatest. In earlier years there was some evidence that women were reported to die of diabetes more often than men after the age of 35 but this trend is no longer evident. Mortality under 25 years is extremely small, a reflection of the success of insulin therapy in IDD.

The standardized mortality ratios (SMRs) for diabetes, based on the 1968 population, are given in Table 25.4 for England and Wales by sex for the years 1966–78. In both sexes there were increases in reported mortality until 1974 for men and 1972 for women. Since 1972 there has been a decline in SMR in women to the levels of 10 years earlier, a downward trend is also found for men since 1974. Analysis of age-specific rates suggests that the rise in the male SMR was due principally to increases in mortality in people over 65 years of age.

Table 25.4. Standardized mortality ratios for diabetes mellitus, England and Wales, 1966–78, with 1968 as base year.

	Year 1966	1967	1968	1969	1970	1971	1972	1973	1974	1975	1976	1977	1978
Men	91	89	100	100	97	100	108	109	111	109	109	106	104
Women	99	95	100	101	100	103	110	102	100	97	95	89	88

There has been a change in mortality from diabetes by social class between the decennial analyses of 1921–23, when the SMR for Social Class I was twice that of Social Class V, and 1970–72, when the gradient was reversed. The reasons for this may lie in the increase in consumption of carbohydrate and fats by the population, affecting the poorer sections of the population relatively more than the wealthier. Other explanations are clearly possible and none is suggested as overriding.

Morbidity

There have been many studies of the prevalence of diabetes in populations throughout the world. Comparison of the rates must be made cautiously because of the great variety of diagnostic criteria used, but some examples may give an idea of the size of the problem. With the new criteria the rates would in most cases be lower.

Studies done among Whites in North America and Europe have given age-adjusted prevalence rates of known diabetes from 5–15 per 1000. The rates for known and unknown diabetics together would be at least twice as large and probably substantially more. In Bedford, United Kingdom, extrapolation of data obtained from a random sample of adults who underwent glucose tolerance tests (GTTs) provided an estimated prevalence rate of 12–14 %. In Birmingham, United Kingdom, the prevalence of known diabetics in 10 General Practices was only 0.64 %, and in those with glycosuria, diabetes was discovered by GTT in 0.69 %. However, GTTs carried out in non-glycosuric individuals suggested that, over the age of 50, 20 % were diabetic and a further 28 % had abnormalities of glucose tolerance. These figures indicate first that diabetes becomes more frequent with increasing age–an observation made in many surveys–and secondly, that it may be a much more prevalent condition than is generally realized.

Early studies showed that diabetes was a disease of affluence as it rarely occurred in primitive people and only at low rates in populations in developing countries. A series of studies using identical methods reported prevalence rates of 2–4% in East Pakistan, Malaysians and Central American populations, compared with 7% in more affluent Uruguayan and Venezuelan groups, and 15% in the USA. It also became clear that some populations which might have been expected to have low diabetes rates had the reverse, among whom are the Pima and Cherokee Indians (and many other tribes), some Pacific Islanders, Africans in the Cape Peninsular and Australian Aborigines[6]. 3 'Sucrose Rules' were propounded, to be met before diabetes becomes common in a population – a high refined sugar intake for 20 years, an annual per capita intake of sugar of 70 lbs and 20% of calories as sugar in low calorie diets.

Although the emergence of diabetes in several populations fits the sucrose rules, there are sufficient examples of populations from the USA, Europe, Israel and the Pacific Islands, which are not consistent, so some other hypothesis is required. High prevalence rates tend to occur in populations which have rapidly altered their way of life – for example many of the American Indian tribes have relatively recently been moved from their original homelands to reserves defined by others. The change has brought a more sedentary life, often an adequate and well-balanced diet but sometimes an excess of either starch or fat. Under these conditions of rapid change it is possible that a 'thrifty gene' which permitted survival during continual semi-famine has disadvantages in times of plenty.

The majority of new diabetes found in surveys is NIDD, since IDD runs a rapid and striking course without treatment. Some estimates of prevalence of diabetes in childhood have been made and these include cases of both types, possibly in the ratio of 1 : 1. In the United Kingdom under the age of 19 years the prevalence rate is of the order of 5–10/10 000 or approximately 1 or 2 in an average sized single-handed General Practice[7,8].

Risk factors

Factors which predispose to diabetes mellitus are relatively few compared with those for ischaemic heart disease for example, but some have given considerable insight into the aetiology of the disease.

Age

In all populations where diabetes is moderately or very common, its prevalence increases with age. In the Oxford Massachusetts, USA, study the rate varied from 2/1000 in 25–34 year olds to 45/1000 at 55–74 years, and nearly 100/1000 over 75 years[6]. Incidence is also positively related to age in the majority of studies which have attempted to make this measurement.

Sex

NIDD has been associated with women in the past, based principally on clinical data, but more recent observations, both clinical and epidemiological, indicate no clear differences between the sexes.

Obesity

NIDD is more common in obese people[9]. Obesity is probably the most important factor in the high prevalence of diabetes in American Indians and some Pacific Islanders (e.g. Nauru, Tonga), although not unique, as diabetes is also found in lean members of these populations. It is possible that hyperglycaemia occurs in obesity because of the smaller density of receptor sites for insulin on adipose than on muscle tissue.

Viral infections

IDD of sudden onset has been found in some cases to be associated with recent viral infections such as mumps or rubella. In addition, from antibody studies, Coxsackie B4 virus infection seems to be unusually associated with new cases of diabetes, but other viruses are implicated as well. IDD in children has a seasonal incidence (defined as the time when first detected rather than when onset occurred) with higher rates in the winter and peaks shortly after the dates for return to school in January and September, observations which fit the hypothesis that viral infections may damage pancreatic islet cells in predisposed individuals[10].

Dietary fibre

Diabetes has been classed as a possible fibre-deficiency disease. Lower blood – glucose responses are found after meals in which whole apples or potatoes are eaten than after equivalent refined carbohydrate. Insulin responses are also lower after whole apples than after purée. Other substances containing fibres also reduce the glycaemic response, including wheat bran and viscous fibres. The possible mechanism is that the fibres, particularly viscous ones, retard the rate of absorption of carbohydrate rather than reduce the total absorbed.

Genes

The role of inheritance in diabetes has become clearer in the last few years. Identical twins with NIDD are much more frequently concordant for the disease than are twins with IDD[11]. NID diabetics taking chlorpropamide are much more likely to show facial flushing after alcohol—chlorpropamide alcohol flushing (CPAF)—than ID diabetics[12]. This reaction can be found in families of NID diabetics, including twins discordant for clinical diabetes, and has been traced through 3 generations. Family histories suggest an autosomal dominant trait associated with CPAF. As not all NIDD is associated with CPAF there remains a group of diabetics for whom there is no defined genetic propensity for the disease.

ID diabetes is also in part genetically determined. These diabetics tend to have human leucocyte antigens (HLA) A8 and Bw15 (as well as Dw3 and Dw4) more frequently than non-diabetics or NID diabetics[13,14]. The genes for these antigens occur on chromosome 6 in the major histocompatibility complex. These associations between diabetics and the antigens may be due to a diabetic gene in linkage disequilibrium with the HLA genes, or to the effects of immune-response genes related to HLA or possibly to activation by viral infection, or due to a direct effect of the HLA antigens themselves.

Other factors

Other factors which may lead to IDD due to direct effects on the pancreas include alcohol, cassava (possibly due to components derived from a cyanide-containing glycoside in the tuber) and the rodenticide N-3-pyridylmethyl-N-P-nitrophenylurea (PNU), a substance similar to streptozotocin and alloxan[15].

Vascular disease

Clinical and post mortem studies carried out over the past 50 years have shown that diabetics with both IDD and NIDD have more atherosclerotic disease than non-diabetics and those with clinically evident atherosclerosis frequently have abnormalities of glucose tolerance. Female diabetics have the same prevalence of arterial disease as male, in contrast with non-diabetics in whom the prevalence of clinical atherosclerosis is 2 to 4 times greater in men. Epidemiological studies in Bedford, United Kingdom, Framingham and Tecumseh, USA, Busselton, Western Australia, and Israel, among others, have confirmed the association. The prevalence of atherosclerotic disease in diabetics varies according to the prevalence in the general population to which they belong – it is high in Western countries but low in India, Japan and in indigenous Africans. The relative frequency of clinical manifestations also differs between countries: ischaemic heart disease predominates in many, but in Japan and Taiwan and possibly India death from stroke is more common[10].

Diabetes is also associated with characteristic microvascular disease affecting particularly the retina and kidney. This complication is found worldwide and shows less variation from one country to another than macrovascular disease.

Intervention

Studies of the effectiveness with which hypoglycaemic therapy prevents the long term sequelae of diabetes are difficult because of the large numbers of patients required to obtain statistically valid results, the length of time before the outcome can be assessed and the need for continuing rigorous observance of rules laid down at the start. It is thus not surprising that only a few such studies have been carried out.

In the Bedford study, 248 borderline diabetics found in a cross-sectional survey were randomly allocated to 2 groups, 1 to be treated with tolbutamide, a sulphonylurea oral hypoglycaemic agent, and the other with placebo[16]. The participants were examined at 6 month intervals. Significant end points taken were death from cardiovascular causes or the occurrence of various specified arterial events during 7 years of follow-up (1962–69). Of those taking tolbutamide, 27.2% had an arterial event compared with 37.4% in the control group ($p < 0.10$). When the 2 groups were further divided into those with and without arterial disease at entry to study, no effect of tolbutamide was found in those with initial disease, but of those without disease only 15.5% taking tolbutamide had subsequent events compared with 30.3% of those on placebo ($p < 0.05$). These results on relatively small numbers of patients suggested a protective effect of tolbutamide.

At about the same time, the University Group Diabetes Program in the USA was examining in much the same terms the effect of 4 treatments randomly allocated to more than 1000 patients attending 12 cooperating clinics[17]. All treatments included a diet to which was added tolbutamide, insulin in fixed dose, variable-dose insulin or placebo. The follow-up period lasted about 8 years. Contrary to the Bedford finding, the UGDP showed a significantly greater mortality from cardiovascular events in those taking tolbutamide than in the other groups (12.7% compared with about 6% on the insulin treatment and 4.9% on diet with placebo). Analysis according to cardiovascular risk factors at entry indicated that in their absence mortality was higher among those taking tolbutamide, whereas when present, mortality was higher in all drug-treated groups than the placebo groups. The effect of phenformin, another oral hypoglycaemic agent, was also tested but over a shorter period[18]. Those taking phenformin had a higher mortality than those on insulin or placebo. A wide range of criticisms of this study has been published, sufficient to suggest caution in acceptance of the results at face value[19].

A third study, in 204 Whitehall (United Kingdom) civil servants, has shown that after 5 years of follow-up, borderline diabetics randomly allocated to 4 groups defined according to treatment by diet or no diet and phenformin or placebo, there was no significant association between phenformin and increased mortality nor, contrary to the UGDP study, between phenformin and increased blood pressure[20].

Despite the enormous amount of work involved in these studies, their conflicting results do not resolve in any clear way the clinical problem of treatment. However, the success of diet treatment alone shows that this approach is to be favoured and that drug treatment should only be considered when diet has failed to control hyperglycaemia.

Primary prevention studies have not been carried out, but all the clinical and epidemiological evidence points to the prevention of obesity as paramount in the prevention of NIDD.

Screening

Tests for glycosuria are commonly used in case finding or screening for diabetes. Despite their popularity, their lack of sensitivity and inadequate specificity, preclude their serious use. In general populations they yield only a small proportion of true cases – of 18 532 subjects in Birmingham, United Kingdom, who tested their urine postprandially, only 55 with positive tests were ultimately found to be new cases of definite diabetes (0.3 %)[21]. The number of cases missed may have been substantially more than those found.

Single blood tests vary in their sensitivity. A fasting capillary whole blood specimen over 7.8 mmol/l usually indicates diabetes and the disease is suspect if the value is over 6.7 mmol/l. The most discriminating single observation is that made 2 hours after an oral glucose challenge. Levels above 6.7 mmol/l are conventionally taken to be diabetic although in the Birmingham survey 7.5 mmol/l seemed more realistic. A level of 11.1 mmol/l or more is definitely diabetic. Table 25.1 indicates that values between 7.8 and 11.1 mmol/l imply impaired glucose tolerance and may need follow-up, and values over 11.1 mmol/l are strong evidence of definite diabetes.

The main problem with any screening programme is the large number of borderline diabetics found relative to definite diabetics. Cohort (a segment of the population born around the same time period) studies show that less than a quarter of those with doubtful abnormalities go on to have diabetes. There is thus a danger of creating patients out of people who have no more than a harmless abnormality of glucose tolerance. The new criteria and classification are designed to reduce this danger.

Because of the low sensitivity of some tests and the lack of customer appeal of the more time-consuming tests (e.g. 2 hour post-challenge test), population screening is likely to be unrewarding. Screening within high risk groups is more appropriate: high risk groups may be defined by those aged between 45 and 70, those with a family history of diabetes and those women who have a history of gestational diabetes or the birth of a l large infant.

Before a screening programme is introduced, one must ensure that there are adequate facilities and services to cope with the newly discovered patients.

Conclusion

The literature on the epidemiology of diabetes is vast, so awareness of the difficulties of defining the disease is essential to understanding the limitations of the research and of the comparability of findings between studies. Understanding of the aetiology of diabetes is advancing rapidly: it is now clear that primary diabetes is a mixture of diseases determined by a variety of genetic and environmental factors which lead to common disturbances of glucose metabolism. Prevention of insulin dependent diabetes (IDD) is not within our grasp, but non-insulin dependent diabetes (NIDD) could be substantially reduced by the conceptually simple expedient of preventing obesity.

References

1. National Diabetes Data Group. Classification and diagnosis of diabetes mellitus and other categories of glucose intolerance. *Diabetes* 1979; **28**: 1039–57.
2. Rushforth NB, Bennett PH, *et al*. Diabetes in Pima Indians. Evidence of bimodality in glucose tolerance distributions. *Diabetes* 1971; **20**: 756–65.
3. Zimmet P, Whitehouse S. Bimodality of fasting and two-hour glucose tolerance distributions in a micornesian population. *Diabetes* 1978; **27**: 793–800.
4. Florey C du V, McDonald H, *et al*. The prevalence of diabetes in a rural population of Jamaican adults. *International Journal of Epidemiology* 1972; **1**: 157–66.
5. Fitzgerald MG. Keen H. Diagnostic classification of diabetes. *British Medical Journal* 1964; **i**: 1568.
6. Miller M, Bennett PH, eds. *International studies in the epidemiology of diabetes*. Advances in Metabolic Disorders. No 9. London: Academic Press, 1978.
7. Wadsworth MEJ, Jarrett RJ. Incidence of diabetes in the first 26 years of life. *Lancet* 1974; **iii**: 1172–4.
8. Calnan M, Peckham CS. Incidence of insulin-dependent diabetes in the first sixteen years of life. *Lancet* 1977; **i**: 589–90.
9. Editorial. Obesity and Diabetes Mellitus *Lancet* 1971; **i**: 381–2.
10. International Diabetes Federation. *Epidemiology of diabetes and its vascular complications*. Proceedings of satellite meeting of IXth International Diabetes Federation Meeting, Bombay, 1976.
11. Tattersall RB, Pyke DA. Diabetes in identical twins. *Lancet* 1972; **ii**: 1120–5.
12. Leslie RDG, Pyke DA. Chlorpropamide-alcohol flushing: a dominantly inherited trait associated with diabetes. *British Medical Journal* 1978; **ii**: 1519–21.
13. Perkins HA. The human major histocompatibility complex (MHC). In: Fudenberg HH, Stites DP, eds. *Basic and clinical immunology*. Los Altos, California: Lange Medical Publications, 1976: 165–74.
14. Cudworth AG, Festenstein H. HLA genetic heterogeneity in diabetes mellitus. In: Bodmer WF, ed. The HLA system. *British Medical Bulletin* 1978; **34**: 285–9.
15. Editorial. Diabetes, cyanide and rat poison. *Lancet* 1979; **ii**: 341.
16. Keen H, Jarrett RJ. The effect of carbohydrate tolerance on plasma lipids and atherosclerosis in man. In: Jones RJ, ed. *Atherosclerosis, Proceedings of the second International Symposium*. Berlin: Springer-Verlag, 1970: 435–44.
17. The University Group Diabetes Program. A study of the effects of hypoglycaemic agents on vascular complications in patients with adult-onset diabetes. I: Design, methods and baseline results. II: Mortality results. *Diabetes* 1970; **19** (2): 747–830.

18. The University Group Diabetes Program. A study of the effects of hypoglycaemic agents on vascular complications in patients with adult-onset diabetes. V: Evaluation of phenformin therapy. *Diabetes* 1975; **24** (1): 65–184.
19. Whitehouse FW, Arky RA, *et al.* Policy statement. The UGDP controversy. *Diabetes* 1979; **28**: 168–70.
20. Jarrett RJ, Keen H, *et al.* Treatment of borderline diabetes: controlled trial using carbohydrate restriction and phenformin. *British Medical Journal* 1977; **ii**: 861–5.
21. Malins JM. Screening for disease. Diabetes. *Lancet* 1974; **ii**: 1367–8.

Further reading

West KM. *The epidemiology of diabetes and its vascular lesions.* New York: Elsevier, 1978.

Chapter 26 · Thyroid disease

P O D PHAROAH

The epidemiology of the thyroid gland may be conveniently considered in the following groups:
1   abnormalities associated with a physiological enlargement of the gland, i.e. endemic goitre and endemic cretinism;
2   conditions in which there is a hypofunctioning of the gland, i.e. sporadic cretinism and myxoedema;
3   conditions with hyperfunctioning of the gland;
4   neoplastic conditions.
From an international perspective, endemic goitre is the most prevalent thyroid disorder. However, it has now largely disappeared from the more affluent countries though it remains a significant problem in many developing countries[1]. Table 26.1 presents a parochial perspective of mortality and morbidity from thyroid disease as shown by England and Wales data.

The thyroid gland and nutritional iodine deficiency

Goitre

Historically, recognition of endemic goitre goes back 4000 years and, even at that time, seaweed and animal thyroid preparations were recommended for treatment. The geographical distribution has also been recognized since the pre-Christian era. The poet Juvenal in the first century BC remarked 'Who wonders at a swelling of the neck in the Alps?'[2].

Areas with a high prevalence are determined by certain geological features. These are:
1   mountainous regions, e.g. the Alps, the Andean cordillera, the Himalayas and the mountain range extending through Burma, Indonesia, New Guinea and the Philippines;
2   alluvial plains that have recently been the site of quarternary glaciation, e.g. the Great Lakes Basin of Canada and the USA;
3   areas where water supplies permeate through limestone, e.g. the Peak District of England.
Fig. 26.1 is a composite of several maps from a previous review of the prevalence of endemic goitre and shows where goitre has been found[3]. However, the map does not indicate the severity of the endemic, neither does it reveal the current

318

Table 26.1. Mortality and morbidity from disease of the thyroid, England and Wales[2].

Disease		Number of deaths 1979	Hospital discharges and deaths 1976
Carinoma	Male	112	1750
Thyroid	Female	282	
Myxoedema	Male	53	2980
	Female	305	
Thyrotoxicosis	Male	27	5960
	Female	144	
Simple & non-	Male	4	5830
toxic nodular	Female	16	
goitre			
Thyroiditis	Male	2	580
	Female	14	
Congenital	Male	0	130
cretinism	Female	0	
Other	Male	0	660
	Female	2	

situation because changing socio-economic conditions and specific preventive measures have altered the global picture.

It is now generally accepted that dietary iodine deficiency is the major cause of endemic goitre. Evidence supporting this comes from several lines of investigation. Goitre occurs in areas of low soil iodine content and an inverse relationship can often be demonstrated between the level of soil iodine and goitre prevalence. Urinary iodine excretion is low in areas of endemic goitre. Experimental goitre can be produced in animals fed on a low iodine diet. Iodine is successful in both preventing and treating goitre. However, in some areas other factors, e.g. dietary goitrogens, may enhance the effect of iodine deficiency[4].

Surveys to establish the prevalence of goitre are usually based on a grading of thyroid gland enlargement of which there are several schemes.

A generally accepted classification is that proposed at a Pan American Health Organization meeting in 1963 and reaffirmed in 1974[5,6]. It is a slight modification of the system of Perez *et al.*[7] and is as follows.

Grade Oa: no goitre;
Grade Ob: goitre detectable only by palpation and not visible even when the neck is fully extended;
Grade 1: goitre palpable, but visible only when the neck is fully extended;
Grade 2: thyroid visible when the head is in normal position; palpation is not needed for diagnosis;
Grade 3: very large goitre which can be recognized at a considerable distance (Fig. 26.2 p. 322).

Endocrine Diseases

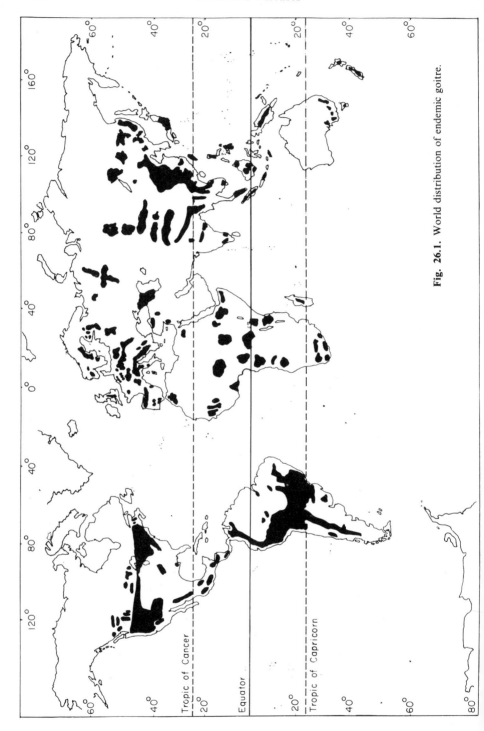

Fig. 26.1. World distribution of endemic goitre.

It is recommended that, in cases of doubt between any 2 stages, the lower be recorded. The enlarged glands may be subclassified depending on whether the enlargement is diffuse or nodular.

For survey purposes, even this classification may be considered unnecessarily complex as the distinctions between grade Ob and 1 and between grades 2 and 3 are not precise.

The prevalence of endemic goitre in a community correlates with the degree of iodine deficiency present. The evidence for this is covered in a previous review of the aetiology of endemic goitre[8]. Characteristically, those at greatest risk of developing goitre are women during the childbearing period and, indeed, there may be an increase in glandular size with successive pregnancies. Adolescent males and females are the next most vulnerable group. The variation in vulnerability amongst different age groups is due to differences in the physiological requirements for iodine. In severely affected areas almost everyone including infants may have a goitre; a prevalence of 92 % has been described in some Nepalese villages[9]. In regions with a borderline iodine nutrition, the more vulnerable sections of the community will be affected and significant age and sex differentials in the prevalence of goitre will be present[10].

The effectiveness of iodine in preventing goitre had been widely demonstrated. The important definitive trial of iodine was that by Marine and Kimball among schoolgirls in Akron, Ohio[11]. Active preventive measures by iodine supplementation have been instigated in several countries. The most common method is by the iodization of salt; recommended levels suggest iodine salt ratios ranging from 1 : 200 000 to 1 : 10 000. In some countries statutory requirements for the iodization of salt have been imposed.

More recently supplementation using an intramuscular depot preparation of iodized oil under trial conditions has been shown to be effective[12] and a single injection has been found effective for at least 5 years. This method of iodine supplementation has proved particularly successful in remote areas where the distribution of iodized salt is haphazard and often least likely to reach those areas where the deficiency is greatest. Other methods of supplementing dietary iodine have included the iodization of bread, water supplies, milk and even chocolate[13]. A goitre often shows a dramatic reduction in size after iodine is given.

Endemic cretinism

There are 2 types of endemic cretinism – neurological and myxoedematous – and they are distinguishable by their clinical characteristics. The relevant
The direct significance of endemic goitre as a health problem is largely cosmetic. Of far greater importance is endemic cretinism which occurs in geographical association with goitre and is also a consequence of iodine deficiency.

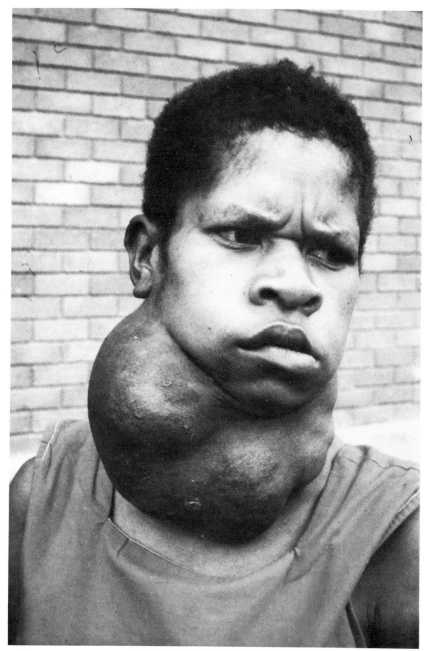

Fig. 26.2. An example of a large goitre.

features of the neurological variety are mental retardation, deaf-mutism, spastic diplegia, strabimus. Clinical hypothyroidism is not evident. The myxoedematous variety has, as the name suggests, the signs and symptoms associated with an inadequate synthesis of thyroid hormone.

The Pan American Health Organization definition[5] of the endemic cretin is 'an individual with irreversible changes in mental development, born in an endemic goitre area and exhibiting a combination of some of the following characteristics not explained by other causes:

1 irreversible neuromuscular disorder;
2 irreversible abnormalities in hearing and speech leading in certain cases to deaf-mutism;
3 impairment of somatic development;
4 hypothyroidism.

While this is all-embracing and includes the clinical manifestations of both varieties of the disorder, it fails to underline the predominance of one variety over the other that tends to be seen in different countries. The hypothyroid variety is more common in some Central African countries whereas the neurological variety predominates elsewhere. These geographical differences have been reviewed[14].

The results of a controlled trial using intramuscular iodized oil established that the defects of neurological cretinism are the consequence of maternal iodine deficiency damaging the fetus during early development[15]. The pathogenetic mechanism is yet to be determined. The effectiveness of iodine as a prophylactic has received support elsewhere[16] and it has also been observed that the withdrawal of a rich source of dietary iodine was associated with a sharp rise in the incidence of the syndrome[17]. Neither treatment with iodine nor thyroid hormones has any effect on the established disorder.

Although the results are as yet inconclusive, preliminary findings suggest that iodine is also an effective prophylactic for myxoedematous cretinism[18]. Furthermore, the symptoms and signs can be alleviated by thyroid hormones. One speculation is that a dietary goitrogen in conjunction with iodine deficiency acting during the late fetal and early postnatal periods is aetiologically responsible.

Even in endemic areas, the prevalence of goitre and cretinism may change sharply from one village to the next and a prevalence of cretinism as high as 15 % has been reported in some villages[19]. Generally a strong positive association between the prevalence of goitre and cretinism is observed[20,21,22].

New cases of endemic cretinism are only found in the developing countries, the disease having been eradicated from most industrialized societies. In many countries a declining incidence has been documented prior to any formal measure of iodine supplementation and is associated with general socio-economic improvement[21].

Hypofunction of the thyroid

Sporadic cretinism

This may be due to dysgenesis of the thyroid gland, an enzyme defect which impairs synthesis of the thyroid hormones, or damage to the gland, for example by radioiodine.

The incidence of congenital hypothyroidism has been determined in 2 national surveys. The Dutch Paediatric Association recorded 97 cases (38 boys, 59 girls) born in the years 1972–74, giving an incidence of 1:6260. Only 11% of the cases were diagnosed within the first 3 weeks of life and 53% were diagnosed by the age of 3 months. 16% were not diagnosed until after 1 year of age[23].

In Sweden there were 112 children (45 boys and 67 girls) with congenital hypothyroidism born during the 7 year period 1969–75, an incidence of 1:6900 live births. Diagnosis was made before the age of 3 months in 54 cases (48%)[24]. The follow-up at 7 years of age of the 1958 cohort in the National Child Development Study found 3 cretins among the 16606 children examined, a prevalence of 1:5535[25].

The earlier that treatment is started, the better the mental prognosis[26] so that the potential for a newborn screening programme is great and, currently, neonatal screening for hypothyroidism is in the vanguard of development. Initially measurement of serum thyroxine (T_4) was the screening test of choice; its main advantage lay in that it could be performed on the same blood spot collected for the Guthrie screening test for phenylketonuria. This greatly simplified the logistics of a screening programme with a concomitant reduction in cost. The disadvantage lay in the high false positive rate necessitating a recall of infants who then required further investigation. The problem of false negatives also arose, particularly among infants with an ectopic thyroid. While such infants have normal thyroid function tests initially, they often subsequently develop severe hypothyroidism. More recently, measurement of serum thyrotrophin (TSH) has superceded serum T_4 as the test of choice because it also can now be carried out on a filter paper blood spot. False positives are less of a problem than with T_4, particularly if the screening test is delayed until the end of the first week to avoid the surge of TSH which occurs soon after birth. False negatives are found with secondary hypothyroidism, but this is a rare disorder and the presenting clinical abnormalities differ from primary hypothyroidism.

Reports from several screening programmes indicate an incidence of congenital hypothyroidism of about 1:3500[27] which is almost twice as great as the observed incidence in the national surveys mentioned earlier. The discrepancy between well-documented surveys and screening series raises several questions. It may be that there are unrecognized and potentially treatable cases of congenital hypothyroidism in the community; that some cretins are dying in early childhood; that there are false positives following screening even after full investigation; or that there is a transient hypothyroidism in the neonate which subsequently disappears spontaneously and is of little clinical significance.

Screening for congenital hypothyroidism is now in the process of change from research to a service commitment and, as such, it is imperative that there is a full and proper evaluation of every programme that is started. It is well recognized that maternal thyroid hormone does not cross the placenta in significant amounts and that some clinical features of hypothyroidism, for example delay in the formation of epiphyseal centres, are evident at birth in many cases. It is likely that there is also some degree of mental retardation present so that even with early treatment, the mental potential may not be realized.

Myxoedema

The prevalence of myxoedema is generally underestimated due to the insidiousness of its onset and the chronicity of its natural history. Thus there is a wide variation in its severity so that there is an inherent difficulty in defining the syndrome for epidemiological purposes.

A community survey of 2779 adults in Whickham in North East England found overt clinical and biochemical hypothyroidism in 14 per 1000 women and 1 per 1000 men. The hypothyroidism was previously untreated in 3 per 1000 women. One-third of those with treated hypothyroidism had previously had surgery and/or radio-iodine for thyrotoxicosis, indicating a significant iatrogenic component[28].

Evered and Hall[29] have proposed a classification of hypothyroidism to include minor degrees of the disorder as follows:
1   presence of thyroid antibodies with an elevated TSH but normal circulating thyroid hormones;
2   subclinical hypothyroidism with an elevated TSH and equivocal thyroid hormone levels;
3   mild clinical hypothyroidism with an elevated TSH and equivocal thyroid hormone levels;
4   obvious clinical and biochemical hypothyroidism.

There have been several population surveys examining the prevalence of thyroid antibodies[30]. The prevalence varies with the test being used for determining the thyroid antibody titre. Consistently it is found that there is at least a 4-fold higher rate in women compared with men and an increased frequency with age. Up to 15 % of women at age 75 have antibodies. Mortality rates for myxoedema show a striking female preponderance and a sharp rise in the rate with increasing age (Fig. 26.3). Hospital discharge data are of limited value because many patients do not require admission but are investigated and treated as out-patients.

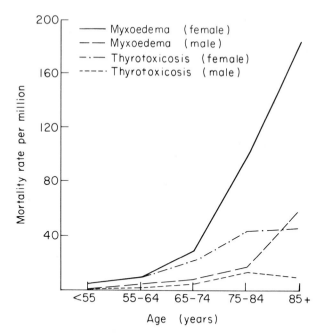

Fig. 26.3. Mortality rates for myxoedema and thyrotoxicosis by age and sex, England and Wales, 1977.

Hyperthyroidism

Hyperthyroidism most commonly occurs with a diffuse enlargement of the gland but may also result from a toxic nodule. Clinical reports suggest that occasionally it is a transient phenomenon, as in the early phase of Hashimoto's thyroiditis in which the natural history is a progression to hypothyroidism. However, data indicating how frequently this occurs are not available.

In some areas of endemic goitre, an increase in the prevalence of thyrotoxicosis has followed an increase in the dietary intake of iodine. For example, during the period 1960–63 in Northern Tasmania, 20–25 cases were treated each year for thyrotoxicosis. Following the introduction of iodophors into the dairy industry and the iodization of bread, there was an increase in the number of cases which reached a peak of 105 in 1967 and declined subsequently. The increase occurred predominantly among those aged 45 or over with a nodular goitre[31].

The limitations of the data on hypothyroidism apply also to hyperthyroidism with the added problems imposed by the naturally relapsing and remitting course of the disease. The data in Fig. 26.3 shows that the increase in mortality with age is not so striking as that for myxoedema though the female predominance is still evident.

The Whickham community survey found a 1.1 % prevalence of overt hyperthyroidism with a further 0.5 % of possible cases. Thus, in the community it is more common than hypothyroidism and differs in this respect from mortality data. Presumably this reflects the natural remission that occurs in many cases of hyperthyroidism.

Carcinoma of the thyroid

This is one of the rarer malignant neoplasms and accounts for approximately 400 deaths (0.3 % of all deaths due to neoplasms) and 1500 admissions to hospital in England and Wales each year. National cancer registration data show an incidence of 0.7 and 1.8 per 100 000 per annum for men and women respectively. There is an increasing incidence with age and the 2-or 3-fold female/male preponderance is present throughout the age range as shown in Fig. 26.4. This preponderance is also found in deaths due to the disease.

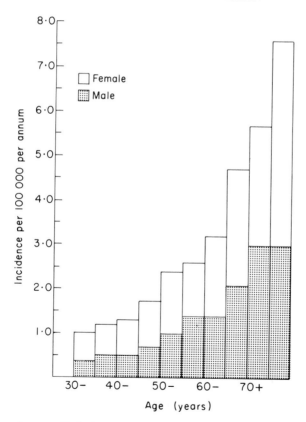

Fig. 26.4. Sex- and age-specific incidence of carcinoma of the thyroid per 100 000 per annum, England and Wales, 1963–66[32].

Histologically, the carcinomas may be classified into undifferentiated and differentiated varieties and the latter is subclassified into papillary, follicular and medullary types.

The female/male sex ratio is greater for the undifferentiated than the differentiated tumours. Papillary carcinoma occurs typically in children, follicular in older age groups, while the undifferentiated variety is most frequent in those over 60 years.

The evidence associating areas of endemic goitre with an increased incidence of thyroid carcinoma is conflicting. In part this is because of the rarity of the condition and also because, in those areas where goitre is highly prevalent, mortality data tend to be incomplete and inaccurate.

References

1. Office of Population Censuses and Surveys. *Mortality Statistics 1979*. Series DH2. No 6. London: HMSO, 1980, and *Hospital In-patient Enquiry 1976*. Series MB4. No 7. London: HMSO, 1980.
2. Langer P. History of goitre. *WHO Monograph Series* 1960; **44**: 9–25.
3. Kelly FC, Snedden WW. Prevalence and geographical distribution of endemic goitre. *WHO Monograph Series* 1960; **44**: 27–233.
4. Delange F, Ermans AM. Endemic goitre and cretinism. Naturally occurring goitrogens. *Pharmacy and Therapeutics. Part C* 1976; **1**: 57–93.
5. Pan American Health Organization. *Report of the Scientific Group on Research in Endemic Goitre*. Washington: PAHO, 1963.
6. Pan American Health Organization. *Report of the Technical Group on Endemic Goitre*. Washington: PAHO, 1974.
7. Perez C, Scrimshaw NS, Munoz HA. Technique of endemic goitre surveys. *WHO Monograph Series* 1960; **44**: 369–84.
8. Roche J, Lissitzky S. Etiology of endemic goitre. *WHO Monograph Series* 1960; **44**: 351–68.
9. Ibbertson HK, Pearl M, *et al*. Endemic cretinism in Nepal. *Institute of Human Biology, Papua New Guinea. Monograph Series* 1971; **2**: 71–88.
10. Clements FW. Health significance of endemic goitre and related conditions. *WHO Monograph Series* 1960; **44**: 235–60.
11. Marine D, Kimball OP. The prevention of simple goitre in man. *Archives of Internal Medicine* 1920; **25**: 661.
12. McCullagh SF. The effectiveness of an intramuscular depot of iodized oil in the control of endemic goitre. *Medical Journal of Australia* 1963; **1**: 769–77.
13. Holman JCM, McCartney W. Iodized salt. *WHO Monograph Series* 1960; **44**: 411–41.
14. Pharoah POD. Geographical variation in the clinical manifestations of endemic cretinism. *Tropical and Geographical Medicine* 1976; **28**: 259–67.
15. Pharoah POD, Buttfield IH, Hetzel BS. Neurological damage to the fetus resulting from severe iodine deficiency during pregnancy. *Lancet* 1971; **i**: 308–10.
16. Ramirez I, Fierro-Benitez R, *et al*. The results of prophylaxis of endemic cretinism with iodized oil in rural Andean Equador. *Advances in Experimental Medical Biology* 1972; **30**: 223–37.
17. Pharoah POD, Hornabrook RW. Endemic cretinism of recent onset in New Guinea. *Lancet* 1974; **ii**: 1038–40.
18. Thilly CH, Delange F, *et al*. Strategy of goitre and cretinism control in Central Africa. *International Journal of Epidemiology* 1977; **6**: 43–54.
19. Pharoah POD. *Endemic cretinism in the Jimi Valley*. MD Thesis. University of London, 1972.

20. Eugster J. *Endemic goitre and cretinism*. Transactions of the 3rd International Goitre Conference. 1938: 130.
21. Trotter WR. Deafness and thyroid dysfunction. *British Medical Bulletin* 1960; **16**: 92–8.
22. Buttfield IH, Hetzel BS. Endemic cretinism in Eastern New Guinea. *Australasian Annals of Medicine* 1969; **18**: 217–21.
23. DeJonge GA. Congenital hypothyroidism in the Netherlands. *Lancet* 1976; **ii**: 143.
24. Alm J, Larsson A, Zetterstrom R. Congenital hypothyroidism in Sweden. *Acta Paediatrica Scandinavica* 1978; **67**: 1–3.
25. Davie R, Butler N, Goldstein H. *From birth to seven*. London: Longmans, 1972.
26. Raiti S, Newns GH. Cretinism: early diagnosis and its relation to mental prognosis. *Archives of Diseases in Childhood* 1971; **46**: 692–4.
27. Smith P, Morris A. Assessment of a programme to screen the newborn for congenital hypothyroidism. *Community Medicine* 1979; **1**: 14–22.
28. Tunbridge WMG, Evered D, *et al*. The spectrum of thyroid disease in a community: the Whickham survey. *Clinical Endocrinology* 1978; **7**: 481–93.
29. Evered D, Hall R. Hypothyroidism. *British Medical Journal* 1972; **i**: 290–3.
30. Tunbridge WMG. The epidemiology of hypothyroidism. *Clinics in Endocrinology and Metabolism*. London: WB Saunders. 1979; **8** (1): 21–7.
31. Stewart JC, Vidor GI, *et al*. Epidemic thyrotoxicosis in Northern Tasmania: studies of clinical features and iodine nutrition. *Australia and New Zealand Journal of Medicine* 1971; **1**: 203–11.
32. Office of Population Censuses and Surveys. *Studies on medical and population subjects. No 24*. London: HMSO, 1972.

SECTION 7 · LOCOMOTOR AND NEUROLOGICAL DISEASES

Chapter 27 · Rheumatic Disorders

P H N WOOD AND E BADLEY

'Rheumatism and arthritis' is a colloquial designation for rheumatic disorders, the latter term being more indicative of the scope because there are over 200 identifiable afflictions of the musculoskeletal system and connective tissue. These conditions can conveniently be considered under 5 main groups – arthropathies, back troubles, nonarticular rheumatism, other rheumatic disorders and soft tissue injury (Table 27.1).

The common feature shared by the rheumatic conditions is that the connective or supporting tissues are presumed to be the seat of pathological dysfunction. In addition, most rheumatic disorders are characterized by pain and by difficulty in moving the parts of the body; swelling is also a common feature. Chronic inflammatory changes are prominent in the more serious, such as rheumatoid arthritis, but the pathological lesions in many of the other disorders, including much back pain, are much less definite. Another notable feature of many rheumatic complaints, particularly the more common ones, is that they are variable in their course. Thus gout, many forms of nonarticular rheumatism and a great deal of back pain, present as episodes of suffering that appear to remit, perhaps to be followed months, or even years, later by a recurrence. In the intervening period, the individual may lack any stigmata of disease. Other rheumatic disorders have a more sustained course, for example, an individual with rheumatoid arthritis is relatively unlikely to become completely symptom-free. However, even with conditions such as this, the pattern of illness commonly fluctuates in severity.

Prevalence

One of the fundamental yields from epidemiological enquiry is an estimate of prevalence; this provides a measure of the burden of suffering in the community, an indication of the relative importance of the condition, and the principal challenges confronting those attempting to plan appropriate health services. The rheumatic disorders have tended to be neglected because they have been incompletely perceived. Important reasons for this have been that the number of cases ascertained from any one source of data tends to be relatively limited. Furthermore, the conditions are not necessarily grouped in a way that corresponds to the interests of a particular patient group or medical speciality. The structure of the World Health Organization's International Classification of Diseases (ICD) has contributed to the latter difficulty.

Table 27.1. Measures of the frequency of experiences with rheumatic disorders (expressed as rates per 1000 population at risk for the year 1971*.)

Rheumatic disorder	International Classification of Diseases (ICD) 8th revision	GP† consultations (home population)	
		Consultations	Episodes
Arthropathies		79.9	35.6
Gout	274	*3.8*	*1.8*
Rheumatoid arthritis (incl. AS)	712	*18.9*	*5.9*
Spondylosis	713.1	*13.7*	*7.6*
Other osteoarthrosis	rest 713	*43.5*	*20.3*
Other arthritis	rest 710–715	–	–
Connective tissue diseases	716 & 734	–	–
Back troubles		68.0	36.1
Sciatica	353	*3.3*	*1.7*
Lumbago	717.0	*15.3*	*9.1*
Displacement of intervertebral disc	725	*17.5*	*6.4*
Vertebrogenic pain	728 excl. 728.9	*10.9*	*5.4*
Other back pain	728.9	*21.0*	*13.5*
Nonarticular rheumatism		60.3	40.3
Frozen shoulder	717.1	*3.2*	*1.8*
Other rheumatism	rest 717 & 718	*14.3*	*9.9*
Other arthritis and rheumatism	rest 710–718	*9.2*	*5.9*
Bursitis and synovitis	731	*12.0*	*7.6*
Symptoms referred to limbs	787	*21.6*	*15.1*
Other rheumatic disorders		31.7	18.8
Rheumatic fever and rheumatic heart disease	390–398	*4.5*	*1.4*
Internal derangement of joint	724	*6.4*	*3.3*
Hallux valgus and varus	737	*1.3*	*0.9*
Other musculoskeletal disorders	rest 720–738	*19.5*	*15.2*
Soft tissue injury	N840–N848	46.6	32.5
(Sprains and strains)			
All rheumatic disorders		286.5	163.3
All diseases and conditions§		3009.6	1808.6 (671.7)**

AS Ankylosing spondylosis.

* Sizes of populations for computation of national experience in Great Britain (England, Wales and Scotland)—multiply rate shown by home population, 54.3 × 10³; insured population, 19.5 × 10³; or adult population, 40.99 × 10³; as appropriate. Population < 15y:12.74 × 10³. (all population figures quoted are in thousands).

† General Practice.

‡ The total of impaired persons with all rheumatic disorders is less than the sum of the individual rates

Sickness incapacity certifications (insured population)		Admissions to hospital (home population)	Impaired persons (adults, ≥ 16 years)		Deaths (home population)
Spells	Days lost		All degrees	Severe and very severe	
6.77	813	1.35	22.10	4.30	0.04
0.74	15	0.02	–	–	0.0008
0.46	168	0.50	3.44	1.29	0.02
}2.17	}261	}0.67	}3.56	}0.52	}0.009
3.40	369	0.11	15.10	2.49	0.002
–	–	0.05	–	–	0.006
18.79	586	0.70	2.00	0.20	0.0005
3.01	99	0.07	0.34	0.01	0.00006
5.74	107	–	–	–	0
3.93	236	0.30	1.66	0.19	0.0003
2.35	66	0.33	–	–	
3.76	78	–	–	–	0.0001
15.62	342	0.58	–	–	0.0004
}10.81	}241	}0.07	–	–	}0.0004
–	–	–	–	•	0
2.04	45	0.29	–	–	0.00002
2.77	56	0.22	–	–	0
2.10	202	1.79	3.23	0.36	0.16
0.22	68	0.41	0.19	0.02	0.14
0.70	32	0.26			0
}1.18	}102	0.19	}3.04	}0.34	0
		0.93			0.02
18.03	330	0.14	0.81	0.09	0.0002
61.31	2272	4.56	27.77‡	4.91	0.20
442.76	16147	103.80††	77.99	12.66	11.61

because more than one disorder was present in a proportion of people.
§ Including all medical and surgical conditions, shown here for purposes of comparison.
** The rate for episodes for all diseases and conditions is inflated by persons experiencing more than one episode, due to different causes; the rate in parenthesis is that for patients consulting and is more useful for comparison with the individual rates shown.
†† Hospital admissions for all diseases and conditions exclude maternity admissions and those to psychiatric hospitals.

These problems may be overcome by juxtaposing aggregated data from different sources (Table 27.1), from which the following points are of particular note.

1 Rheumatic disorders contribute a high proportion of the work load in General Practice. They account for almost 10% of all consultations and are present in some form in nearly a quarter of all patients consulting. They are the cause of more than 12% of recorded sickness incapacity.

2 They are seen relatively infrequently in hospital practice, being the reason for 4% of hospital admissions.

3 Less than 2% of all deaths are attributed to a rheumatic disease; the majority of these are from rheumatic fever and its resultant heart disease.

4 Amongst persons who are impaired or severely disabled, more than one-third are individuals suffering from one of the rheumatic disorders. 1% of the population have sufficient disability from rheumatism and arthritis to need assistance in the activities of daily living.

5 Of the 5 major groups, the arthropathies are both one of the more frequent and also the most serious (as reflected in Table 27.1 by days lost from work and the hospital admission and impairment rates).

Specific studies

With the exception of the arthropathies, little attention has been devoted to elucidation of the epidemiology of most of the rheumatic disorders. Many of them have not attracted much interest because they are regarded as trivial in themselves. However, because of the frequency with which they occur their overall contribution to the totality of rheumatic morbidity is considerable; for example, almost two-thirds of the days lost from work from rheumatic conditions are attributable to ill-defined conditions. Even when enthusiasm for investigations exists, there are methodological difficulties, particularly the unsatisfactory clinical criteria used to diagnose these complaints. Their generally benign nature and brief duration give rise to uncertainty about the moral justification for invasive investigation, such as tissue biopsy. As a result, little more is known of their pathology than that notions such as 'fibrositis' are unwarranted and the existence of entities such as 'panniculitis' remains unsubstantial.

A further problem arises out of the fact that a key feature of rheumatic complaints is their subjective nature; this increases the variation in response to them. There is no objective method for establishing the presence of pain and in many of these conditions there are few relevant physical signs to confirm or refute a diagnosis. Furthermore, subjective conditions are especially vulnerable to variations in sickness behaviour, and the latter is as likely an explanation for observed secular changes in sickness absence experience as is alteration in disease incidence.

There are 3 types of disorder about which a little more can be said. Polymyalgia rheumatica is a generalized form of nonarticular rheumatism. The condition is more common than is often realized, its prevalence in the elderly probably approaching 1 %. Prodromal features are often identical with those of temporal (giant cell) arteritis, and many regard the 2 disorders as part of the same disease spectrum. Certainly polymyalgia rheumatica also carries with it an appreciable hazard of blindness, and both diseases appear to be controlled fairly satisfactorily by corticosteroid therapy. Recent work has tried to tackle the problem of how polymyalgia rheumatica might be identified in a reproducible manner[2].

Acute rheumatic fever is still a serious problem in the world despite the fact that effective measures for primary prevention are well known. There are interesting differences in the manner in which this condition expresses itself in various parts of the world. For example, 2 major features – chorea and polyarthritis – appear to be encountered much less frequently on the Indian subcontinent, an observation that seriously limits the value for universal application of the standard Duckett Jones diagnostic criteria.

Most detailed studies have been concerned with the arthropathies, particularly rheumatoid arthritis, ankylosing spondylitis, osteoarthritis and gout; these are considered later. With the other forms of rheumatic disorder, the following aetiological influences have been identified.

Trauma

The importance of trauma in soft tissue injury is self-evident. The major outstanding questions concern the possibility of its prevention and whether more effective means of treatment can be developed to prevent disability.

Occupation

Many forms of nonarticular rheumatism have higher incidences in certain occupations. They appear to be the result of the way in which parts of the body are used. Occupational disorders include various types of bursitis, vibration-induced white finger, chronic crepitant synovitis (e.g. of the wrist), and some of the enthesopathies (lesions of musculotendinous attachments such as tennis elbow).

Microbial agents

Some of the rheumatic disorders have been shown to be associated with infection by certain microbial agents. The link between the streptococcus and acute rheumatic fever is well-documented. Certain polyarthritides follow viral infections, for example, that associated with rubella. Other forms of rheumatic disorders (e.g. Lyme arthritis and chikungunya) appear to involve an insect vector.

Environmental exposures

These are also relevant, giving rise to conditions such as skeletal fluorosis and saturnine gout. Some industrial intoxicants, such as polyvinyl chloride, can also have a harmful effect on the musculoskeletal system.

Genetic factors

These contribute to familial joint laxity and congenital dislocation of the hip, as well as the Marfan, Hurler and Ehlers – Danlos syndromes.

Gout

This disorder provides 2 examples of the way in which epidemiological rigour can clarify our knowledge.

The first concerns apparent differences in disease frequency, which are of great potential value in identifying possible aetiological factors. Some years ago an apparently high frequency of gout was reported from parts of the Cotswolds in England. A large survey, extending over 18 months, appeared to confirm that the prevalence was unusually high. However, when the results were compared with those from one of the few well-executed studies in populations of similar ethnicity, in Sudbury, Massachusetts, after standardization for age, the apparent excess in the Cotswolds was not substantiated[3].

Secondly, there have been reports of an association between gout and diabetes. Such a link would be very interesting biologically, but when the serum uric acid and blood–sugar levels of the population of Tecumseh, Michigan were examined, no correlation between the two could be demonstrated. The reported clinical association may have been a selection artefact in Caucasian patients presenting for medical care. However, in an ethnically different group from Polynesia, a relationship between diabetes and gout, and their associated blood abnormalities, did hold true. A combination of genetic susceptibilities and environmental exposures appears to have determined the link.

The refutation of an hypothesis can be frustrating but it is only by disposing of false leads in this manner that the factors that are relevant can be identified. Rheumatological epidemiology often leads to such negative conclusions; this may be attributable to poverty of aetiological hypotheses and confusion over the characteristics of the condition under study. An inescapable feature of gout is the trend towards increase in frequency since the last war. As with diabetes, this is usually explained in terms of a more abundant diet, although rigorous proof of this proposition is lacking.

Osteoarthrosis

Arthrosis is the commonest form of joint disorder. Its frequency increases with age to a greater extent than with any other rheumatic disease. The interpretation of this age distribution is difficult. If the pathological joint changes are an integral part of the ageing process they should be consistent and universal. If not, then the association may reflect a relatively non-specific concomitant of age, such as greater exposure to wear, or it may be the consequence of a more specific and nonuniversal pathological process which is itself more common in those of greater age. Osteophytes are commonly regarded as an essential feature of arthrosis, but they are probably a non-specific accompaniment of age. The other changes in osteoarthrosis are more likely to reflect the disease process[4].

Despite attention devoted to the epidemiological study of arthrosis, the significance of the results is confounded by uncertainty about the nature of the condition. The term 'arthrosis' is used to identify radiographic changes, morbid anatomical features and the clinical state of a patient complaining of pain in a joint. The importance of each of these characteristics is different and their inter-relationships are far from straightforward. This is illustrated in Table 27.2, which shows the imperfect association between symptom experience, itself often rather non-specific, and other evidence of the condition. The difficulties arise from the problem of trying to interpret patients' complaints presumed to originate from deep and often remote structures, and from the confusion in concepts.

Table 27.2. Symptoms and radiographic changes of arthrosis[5].

Symptom	Radiographic changes	% Symptom positives who are radiographic positives (Sensitivity)	% Symptom negatives who are radiographic negatives (Specificity)
Pain in hip	Arthrosis of hip	39	92
Pain in knee	Arthrosis of knee	68	88
Cervicobrachial pain	Spondylosis–cervical disc degeneration	50	65
Back/hip/sciatic pain	Spondylosis–lumbar disc degeneration	59	55

Similarity between the pathological changes that are seen in different joints has encouraged the notion that osteoarthrosis is a general phenomenon. This has led to problems, particularly when studies include all degrees of change as cases. In this way it has been shown that arthrosic radiographic abnormalities of at least mild degree occur in almost all individuals aged 65 years or more. However, to treat arthrosis as if it were a single entity, when it includes changes in different anatomical sites, both conceals important differences between sites and leads to erroneous estimates of the magnitude of the populations at risk of developing these changes[6].

The fact that osteoarthrosis does not develop in all individuals in the same joint allows cautious optimism that preventive intervention in susceptible individuals may be possible. Evidence to support such a view comes from epidemiological analysis of the contrast between localized and multiple osteoarthrosis[4], and from more recent findings on metabolic abnormalities in some patients with this disorder. The implications of these observations are to challenge the notion of arthrosis being a degenerative condition.

Ankylosing spondylitis

Currently, there is a great deal of interest in the human leucocyte antigens (HLA) as genetic markers. An association between ankylosing spondylitis and HLA-B27 has been demonstrated but the associations of gene products with other rheumatic disorders are less impressive. However, there is a tendency to oversimplify the interpretation of HLA associations[1]. These antigens are not disease markers. They provide some indication of genetically determined susceptibility or diathesis, but probably only incompletely, because other inherited forces are also likely to influence susceptibility.

Identification of the association between HLA-B27 and ankylosing spondylitis has altered our understanding in 3 ways. Firstly, it has led to controversy over whether or not the disease is more frequent than had previously been calculated from population surveys. Underlying the controversy is an element of circular reasoning because recourse is made to ill thought-out attempts to redefine the disease in terms of the antigenic status of individuals. The most extreme expression of this view postulates a new concept of HLA-B27 positive rheumatic disease.

A second, and much more significant, development is that with a marker for susceptibility, albeit only partial, the causal factor should be easier to identify. Rather than trying to detect pathogenic associations that are diluted amongst a majority of non-susceptible individuals and that obscure relationships, it is now possible to examine whether susceptible individuals respond in some unusual way to a microbe. The Klebsiella species are currently favoured as a causal factor by some workers. If the aetiological determinants of ankylosing spondylitis can be established in this way, then primary or secondary control of the disease might be possible.

A third way in which progress is being made depends on the use of antigen status as a measure of commonality in exploring the relationship between ankylosing spondylitis and other diseases. Clinical observers have for long been perplexed by the significance of spondylarthropathy developing in association with psoriasis, Reiter's disease, and inflammatory conditions of the bowel, such as ulcerative colitis and regional enteritis (see also Chapter 17). The unifying concept of the seronegative spondylarthropathies scarcely advances our understanding of the diseases, but the observation that there is also an increased frequency of HLA-B27 in patients with these other diseases has provided the basis for further exploration. The problem, which is common to most HLA associations, is that the degree of association tends to be less strong than in ankylosing spondylitis alone. The significance of this weaker relationship is much more difficult to determine.

Connective tissue diseases

Most of the disorders considered so far have been studied in population samples. The considerably lower frequency of conditions like systematic sclerosis, polymyositis, dermatomyositis, and polyarteritis nodosa, means that epidemiological studies must start from defined cases, and then try to identify the population from which they are drawn. Estimates of incidence and prevalence derived in this way have been reviewed by Wood[1].

Systematic lupus erythematosus (SLE) deserves more comment. As with the other collagen diseases there have been marked changes in diagnostic sensitivity over the last 30 years. This has led to increased case ascertainment, especially since the discovery of the lupus erythematosus (LE) cell marker and more recent tests. Appreciation of the spectrum of disease severity has been extended as a result. The reported higher prevalence in the USA is questionable. The disease appears to have predilection for women and for non-White Americans.

The nature of associations with drug exposure is difficult to assess. Precise measures of the frequency of a relatively uncommon condition are not easy to derive, and comparative estimates of the drug-induced state are even less accurate, particularly as it is not possible to challenge all the population at risk with the drug. Thus, whereas some of the mechanisms in thiazide-induced gout are clear, with drug-induced SLE it is uncertain whether the drugs cause a distinct and specific entity in a susceptible subpopulation, or whether they alter the threshold at which occult disease expresses itself.

Rheumatoid arthritis

Rheumatoid arthritis has been the subject of extensive epidemiological enquiries[7,8,9,1].

The principal frequency estimates are presented in Table 27.3.

Table 27.3. Estimates of the frequency of occurrence of various rheumatic disorders in the population of Great Britain (estimates in parenthesis are tentative; abridged from Wood[9]).

Rheumatic disorder	International Classification of Diseases (ICD) 8th revision	Prevalence per 100 population	Incidence per 100 persons per year
Rheumatoid arthritis	712.3	1.0	> 0.02
Osteoarthrosis	713	12.8	—
Gout	274	0.3	< 0.1
Ankylosing spondylitis	712.4	0.1	—
Connective tissue diseases	447, 716, 734, 734.1	0.02	0.0015
Back troubles	353, 717, 725, 728	(> 20.0)	(> 6.0)
Nonarticular rheumatism	717 (part) and 731 (part)	—	5.2
All		(> 35.0)	—

Rheumatoid factor

The discovery of the auto-antibody, rheumatoid factor (RF), raised hopes that it might be useful in screening for rheumatoid arthritis (RA). It appears to work reasonably well clinically. However, there are limitations when it is used in population studies, because a minority of people who are RF-positive have rheumatoid arthritis.

Rheumatoid factor is present in 75% of patients with rheumatoid arthritis (RA) and 5% of hospital non-RA patients. If these rates are applied to the general population:

In a sample of 1000 people—

2% or 20 have RA, so RF at 75% will be present in 15 people;

98% or 980 do not have RA, so RF at 5% will be present in 49 people.

The total with rheumatoid factor is 64.

Thus only 23% of RF-positive individuals will have rheumatoid arthritis.

The significance of this observation is that any biological explanation for the occurrence of rheumatoid factor has to reconcile its non-specificity with the disease-orientated hypotheses developed by clinical investigators.

Diagnostic criteria

Initial attempts at formulating diagnostic criteria for rheumatoid arthritis were based on the selection of characteristic clinical features of the disease. These neglected the potential distortion caused by duplicated information, which led to undue weight being attached to some aspects. This distortion can be avoided by selecting different classes of information. For example, 3 qualities of evidence go to the making of a clinical diagnosis of rheumatoid arthritis: clinical features in the joints – inflammatory polyarthropathy (IP); radiographic changes – erosive arthritis (EA); and serological characteristics – the presence of rheumatoid factor (RF) (Table 27.4). Once again, there are problems of non-specificity in population studies.

What is observed in Table 27.4 is a variable overlap in features, which can be represented by a Venn diagram (Fig. 27.1). The critical difficulty relates to what criteria or combination of criteria are necessary and sufficient to justify a diagnosis. Depending on how this is resolved, requiring 1, 2, or 3 of the features in Table 27.4, the prevalence of rheumatoid arthritis varies between less than 1 % and over 10 %. Some of the reasons for the discordance are fairly obvious. For example, certain of the 'objective' signs, such as radiographic changes, lag behind other developments in the disease process. However, these time differentials are not sufficient to account for the degree of discordance that is observed.

Table 27.4. Occurrence of features of rheumatoid arthritis (in the Leigh and Wensleydale population samples[10]).

		Number of respondents	Proportion of respondents (%)
No features		1968	89.6
1 feature	inflammatory polyarthropathy (IP)	100 ⎫	
	erosive arthritis (EA)	21 ⎬	8.7
	rheumatoid factor (RF)	70 ⎭	
2 features	IP & EA	8 ⎫	
	IP & RF	11 ⎬	1.0
	EA & RF	2 ⎭	
3 features	IP & EA & RF	15	0.7

Geographical variation

At first sight the marked differences in prevalence between countries appear interesting (Table 27.5). However, the variable sex ratio and the contrasting patterns of reported mortality raise doubts about the comparability of these data. Closer examination reveals that most of the variation in prevalence is contributed by individuals in whom the diagnosis was uncertain – 'probable cases' according to the nomenclature of the American Rheumatism Association (ARA). If only the definite cases are included then the prevalence of rheumatoid arthritis throughout the world appears to be uniform at about 1–2 % of the population. This lack of geographical variation is both unhelpful in providing clues to an aetiology, and biologically implausible.

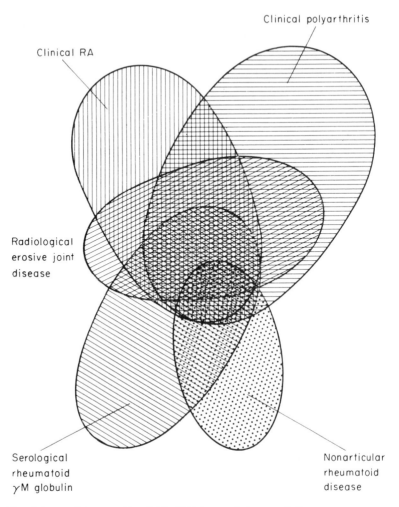

Fig. 27.1. Schema of rheumatoid arthritis (RA) in population sample[11].

Outcome and treatment

Many of the more important rheumatic disorders follow a chronic course and are a major cause of morbidity and disablement. 2 main classes of pharmacological agents are widely used in treatment. Non-steroidal anti-inflammatory drugs probably exert their principal action on the exudative component of the inflammatory process. In so doing, they make the patient more comfortable but the long-term outcome is probably not much influenced. A high frequency of adverse effects is encountered and anti-rheumatic drugs make a considerable contribution to therapeutic misadventures.

Table 27.5. Estimates of rheumatoid arthritis in different countries[12].

Country	Prevalence		Mortality	
	Probable & definite cases by ARA criteria (%)	Ratio of rates in the sexes (M:F)	Standardized death rate	Ratio of rates in the sexes (M:F)
Finland	7.5	1:2.5	46.9	1:3.2
German Federal Republic	5.7	1:0.5	33.2	1:2.4
UK	4.0	1:2.1	27.5	1:2.8
USA (Tecumseh)	2.5	1:4.7	13.6	1:2.1
Czechoslovakia	1.3	1:1.5	20.1	1:3.8
Japan	0.4	1:13.8	41.4	1:2.8

ARA American Rheumatism Association.

A different class of therapy is represented by the disease modifying drugs, such as penicillamine. These are likely to temper the proliferative component of inflammation and because of this they can improve the ultimate outcome of the disease. If these suppositions are correct, then there is a case for earlier and more aggressive use of such drugs. Epidemiologists have a part to play in 2 aspects of this situation. Clinicians have to balance the well-recognized hazards of therapy against the benefits that may be achieved. This requires a surveillance system to monitor adverse effects and a means of assessing benefits – to which epidemiological studies of disablement as an outcome measure can make an important contribution[13]. One then has to have a means of making choices, which may be illustrated by epidemiological approaches to prediction and therapeutic decision-making in relation to thromboembolism after hip replacement surgery[14].

References

1. Wood PHN. Epidemiology of rheumatic disorders, and nomenclature and classification in rheumatology. In: Scott JT, *Copeman's textbook of the rheumatic diseases*. 5th ed. London: Churchill Livingstone, 1978, Chapters 2 & 3.
2. Bird HA, Esselinckx W, *et al*. An evaluation of criteria for polymaglia rheumatica. *Annals of the Rheumatic Diseases* 1979; **38**: 434–9.
3. Badley EM, Meyrick JS, Wood PHN. Gout and serum uric acid levels in the Cotswolds. *Rheumatology and Rehabilitation* 1978; **17**: 133–42.
4. Wood PHN. Osteoarthrosis in the community. In: Wright V, ed. Osteoarthrosis. *Clinics in Rheumatic Diseases*. London: WB Saunders, 1976; **2** (3).
5. Wood PHN. Radiology in the diagnosis of arthritis and rheumatism. *Transactions of the Society of Occupational Medecine* 1972; **22**: 69–73.
6. Wood PHN. Rheumatic complaints. In: Epidemiology of non-communicable disease. *British Medical Bulletin* 1977; **27**: 82–8.

7. Bennett PH, Wood PHN, eds. *Population studies of the rheumatic diseases*. International Congress Series. No 148. Amsterdam: Excerpta Medica Foundation, 1968.

8. Lawrence JS. *Rheumatism in populations*. London: Heinemann Medical, 1977.

9. Wood PHN, ed. *The challenge of arthritis and rheumatism—a report in problems and progress in health care for rheumatic disorders*. London: British League against Rheumatism, 1977.

10. Kellgren JH. Joseph J Bunim memorial lecture—epidemiology of rheumatoid arthritis. *Arthritis and Rheumatism* 1966; **9**: 658–74.

11. Kellgren JH. Epidemiology of rheumatoid arthritis. In: Duthie JJR, Alexander WRM, eds. *Rheumatic diseases* Edinburgh: University Press, 1968: 8–17.

12. Wood PHN, Benn RT. Statistical appendix, digest of data on the rheumatic diseases 3: handicap and disability, and international comparisons of morbidity and mortality. *Annals of the Rheumatic Diseases* 1972; **31**: 72–7.

13. Wood PHN. In: *International classification of impairments, disabilities and handicaps—a manual of classification relating to the consequences of disease*. Geneva: World Health Organization, 1980.

14. Kelsey JL, Wood PHN, Charnley J. Predictions of thromboembolism following total hip replacement. *Clinical Orthopaedics* 1976; **114**: 247–58.

Chapter 28 · Multiple Sclerosis

EMER SHELLEY and G DEAN

Multiple sclerosis (MS) is the commonest chronic neurological disease of young adults in Europe and North America. The most frequent presenting symptoms, which may occur alone or in combination, are motor weakness, retrobulbar neuritis, paraesthesiae, unsteadiness in walking, double vision, vertigo and vomiting, and disturbance of micturition[1a]. When there is a classical history of relapse and remission of symptoms, clinical diagnosis rests on the demonstration of physical signs at 2 or more distinct sites in the central nervous system(CNS).

The causal agent or agents of MS are unknown. It is a demyelinating disease, with loss of the myelin sheath which normally coats nerve cells. Lesions are confined to the CNS, in which there are distinct sites of predilection and there is a more than chance tendency to symmetry of lesions. In early lesions, in addition to 'slender perivenular sleeves of selective demyelination'[1b], there are plasma cells, lymphocytes and microglia (the CNS macrophages) situated in cuffs around the small blood vessels.

Morbidity and mortality data problems

In order to appreciate the lack of completeness of ascertainment inherent in studies of the point prevalence rate of MS, it is necessary to have some knowledge of the varying course and prognosis of the disease. In any large series, 10 % of cases have no remission of symptoms following initial presentation. However, in a series of 586 cases '1 patient in 20 did not relapse until 15 or more years after the onset. In 4 cases the latent interval lasted over 30 years, the longest being 37 years'[1c]. A long latent period can lead to diagnostic difficulties. Some cases of MS may be asymptomatic and be revealed for the first time at post mortem examination.

In a population based survey of MS the majority of cases may be diagnosed with confidence, but in a sizeable minority less certainty may be attached to the diagnosis. Criteria have been specified for the categorization of cases into definite, probable or possible MS[1d], or alternatively, since some would argue that the diagnosis is only definite at autopsy, into 2 categories–probable and possible. Opinions differ among epidemiologists as to whether 'possible' disease should be included in epidemiological comparisons[2a]. Such difficulties may be reduced in the future by the inclusion of results of laboratory investigations in the categorization process, thereby increasing the probability of correct diagnosis.

The pattern of alterations in the cell content, total protein and immunoglobulin levels in the cerebro-spinal fluid (CSF), while not specific, is highly suggestive of MS[3a]. Noninvasive techniques may be used to confirm lesions in the CNS, or to demonstrate asymptomatic and clinically unsuspected lesions. For example, a black and white checker-board pattern presented to a subject causes a volley of impulses to travel from the retina along the optic pathways. The resulting 'visually evoked potentials' may be recorded over the occipital cortex and give information about the integrity of the visual pathways. Lesions demonstrated by techniques such as this may support a clinical diagnosis of MS.

'Population-based surveys' may convey images of a door-to-door search for diseased individuals. In practice, such surveys focus attention on those who have presented with symptoms which could have been caused by MS. The completeness of ascertainment depends on the willingness of the general population to seek medical advice, the level of medical care, the number of trained neurologists, the standard of medical records and the enthusiasm of the investigators[4a]. In MS, incidence rates are rarely used because the numbers are so small and because almost all such incidence rates have been retrospectively calculated from prevalence data. Case registers for MS have been kept, such as those in Denmark, Northern Ireland and Rochester, Minnesota[4a]. These registers have yielded valuable data on incidence and prevalence of MS. The register in Rochester has shown that while the incidence of MS has remained constant over 60 years, the prevalence of MS has doubled. This is probably a reflection of an improvement in the treatment of complications of MS.

Mortality data underestimate the number of persons dying with MS[1e]. An intercurrent condition or a complication of MS may be the immediate cause of death. For comparative epidemiology it is necessary to ensure that mortality data includes cases where MS was a contributory cause of death in addition to deaths caused primarily by MS. In approximately 30 % of diagnosed cases of MS, the diagnosis is not mentioned on the death certificate.

Incidence and prevalence

Age and sex

The risk of developing the disease rises in adolescence, reaches a peak in the early 30s and falls away in the 60s, largely irrespective of incidence or prevalence rates. Women are affected more frequently than men, with a ratio of 3:2, and at a younger age (Fig. 28.1).

World distribution

Using information from many different studies it is possible to divide the world into zones of high, medium and low risk for MS, with prevalence rates of ≥ 40,

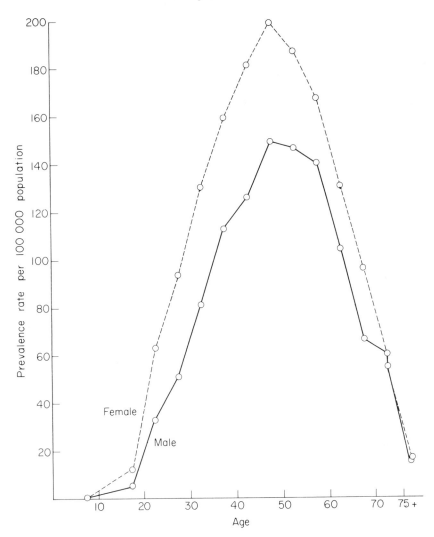

Fig. 28.1. Age- and sex-specific prevalence rates of probable multiple sclerosis in Ireland, Census Day 1971. A total of 1951 cases (818 men, 1133 women) gave a crude prevalence rate of 65.5 per 100 000 population. (Brady R, Dean G, *et al.* Multiple sclerosis in the Republic of Ireland. *Journal of the Irish Medical Association* 1977; **70**: 500–6.)

20–39 and < 20 per 100 000 respectively[5]. When data first appeared it was thought that there was a relationship between prevalence rates in an area and latitude north and south of the equator. While there seems to be a reasonably clear separation into 3 zones of MS risk, latitude alone is insufficient to explain the location of these zones in Europe and in America, while the relationship between prevalence rates and latitude is even less clear in Asia and the Pacific[2b].

In Europe, the high risk zone extends from 45° to 65° North latitude. Iceland, the British Isles, northern France, Holland, Belgium, Germany and Poland lie within the high risk zone. Very high prevalence rates (greater than 1 per 1000) have been reported from the Orkney and Shetland islands and North-East Scotland. The Scandinavian countries have a high risk except along the Atlantic coast of Norway and in the extreme north, which are medium risk zones.

Low rates have been reported from Italy, and intermediate rates from southern France and southern Switzerland. The high prevalence of MS among Italian immigrants hospitalized in the Greater London area[6] suggests, however, that the prevalence in Italy as a whole is not greatly different to that in the United Kingdom. No MS patients were found among the immigrants from Malta, although the expected number at the United Kingdom-born rate was 9.7. Recent studies found a high MS prevalence rate in Enna city, Sicily (53 per 100 000)[7], but a very low rate in the neighbouring islands of Malta (4 per 100 000)[8]. Thus the Mediterranean region acts as a border area between zones of high–medium MS risk and low risk zones.

Details of the distribution of MS on a world-wide basis are contained in accounts by Acheson[5] and Kurtzke[2b]. Briefly, in North America, the prevalence of MS increases as one moves from New Orleans to Winnipeg. Furthermore, both North and South, MS was found to be less frequent in American Blacks than in Whites. Mexico, South America and all of Asia appear to be areas of low MS risk. Careful studies have confirmed that MS is rare in Japan. Australia and New Zealand are medium risk zones.

Migration

Studies of groups of migrants have yielded useful results. South Africa is an area of low risk for MS. Immigrants to South Africa from northern Europe were found to have a 3 times greater risk of MS than immigrants from the Mediterranean countries, but White immigrants from other African states had a lower risk.[9] However, those who migrated from Europe to South Africa below the age of 15 years had a low risk of developing MS.

In Israel MS was found to be common among immigrants from Europe and rare among immigrants from Afro-Asian countries[4b]. Native Israelis of either European or Afro-Asian ethnic origin had prevalence and incidence rates which were quite similar to those of the European immigrants. Immigrants from Europe who migrate to Israel before the age of 15 have a low MS risk.

In the study of 3970 first hospital admissions for MS in Greater London, there was a marked deficit of cases among those who had emigrated from India (1 Indian), Pakistan (none), Africa (1 African) and New Commonwealth America (the West Indies; 16)[6]. This suggests that these areas have a low incidence of MS, and that the risk of MS was not increased by migration to an area of high risk.

An epidemic of MS

The incidence of MS in any area is thought to be constant over long periods of time. An exception to this was the 'epidemic' which has been reported on the Faröe Islands, with 18 definite cases being diagnosed from 1944 to 1960[10]. In contrast, no case was recorded between 1929 and 1943 and there were only 2 cases with onset between 1960 and 1974. It was suggested that a slow virus with a long incubation period was introduced to the Faröe Islands during the British occupation from 1940–44. It has also been suggested that the epidemic of MS may be related to the severe outbreak of canine distemper which occurred on the islands in the 1940s[11].

Genetic predisposition

MS occurs with increased frequency among close relatives of those who already have MS. Prevalence rates for siblings and for parents of patients with MS have been calculated to be about 8 and 4 times the expectations for the general population[4c].

That the increased familial incidence has a genetic component was confirmed with discovery of the human leucocyte antigen (HLA) system. It is accepted that HLA types A3, B7 and Dw2 are found more frequently in caucasoid patients with MS than in the general population. Dw2 is more strongly associated with MS than is B7 which in turn is more strongly associated than A3. HLA-Dw2 was found in 70 % of Danish MS patients compared with 16 % of the normal Danish population[12]. In some families the development of MS has been shown to segregate with histocompatibility type.

Close to the genes which determine HLA type are genes which code for antigens on B lymphocytes, known as immune region associated antigens (HLA-DR). An association has been found between HLA-DRw2 and MS in caucasoids[12]. Further, a locally defined antigen BT101, closely related to DRw2, was significantly associated with an increased risk of developing MS in patients with isolated optic neuritis.

There is a steady decrease from Northern to Southern Europe in the strength of the association between MS and HLA-A3, B7, and Dw2 and DRw2. Specifically different associations are found in Mediterranean and Japanese populations of MS patients.

The mechanism whereby genes determining histocompatibility type leads to increased susceptibility to MS is unknown. The animal model for human MS is experimental allergic encephalomyelitis (EAE). Repeated injections of aqueous solutions of rabbit brain into monkeys produce a diffuse encephalomyelitis, the antigen responsible being a basic protein of the myelin sheath. In the rat, susceptibility to EAE has been shown to be under the control of immune response genes, closely linked to the major histocompatibility locus.

Environmental factors

An infectious agent?

Why does migration from a high to low risk zone before the age of 15 lead to a reduction in the risk of developing MS? It has been suggested that the causative agent of MS is a common disease of childhood, possibly a virus gastro-intestinal infection[13]. Those who escape early infection because of a high level of domestic hygiene or a colder climate may, if they are so predisposed, develop the adult form of the disease, that is, MS. Migration to a low risk zone at a young age may increase the probability of contracting the illness in childhood, thereby reducing the risk of developing MS in adult life.

Groups of MS patients have been found to have slightly raised antibody titres to measles virus or to herpes or pox-virus when compared with control groups. In a review of studies of antibody titres in MS, it was concluded that in a study with a large group of patients and controls, possibly only the antibody to measles virus would be increased in MS when compared with controls[14]. This association must be interpreted with caution. It may mean that the measles antibody levels act as a marker of an abnormal immune response to viruses in patients with MS.

Belief in the importance of an infectious agent has been strengthened by the discovery of the 'granulocytopenic factor.' Inoculation of mice with MS tissue produced a granulocytopenia and serum from such mice induced a granulocytopenia in other mice[15]. Cell cultures of mouse fibroblasts have been inoculated with MS material. The cell-free lysate from the 18th passage also produced a granulocytopenia when inoculated into mice. This suggests that a transmissible agent plays a role in the aetiology of MS.

Diet

The high prevalence of MS in the more northern countries may be associated with a high dietary fat intake. Incidence and prevalence is high in inland areas of Norway in contrast to the low risk coastal areas which have a lower fat intake with a higher proportion of polyunsaturated fatty acids. The myelin sheath is mainly composed of lipids and there is a change in the relative proportions of saturated and unsaturated fatty acids in the brain lipids of patients with MS.

It has been reported that vegetable oil supplements taken for more than 20 years, with a low animal fat intake, gave better relapse and survival rates when compared with rates reported in the literature[16]. A double-blind trial of linoleate supplementation in MS patients found that the rate of relapse per patient-year was less for the treated group than for the control group, though the difference was not statistically significant[17]. However, there was a significant reduction in the severity of relapses in the treated group. Serum linoleate is reduced in MS, and oral supplementation produced an increase in serum linoleate. The numbers in this trial were small. Many believe that further large scale trials are justified. In the meantime, it has been suggested that a diet which restricts fat intake to vegetable oils and margarines with a high content of polyunsaturated fatty acids 'may possibly contribute to a more favourable course of MS'[3b].

No other treatment has been shown to be of benefit in MS. It is still controversial whether the use of corticosteriods or corticotrophins is of value, though there is consensus that their use should be limited to short courses during acute exacerbations of MS.

Health care planning for MS patients

Health care planning with regard to MS must concentrate on the alleviation of medico-social problems. The *Manual on MS*[3] issued under the auspices of the International Federation of Multiple Sclerosis Societies, lists the following medico-social needs of those with MS:

1 qualified medical care;
2 continuous active physiotherapy when needed;
3 aids in maintaining employability and protection in the work environment;
4 vocational guidance – re-education to new occupation;
5 occupational therapy;
6 transportation;
7 adaptation of the home to the patient's needs, home help;
8 advice in the management of personal affairs (business matters, personal problems, sex life);
9 information and advice to family members;
10 social contacts and recreational activities;
11 nursing care;
12 economic security.

The requirements of an individual patient will be determined by his disabilities and social circumstances. The Multiple Sclerosis Society* or the Action for Research into Multiple Sclerosis† organization may help by providing home visits or a telephone counselling service[18]. It is hoped that active support of the patient and his family may prolong the period for which home care is possible and postpone the decision to transfer to a nursing home.

Conclusion

There can be no doubt that epidemiological studies have contributed to an understanding of the genetic and environmental factors leading to the development of MS. Recognition of the increased familial incidence of MS, the geographic variations in prevalence, the effects of migration and the possibility of

* Multiple Sclerosis Society, 4 Tachbrook Street, London SWIV ISJ.

† Action for Research into Multiple Sclerosis (ARMS), 71 Grays Inn Road, London WCIX 8TR. Telephone counselling service: 01–568 2255.

an association with a diet high in animal fats, have provided scientists in other disciplines with a framework within which to form and test hypotheses. Progress has been made with the recognition of an association with particular histocompatibility types, in the search for a transmissible agent, and in the study of abnormal lipid metabolism in patients with MS. The co-ordination of knowledge derived from epidemiology, virology, immunology, pathology, biochemistry and other disciplines will continue to be necessary until a clearer understanding is obtained of the aetiology of MS and means are found for its prevention and treatment.

References

1. McAlpine D, Lumsden CE, Acheson ED. *Multiple sclerosis, a reappraisal.* London: Churchill Livingstone, 1972.
   a = p. 135; b = p. 319; c = p. 206; d = p. 202; e = p. 9.
2. Field EJ, ed. *Multiple sclerosis, a critical conspectus.* Lancaster: MTP Press Limited, 1977.
   a = p. 22 & p. 102; b = pp. 83–142.
3. Bauer HJ. *A manual on multiple sclerosis.* Vienna: International Federation of Multiple Sclerosis Societies, 1977.
   a = p. 9; b = p. 42; c = p. 64.
4. Field EJ, Bell TM, Carnegie PR, eds. *Multiple sclerosis, progress in research.* Amsterdam: North Holland Publishing Company, 1972.
   a = p. 230—246; b = p. 196.
5. Acheson ED. Epidemiology of multiple sclerosis. *British Medical Bulletin* 1977; **33** (1): 9–14.
6. Dean G, McLoughlin H, *et al.* Multiple sclerosis among immigrants in Greater London. *British Medical Journal* 1976; i: 861–4.
7. Dean G, Grimaldi G, *et al.* Multiple sclerosis in southern Europe I: prevalence in Sicily in 1975. *Journal of Epidemiology and Community Health* 1979; **33** (2): 107–10.
8. Vassallo L, Elian M, Dean G. Multiple sclerosis in southern Europe II: prevalence in Malta 1978. *Journal of Epidemiology and Community Health* 1979; **33** (2): 111–13.
9. Dean G, Kurtzke JF. On the risk of multiple sclerosis according to age at immigration to South Africa. *British Medical Journal* 1971; iii: 725–9.
10. Kurtzke JF, Hyllested K. Multiple sclerosis: an epidemic disease in the Faröes. *Transactions of the American Neurology Association* 1975; **100**: 213–5.
11. Cook SD, Dowling PC, Russell WC. Multiple sclerosis and canine distemper. *Lancet* 1978; i: 605–6.
12. Batchelor JR, Compston A. McDonald WI. The significance of the association between HLA and multiple sclerosis. *British Medical Bulletin* 1978; **34** (3): 279–84.
13. Dean G. Annual incidence, prevalence and mortality of multiple sclerosis in White South African-born and in White immigrants to South Africa. *British Medical Journal* 1967; ii: 724–30.
14. Frazer KB. Multiple sclerosis: a virus disease? *British Medical Bulletin* 1977; **33** (1): 34–9.
15. Carp RI, Licursi PC, *et al.* Decreased percentage of polymorphonuclear neutrophils in mouse peripheral blood after inoculation with material from multiple sclerosis patients. *Journal of Experimental Medicine* 1972; **136**: 618–29.
16. Swank RL. Multiple sclerosis: twenty years on a low fat diet. *Archives of Neurology* 1970; **23**: 460–73.
17. Millar JHD, Zelka KJ, *et al.* Double-blind trial of linoleate supplementation of the diet in multiple sclerosis. *British Medical Journal* 1973; i: 765–8.
18. Burnfield A, Burnfield P. Common psychological problems in multiple sclerosis. *British Medical Journal* 1978; i: 1193–4.

Chapter 29 · Epilepsy

E M ROSS

The unqualified word 'epilepsy' (epi-*lambano*: Greek—a taking hold of) has no more precision than terms like 'gastritis' or 'chest diseases'. There are many 'epilepsies', the prevalence of which varies at different ages and between the sexes. Adequate prevalence studies have been available for only the last 30 years. Little is known about the epidemiology of epilepsy in underdeveloped countries.

Cerebral seizures have been defined as abnormal, sudden, excessive electrical discharges of neurones (grey matter) which propagate down the neuronal processes (white matter) to affect an end organ in a clinically measurable fashion[1]. The diagnosis of epilepsy demands that seizures be recurrent and unassociated with acute febrile incidents. Febrile convulsions, single seizures and acute manifestations of abnormal metabolic states are not conventionally regarded as epilepsy. Proper epidemiological studies of epilepsy must exclude patients with transient fainting attacks and undefinable 'funny turns', that can easily masquerade as epilepsy and may be misdiagnosed by the unwary doctor. There is, however, no single method by which a totally confident diagnosis of epilepsy can be made. The diagnosis is primarily clinical, and relies on the accurate analysis of contemporary eye witness accounts of attacks. It is not possible to confirm that the person has or does not have epilepsy solely on the basis of an electro-encephalogram (e.e.g.) or on the result of any other diagnostic tests. This means that the diagnosis often cannot be confirmed until the person has had several witnessed attacks.

The epidemiology of epilepsy poses problems because many affected people keep the condition to themselves. Patients tend to consult many doctors, both in hospital and General Practice, in the course of their lives. This makes the study of prognosis very difficult. Therefore, it is not surprising that the prevalence rates of epilepsy derived from different studies vary markedly and are much influenced by study design.

Seizures in the new-born

The incidence of fits in the new-born varies markedly in different series, reflecting both differing definitions and widely varying standards of perinatal care available in different centres. From an analysis of babies with 'cerebral signs' in the first week of life, Chamberlain[2] reported that 0.4% of 16 000 children included in the 1970 British Births Survey had 1 or more seizure. Of these infants one-fifth died, two-thirds of whom weighed under 2.5 kg at birth. Fits in the new-born have many different causes. Metabolic seizures, particularly those due to low serum calcium or sugar, are readily preventable. Neonatal meningitis often presents with seizures and has a poor prognosis. Congenital malformations of the brain affect about 3 per 1000 children and some of these present with seizures.

The role of birth trauma, as a preventable factor in the causation of epilepsy, poses the epidemiologist great problems and remains an important area of debate. In the mid 1950s Lilienfeld and Pasaminick[3] summed up a long held view that fits were part of a 'continuum of reproductive casualty'. In other words, the most severely brain damaged baby dies at birth, those less severely affected may be left with degrees of brain damage, including cerebral palsy and fits, to some extent proportionate to the degree of injury suffered at birth. This theory was based on Mayo Clinic experience. The authors acknowledged that 25 % of cases of epilepsy had no available birth records, which greatly weakens their case.

Mellor[4] studied 128 Aberdeen school children with epilepsy who had no obvious post neonatal causes. 40 children with a strong family history of epilepsy had no greater perinatal risk factors, whereas the 88 without a family history of epilepsy had considerably more adverse features in their perinatal history than had children in a control group matched for sex, social class, age and school attended. Single adverse perinatal events do not seem to play a major role in the cause of epilepsy. As an illustration, of the 64 children at age 11 who had epilepsy in the 1958 perinatal mortality study, 5 had obvious perinatal problems; 2 of these were associated with severe jaundice, a now largely preventable condition. The study showed no greater chance of epilepsy in children whose birth presentation or delivery was abnormal unless it was totally unattended. Low birth weight children tend to have complex coexisting congenital abnormalities. These findings, together with those from other recent series suggest that when good perinatal care is available, seizure disorders directly due to perinatal problems should be rare.

Epilepsy and multiple handicap

Many people with epilepsy have multiple problems. In recent studies[5], 1 in 3 epileptic children have been shown to require education at special schools, mainly because of mental handicap. Patients with demonstrable brain damage are particularly likely to develop epilepsy. When intellectual deterioration occurs it is very difficult to determine whether it has been due to the occurrence of fits or to progressive brain disease.

Diagnosis

The nomenclature of epilepsy gradually expanded through the centuries and led to differences of definition in different countries. In 1969 the International

League Against Epilepsy[6] proposed a standard definition for epilepsy and for its subtypes. They proposed that cases be divided into 'generalized', where the fit affects both sides of the body with equal severity, and 'partial', where part of the body is not affected. The disorders were further divided into those of primary aetiology (unknown cause) or secondary (known cause). A third 'unclassifiable' category is needed to account for those where the cause is uncertain.

Although this classification is still not used universally by clinicians, it forms the basis for comparison of one country's experience with that of another. Unfortunately a wide diversity of definitions has been used in recent epidemiological investigations making great problems in comparing results. As an illustration of these difficulties, Kurland[7], in a 40 year analysis of data derived from the Mayo Clinic included both 'any patient whose seizure has occurred during the 5 years preceding this (prevalence) day as 'active' as well as any patient who had been on anticonvulsant medication within 5 years of the prevalence day even if seizure-free during this period'. Pond et al.[8] in a study of English General Practice populations, defined an epileptic 'as a patient who had had epileptic fits of any sort at some time during the 2 years prior to the time of the survey, or who had been on regular anticonvulsants during this period'. In a study of children aged 5–14 years in the Isle of Wight, Rutter et al.[9] required that 'to be regarded as having epilepsy a child must have had a definite fit since he started school, and during the previous 12 months there must have been either a fit or the child must have taken regular anticonvulsants'.

Prevalence

Clinicians vary amongst themselves in their readiness to label a person as having epilepsy. Most clinical data about epilepsies has been derived from individual case studies largely carried out in the main neurology centres. These centres tend to see only the most severely affected patients. Out-patient studies based on hospital clinics, particularly those in large cities, are not usually able to follow up patients long enough to learn much about prognosis. There is conflicting evidence concerning the value of hospitals for case finding purposes. Crombie[10] who carried out a study under the aegis of the Royal College of General Practitioners, reported that 75 % of patients with epilepsy were entirely treated by their family doctor. In contrast, the Carlisle population study[11] in a similar period, found that 78 % of patients had seen specialists. General Practices tend to exclude the most seriously affected, especially those permanently resident in institutions. Neither type of study has access to those who do not seek treatment. Costeff[12], from an area of Israel well endowed with medical services, reported that many children were never brought to medical attention following fits. This does not seem to apply in the United Kingdom as only 12 parents of 15 000 children in the National Child Development Study reported that their child had seizures but had not been seen by a doctor[5], during their first twelve years.

Epileptic conditions can remit and it is necessary to know when patients can be considered free from their condition. The nature of attacks often changes with the passage of time and these constraints make longitudinal studies both necessary and difficult to interpret. These difficulties account for widely varying opinions about prognosis. An ideal study of people with epilepsy would involve a cohort of several hundred affected persons followed up over an entire life span. A cohort study involving 200 children, the minimum needed to explore some of the less common forms of epilepsy, would require the follow-up of 40 000 births.

There is no shortage of recent prevalence studies from the USA and from Northern Europe, all of which have endeavoured to quantify the size and nature of the problem in child populations. Few studies have been published on adults and old people and there is little reliable information from developing countries or from Eastern Europe.

Rose *et al.*[13] reviewed over 30 prevalence studies of epilepsy in children. Rates varied from 150 per 1000 children, with fits of all types in the tropical island of Guam (although the proportion with afebrile epileptic seizures at 3 per 1000 was no higher than that found by the same workers in the USA), to the lowest figure of 1.5 per 1000 reported in Japanese school children. Rose's own child study, based on postal enquiries to parents, yielded a high rate of epilepsy (16 per 1000) by USA and European standards. Their study illustrates well the fact that both the method used and the definition of epilepsy greatly influence findings.

Since most recent studies have suggested that about 5 per 1000 of the population have a history of some form of epilepsy, it is necessary to study very large yet geographically discrete populations, in order to explore the epidemiology of subgroups in adequate detail. The best example of this approach comes from Iceland[14] where a single enthusiastic neurologist attempted to trace every person with epilepsy among the 200 000 population, even to the extent of conducting neurological examinations and taking histories in fields and freezer factories! Examples of other closed population studies include those in a sparsely populated area of Finland,[15] the Mayo Clinic catchment area in Minnesota, USA[7], in Carlisle, England[11], and among the British child populations of Aberdeen[4], Bedford[16], Bristol[17] and the Isle of Wight[9]. Table 29.1 summarizes the findings from 8 large well conducted studies of non-febrile epilepsy in the age group 10–20 years from developed countries in the Northern Hemisphere.

Epilepsy in developing countries

Reports of high rates of epilepsy have emerged from African, Asian and South American countries[19]. These have been interpreted as suggesting that the epilepsy rate is up to 4–5 times higher than in industrialized countries. However, it is very difficult to undertake true community studies in underdeveloped countries and most of these reports stem from hospital centres thereby presenting

Table 29.1. Prevalence of epilepsy[17].

Investigator		Age group (years)	Population	Number with epilepsy	Rate per 1000
Crombie et al.[10]	England & Wales	10–14	22 336	88	3.9
Gudmundsson[14]	Iceland	10–19	32 872	143	4.3
Cooper[18]	England, Scotland & Wales	11	3 934	23	7.1
Sillanpaa[15]	Turku, Finland	10–15	108 019	340	3.2
Rutter et al.[9]	Isle of Wight	5–14	11 865	86	7.2
Kurland[7]	Rochester, USA	10–19	3 763	13	3.4
Ross et al.[5]	England, Scotland & Wales	11	15 496	64	4.1
Ross[17]	Bristol	11–16	25 165	110	4.3
Total			223 450	867	
Average					3.9

a major problem of definition and interpretation. Poor perinatal services, malnutrition and parasitism are all potent factors in the development of epilepsy which can be used as a marker of the quality of health. The high price of anticonvulsants and lack of skilled diagnostic services together with local taboos and prejudices greatly worsen the lot of affected people.

Cohort studies

2 cohort (segment of the population born around the same time period) studies have been reported from the USA. The first[20] involved children of subscribers to a pre-paid health care scheme, from birth to age 6. The second[21] followed 50 000 children from birth in University towns for 7 years. A further 2 studies from England, Scotland and Wales used 1 week national birth cohorts in 1946[18] and 1958[5] as a basis for studies of epilepsy in childhood through to adolescence.

National Child Development Study

The National Child Development Study[5] included questions about fits in a detailed review of health, social welfare and educational progress at ages 7, 11 and 16 (Table 29.2). It was supplemented by extra questionnaires completed by general practitioners and hospital doctors for children who developed epilepsy in their first 11 years. Although 8 % of children in the study had at least 1 recorded attack of altered consciousness or possible seizure during their first 11 years, the great majority of these were transient events such as breath holding attacks or faints. Nearly 2 % had a single attack and a further 1 % had repeated febrile convulsions. Despite extensive enquiries, it was difficult to verify the diagnosis of

Table 29.2. Convulsive histories in 14 190 11-year olds[5].

	n	Rate per 1000
Definite epilepsy (a)	64	4.5
Disputed epilepsy (b)	39	2.4
Febrile convulsions	366	26.0
Fits with meningitis only	12	0.8
Breath-holding, tantrums faints etc.	605	46.0

(a) Cases where information returned fulfilled study definition of epilepsy.
(b) Cases where children had been labelled by family doctor as having epilepsy, yet did not fulfil study diagnosis.
n Total number observed.

Table 29.3. Age of onset of convulsive disorders in National Child Development Study[5].

Age of onset (years)	Number	%
1	15	23
1–2	8	12.5
3–4	16	25
5–6	11	17
7+	14	22
Total	64	100

epilepsy in 39 cases (0.24%). One doctor might affirm the diagnosis and another deny it. Such disputed cases, leaving 64 (0.4%) with a definite diagnosis.

Most children destined to develop epilepsy by age 16 had their first fit before the age of 5 (Table 29.3). About 2.5 per 1000 children had seizures between ages 9 and 11 years. Slightly fewer (2.0 per 1000) had an earlier history only.

Of the 64 children with epilepsy, 35 (55%) had generalized seizures of a grand mal type. Of the remainder 18 (28%) had a variable pattern of seizures that could not be allocated to a particular category. 8 (12.5%) had a mixed picture of petit mal (brief seizures associated with momentary blank episodes) and grand mal symptoms but only 1 child had uncomplicated petit mal. 2 children had a history with features of temporal lobe (psychomotor) epilepsy but their features were not entirely characteristic.

Seizures form the most common reason for admission of children to many hospitals. An estimate of the occurrence of fits in child patients of an average sized General Practice (Table 29.4) shows a very low rate per practice for the subtypes of epilepsy. The average general practitioner, thus, gets relatively little day-to-day experience in their management.

Table 29.4. Frequency of fits in children: (National Child Development Study (1958) cohort)[5].

Type of fit	Ever occurred among the 2500 children of a 10 000 patient Group Practice per year	Number of new cases likely in this practice in a year
Any loss of consciousness	250	14
Fits in first week of life	6	< 1
First febrile convulsion	50	3
Repeat febrile convulsion	15	1
Temper tantrums and breath holding	45	2
Infantile spasms	< 1	≤ 1
Non-febrile epilepsy	10	≤ 1
Petit mal	< 1	≤ 1
Grand mal	6	≤ 1
Temporal lobe	< 1	≤ 1
Mixed types	2	≤ 1

The concept of a single cause for epilepsy has long been abandoned. A careful search for known factors that are recognized causes of brain damage largely excluded single perinatal factors, though 5 children had been exposed to them in combination. Only 15 children in 64 were considered to have had a possible definite cause, of which half might now be preventable. (Table 29.5). No possible aetiological factors could be found in three-quarters of cases. This is a challenge to the epidemiologist and future cohort studies may require inclusion of detailed virological and immunological investigations.

The child with epilepsy requires appropriate medical management. Many of the children in the study were on either excessive or inadequate drug regimes. Other studies have shown that many children do not take their drugs in prescribed doses.

Table 29.5. Cause of epilepsy in children: (National Child Development Study (1958) cohort)[5].

Causal agent	*n*	Currently preventable
Congenital disorders	3	0
Birth hazard	5	5
Postnatal infection	4	0
Postnatal accident	2	2
Clear cut role of inheritance	1	?
Sub total	15	7
No aetiological clue	49	
Total	64	

n Total number observed.

Two-thirds of the children attended normal schools. By the age of 16 their educational attainment in reading and mathematics, though inferior, was within 1 standard deviation of the mean for children without epilepsy. Those at special schools had minimal educational achievements and most would need sheltered employment, mainly on account of handicaps other than epilepsy (Table 29.6).

Recent studies have found that those with relatively mild epilepsy may be less well-adjusted and have an inferior self image than those who are more seriously affected. As a group, the National Child Development Study children with severe epilepsy were much more likely to be bullied at school and have prolonged absence, yet less likely to be regarded as aggressive or delinquent than the less affected children.

Table 29.6. Major reasons for special education (11 years): (National Child Development Study (1958) cohort)[5].

Reason	Number of Children
Epilepsy alone	3
Educational backwardness (ESN)	6
Severe retardation (SSN)	3
Deafness	1
Cerebral palsy	2
Behaviour problems (including autism)	3
Other reasons	3
Total	21

Long-term studies

Clinicians often experience difficulties in categorizing epilepsy. Classification has to be reviewed at frequent intervals because clinical features often change as children grow older. Many become fit-free with the passage of time, although freedom from recurrence can never be guaranteed. Few long-term studies of epilepsy from childhood to adult life have been completed and more information is needed. Harrison and Taylor[22] in a 25 year study found that the majority of children with epilepsy grew up to be healthy adults but a quarter either died or spent their lives as multiply-handicapped adults in institutions.

Long-term studies are particularly valuable to the understanding of convulsive disorders with a progressive nature, such as temporal lobe epilepsy, which may take many years to manifest its full extent. Birth injury, congenital hamartomata and febrile convulsions have been incriminated as causes. In a careful long-term study of 106 surgically treated cases in Denmark over a 15 year period, Jensen[23] found that 25 patients became completely seizure free, and the majority showed some improvement.

Prevention

Only a minority of patients who have severe permanent brain damage following meningitis or trauma develop epilepsy. The reasons are not clear and cannot be explained in terms of histology. Kurland[24] from a study of head injuries, found 11.6 % of those with the most severe injuries had post-traumatic seizures in the following 5 years, with much lower rates in those with less serious injury and amongst children. The conventional explanation is that every individual has a personal threshold for the development of seizures which can be lowered by brain damage, fatigue, certain states of mind, fluid and electrolyte retention and raised by anticonvulsant drugs.

Genetic factors have been widely studied and implicated as a cause of seizures. However, they do not obey simple Mendelian rules. The Metrakos[25] studies suggest that certain abnormal e.e.g. patterns are inherited but may not result in expressed disease. The study of family histories presents problems because parents of young children who have had fits may never be told and hospital medical records are often only kept for 7 years. The causes for most epilepsy are not known and primary prevention is rarely possible. The prevention of accidents and effective treatment of brain illnesses will result in the reduction of secondary epilepsies, which tend to be severe and are commonly associated with multiple pathology.

Because there is no effective prophylaxis for epilepsy, screening has little merit. Petit mal is frequently missed and deserves thought during school medical examinations because, untreated, it may result in poor learning. Children with epilepsy need continuing provision of high quality consistent medical and social advice and a preparedness to recognize remission and withdraw treatment.

Implications for planning

The United Kingdom Government sponsored report *People with epilepsy* in 1969[26] suggested that about 300 000 people in England and Wales have epilepsy, though under 20 000 are registered as disabled. In practical terms, about 2–3 per 1000 of the population live in a shadow of attacks. This rate appears to be relatively constant throughout life. The greater mortality of young congenitally handicapped children with epilepsy is counter-balanced by the later development of epilepsy in adolescence following trauma, especially road accidents, and in older patients with arterial degeneration and tumours. It has been estimated[5] that in England, Scotland and Wales there are about 2000–2500 school leavers each year with a history of 2 or more seizures, of whom 650 will require sheltered employment and residential care. Most of the latter group have multiple handicaps, particularly mental backwardness, as well as epilepsy. They have great employment problems and many require sheltered workshops. The need for residential centres for people with epilepsy has been declining since the advent of more effective anticonvulsants and as local community care improves.

Febrile convulsions

The study of epilepsy is complicated by the many young children who have seizures of a typical grand mal type solely in the course of acute febrile illnesses. Febrile seizures have been described as 'the purest form of epilepsy' yet they do not fulfil the usual definition of epilepsy which excludes episodes which have occurred solely in the course of febrile illness. Such seizures are usually brief and innocuous but occasionally children who have a febrile seizure present later with afebrile seizures. It is difficult to place febrile convulsions in a scheme of epilepsies, they are important because they are much more common than afebrile epilepsy, being reported as affecting between 2 and 15 % of all children[27]. They are the commonest single reason for admission to children's medical beds.

Febrile fits terrify parents: 75 % of parents in a recent series thought their child was about to die. The relationship of febrile convulsions to non-febrile epilepsy has been a matter of considerable controversy. A hospital study found evidence of acute viral infection in 83 % of children with febrile convulsions compared with 40 % of control cases with acute gastro-intestinal symptoms[28]. Febrile convulsions tend to run in families, suggesting that they have a lower threshold to the condition, the trigger being acute viral illness. In a study of 1706 children in the USA with a history of febrile seizures[21], those with abnormal or suspect neurological status before their febrile fits were at higher risk of later non-febrile seizures (20 per 1000) than the majority. Those who were normal before their febrile seizures had a susbsequent epilepsy rate of 11 per 1000, only twice that for children who never had febrile fits.

The question is whether these first convulsions are merely misdiagnosed cases of epilepsy or whether febrile convulsions in themselves damage the brain, causing scarring which occasionally acts as a focus for later epilepsy. If the latter is the case, it poses the further question: what is the mechanism? It has been postulated that it could be due to viral damage or hypoxaemia, or a combination of both. The former explanation is probably correct in most instances. Detailed hospital based studies, carried out in Edinburgh and Cardiff[29] have delineated characteristics of children prone to febrile convulsions. It has been widely debated whether these children should be treated with long-term anticonvulsant drugs. Although the febrile seizure rate can be reduced in this way, a review of evidence by the USA National Institute of Health[1] concluded that 'there is no evidence to support the concept that prolonged therapy with anticonvulsants prevents the development of epilepsy or significant neurological defects, though anticonvulsants may be advisable where fits are prolonged, focal or followed by neurological abnormality.

References

1. National Institute of Health. Concensus Statement. Febrile seizures: long term management. *British Medical Journal* 1980; **ii**: 277–9.
2. Chamberlain R. *British births I. The first week of life.* London: Heinemann, 1975.
3. Lilienfeld AM, Pasaminick B. Association of maternal and foetal factors with the development of epilepsy. *JAMA* 1954; **155**: 719–24.
4. Mellor DH, Lowit I, Hall DJ. Perinatal problems and epilepsy in childhood. In: Parsonage MJ, ed. *Prevention of epilepsy and its consequences.* London: International Bureau for Epilepsy, 1973.
5. Ross EM, Peckham CS, *et al.* Epilepsy in childhood. *British Medical Journal* 1980; **i**: 207–10.
6. International League Against Epilepsy. A proposal for an international classification of the epilepsies. *Epilepsia* 1969; **11**: 114–19.
7. Kurland LT. The incidence and prevalence of convulsive disorders in a small urban community. *Epilepsia* (Amsterdam) 1959; **i**: 143–61.
8. Pond DA, Bidwell BH, Stein L. A survey of epilepsy in fourteen General Practices I: demographic and medical data. *Acta Psychiatrica Neurologica Neurochirugia* 1960; **63**: 217–36.
9. Rutter M, Tizard J, Whitmore K. *Education health and behaviour.* London: Longman, 1970.
10. Crombie DL, Cross KW, *et al.* A survey of the epilepsies in General Practice. *British Medical Journal* 1960; **ii**: 416–22.
11. Brewis M, Poskonzi D, *et al.* Neurological disease in an English city. *Acta Paediatrica Scandinavica* 1960; **24**, Supplement.
12. Costeff H. Convulsions in childhood: Their natural history and indications for treatment. *New England Journal of Medicine* 1965; **223**: 1410.
13. Rose SW, Penry JK, *et al.* Prevalence of epilepsy in children. *Epilepsia* (New York) 1973; **14**: 133–5.
14. Gudmundsson G. Epilepsy in Iceland. *Acta Neurologica Scandinavica* 1966; Supplement No 25.
15. Sillanpää M. Social prognosis of children with epilepsy. *Acta Paediatrica Scandinavica* 1973; **237**, Supplement.
16. Holdsworth J, Whitmore K. A study of children with epilepsy attending normal schools. *Development in Medicine and Child Neurology* 1974; **196**: 746–65.
17. Ross EM. Epilepsy in children. In: Rose FC, ed. *Clinical neuro-epidemiology.* Tunbridge Wells: Pitman, 1980: 344–50.
18. Cooper JE. Epilepsy in a longitudinal survey of 5000 children. *British Medical Journal* 1965; **ii**: 1020–2.
19. World Health Organization *The application of advances in neurosciences for the control of neurological disorder.* WHO technical report series. No 629. Geneva: WHO, 1978: 14–20.
20. Van den Berg BJ, Yerushalmy J. Studies on convulsive disorders in young children. *Epilepsia* (New York) 1973; **14**: 298–304.
21. Nelson KB, Ellenberg JH. Predictors of epilepsy in children who have experienced febrile seizures. *New England Journal of Medicine* 1976; **19**: 1029–33.
22. Harrison RM, Taylor DC. Childhood seizures. A 25 year follow-up. *Lancet* 1976; **i**: 945–51.
23. Jensen I. Temporal lobe epilepsy. Etiologic factors and surgical results. *Acta Neurologica Scandinavica* 1976; **53**: 103–18.
24. Kurland LT. Head trauma and sequelae in the Olmsted county. Minnesota population. In: Rose FC, ed. *Clinical neuro-epidemiology.* Tunbridge Wells: Pitman, 1980: 361–5.
25. Metrakos JD, Metrakos K. Genetic factors in epilepsy. *Modern Problems in Pharmacopsychiatry* 1970; **4**: 71–86.
26. Central Health Services Council. *People with epilepsy: a report of a joint subcommittee of the Standing Medical Advisory Committee and the Advisory Committee on the Health and Welfare of Handicapped Persons.* London: HMSO, 1969.
27. Millichap JG. *Febrile convulsions.* New York: MacMillan, 1968.

28. Lewis HM, Parry JV, *et al.* The role of viruses in febrile convulsions. *Archives of Disease in Childhood* 1979; **54**: 869–76.
29. Wallace S. Spontaneous fits after convulsions with fever. *Archives of Disease in Childhood.* 1977; **52**: 192–6.

SECTION 8 · ACCIDENTS AND SUICIDE

Chapter 30 · Accidents

R D T FARMER, A NIXON AND J CONNOLLY

A substantial proportion of the morbidity and mortality experienced by people up to the age of 50 years is the result of injuries sustained following accidents. With increasing age, relatively trivial accidental events can cripple people who had previously led independent lives. The investigation of accidents with a view to their prevention is, therefore, an important field of research. It is also a complicated and difficult area to research.

The principal focus of medical activity is the injury rather than the event that caused it. However, the injury is not an inevitable result of an accident nor is its severity necessarily related to the severity of the accident itself. Accidents are caused by varying combinations of human error, environmental circumstances and chance from which injury may or may not follow. The study of the epidemiology of injuries, whether they are fatal or not, is concerned with particular outcomes of accidents. It will necessarily give incomplete data on accidents themselves.

The study of accidents as such is hampered by the absence of a universally accepted definition which allows all such events to be recognized. Many workers have attempted definitions. All are cumbersome and none is entirely satisfactory. That suggested by Arbous and Kerrick[1] is a good example. It mentions all the essential features but it is difficult to put into operation for research purposes. 'In a chain of events, each of which is planned or controlled, there occurs an unplanned event which, being the result of some non-adjustive act on the part of the individual (variously caused), may or may not result in injury. This is an accident.' Only 1 important feature of an event that is normally registered as an accident is missing from this definition. Most accidents occur suddenly. Without adding the time factor to Arbous and Kerrick's definition it could include many of the industrial diseases. Conversely, it could be argued that many of the industrial diseases should be treated as accidents since they have much in common with them. A full discussion of this taxonomic problem is beyond the scope of this chapter. It is sufficient to say that the distinction is arbitrary rather than real and that it has a practical value at the present time.

Most of this chapter is concerned with the personal injuries that result from accidents and with the inferences that can be drawn from them. This reflects the general direction of research in this field. Notwithstanding the reservations already expressed regarding this approach there are many important lessons to be learned.

Sources of data

Data are not routinely collected on all accidents. Those data that are collected vary according to the circumstances in which the accident occurs, the extent of the injuries sustained, the individual's response to his injuries and the extent to which property is damaged. Each accident that comes to official notice may be viewed in 3 ways. Firstly, the nature of the injury sustained can be classified, for example, a fracture, burns, poisoning. Secondly, the external cause of that injury may be stated, for example, a fall, an explosion. Thirdly, the accident can be classified according to the situation in which it occurred, for example, road, industrial premises, home.

In England and Wales, all deaths that are thought to have been accidental are investigated by a coroner. In most other countries similar systems exist for the investigation of unnatural deaths. After as full an enquiry as he considers necessary, the coroner will give a verdict as to cause, both according to the nature of injury and the external cause of the injury. If after full enquiries it is not possible to say whether the death was accidental or deliberate the coroner may record an 'open verdict'. The place at which the incident occurred is also noted and is supplied to the Office of Population Censuses and Surveys (OPCS). Tables derived from collated data are published annually by the Office of Population Censuses and Surveys.

No data are routinely collected on the numbers of and types of injury that are treated in hospital Accident and Emergency departments without admission to the wards. Similarly, injuries treated exclusively by general practitioners are not recorded routinely. Some sample data from general practitioners are published from time to time as the National Morbidity Survey. The material available from the hospital in-patient enquiry (HIPE) and from hospital activity analysis (HAA) relates to admissions for the treatment of injuries, not to individuals injured. They are classified according to the nature of injury (the World Health Organization International Classification of Diseases (ICD) N list) and are subclassified as road accidents, domestic accidents and other accidents. Industrial accidents are not separately identifiable.

The routinely published morbidity data are less than ideal for epidemiological study for 2 reasons. Firstly, they lack essential detail in the 3 dimensions of study; place of event; cause of injury; nature of injury. Secondly, they relate only to those individuals who sought treatment. The decision to seek treatment is affected by factors other than the nature and extent of the injury sustained, for example, concomitant disease, the possibility of compensation and the ease of access to treatment. In some countries the cost of treatment also affects treatment-seeking behaviour.

In the United Kingdom other routinely gathered morbidity statistics on accidents include sickness absence claims. Although accidents at work are tabulated separately from other types of sickness, episodes of less than 3 days duration do not qualify for benefit and are not, therefore, included.

Only 2 types of accident are likely to be reported irrespective of whether injury occurred. These are road accidents and some types of industrial accident. Even these data are incomplete. The tendency is for those road accidents that involved a possible offence, and those that resulted in injury requiring treatment, to be noted by the police. These represent a biased sample of all road accidents.

The Health and Safety at Work Act (1974) places a statutory obligation on employers to notify the enforcing authorities of all accidental injuries sustained at work. Subsequent regulations (The Notification of Accidents and Dangerous Occurrences Regulations) provide for the notification of some accidents that do not result in injury. The employer must notify the enforcing authorities of any accident causing death or major injury to an employee or to any other person whilst on the premises and of any of a defined list of dangerous occurrences whether or not they cause death or injury. The list of dangerous occurrences is given in the appendix to this chapter. Collated figures of notified industrial accidents are published by the Health and Safety Executive[2].

Secular trends

Despite the many improvements in the environment and in the structure of society, the reduction in mortality from accidents during the past 150 years has been modest. It is salutory to reflect on the comments made by Dr William Farr in his letter to the Registrar General in 1839: 'it must not, nevertheless, be imagined that the number of accidental deaths, injuries and mutilations cannot be reduced in England . . . . It is well known that fewer lives are lost by shipwreck in Her Majesty's service than in emigrant vessels; that less accidents happen in one factory than another; and that men are crushed, burnt or blown to pieces much less frequently in coal mines of certain proprietors than those in others. Many 'accidental deaths' are, therefore, indirectly caused by human agency. Many accidents happen from ignorance and carelessness. The knowledge of the accidents to which people are exposed in different occupations may put them more on their guard against danger . . . . In the metropolis, in 2 years, 142 males and 285 females, died by burns. This is ascribed to the greater combustability of the dresses of females . . . . Many children are burnt from the same cause. It deserves the consideration of manufacturers, whether cotton and linen may not be made . . . . as little liable to take fire as textures of wool.'

When Dr Farr was writing (1839) there were 1058 violent deaths (excluding suicide) per million males per year and 402 per million females. The equivalent figures today are 406 and 301 respectively. The reduction is principally attributable to a reduction in industrial accidents but the pattern has changed in some other respects. The average annual mortality rate for successive 5 year periods for different types of accident are shown in Fig. 30.1. The category 'other accidents' includes most domestic and industrial fatalities. In this category rates have fallen steadily. Road transport accidents form a large category, and have tended to increase. There has been a tendency for poisoning to increase. Similar secular trends to those of England and Wales are seen in most developed countries.

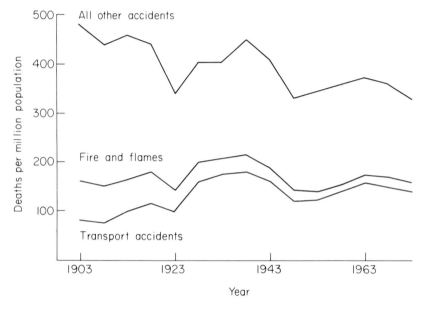

Fig. 30.1. Average annual mortality from accidents for 5 year periods, mid years given, England and Wales (OPCS statistics).

Road accidents

Deaths and injuries caused by accidents involving moving vehicles are not unique to the age of the motor car. Even in the ancient societies of Greece, Egypt and Rome the numbers of moving vehicle accidents gave rise to comment and concern. In Victorian England, particularly during the industrial revolution, the hazards of horse drawn carriages and carts and of the new power driven vehicles were well recognized. In contemporary England and Wales road accidents cause about 6000 deaths each year, a further 77 000 people receive treatment in hospital and an uncounted, but doubtless larger number, are treated as out-patients or receive no treatment.

In all age groups morbidity and mortality from accidents amongst males exceeds that for females. The highest rates are among adolescent and young adult males (Table 30.1). The remarkably high death rate of 15–24 year old males from motor cycle accidents is probably a reflection of the inherent dangerousness of this method of transport coupled with lack of experience and the enthusiasm with which the cycles are used. The highest rates of mortality and morbidity of drivers and passengers are also in this age group. Pedestrian casualties are high in young children at an age when they first begin to walk and are not fully aware of the dangers of the road. The underlying behaviour in road accident casualties in both children and young adults is similar: both are exploring, either their world or their strength, neither are fully appreciative of the hazards and have to learn by their experience. This process of learning is not a new phenomenon, but the dangers of man's environment have increased.

After the middle years of life pedestrian accident casualty rates increase with increasing age. This is likely to be related to a progressive slowing of reaction time rather than because they encounter more accident situations. The fact that the same increase is not seen in motor vehicle driver and passenger accident rates or motor and pedal cycle accident rates is probably due to the proportion of the population at risk being smaller.

The secular trends for each type of road accident fatality differ (Fig. 30.2). There has been a steady fall in the numbers of deaths of pedal cyclists in England and Wales since 1958, possibly because the number of cycles in use in the country has declined. Motor cycle accident deaths fell until the early 1970s and have since

Table 30.1. Mortality and morbidity rates from road accidents in England and Wales, 1978, rates per million population.

Age (years)	Deaths				Hospital admissions All road accidents
	Pedestrians	Pedal cyclists	Motor cyclists	Motor vehicle drivers & passengers	
Male					
0–4	41	3	1	7	935
5–14	54	18	0	10	1977
15–24	33	11	220	173	6168
25–44	20	4	25	92	1888
45–64	49	9	11	79	1130
65–74	113	17	8	87	1015
75+	351	20	4	80	1272
Female					
0–4	26	0	0	12	494
5–14	28	4	1	7	1033
15–24	20	4	22	57	1892
25–44	8	2	2	32	733
45–64	33	3	1	32	612
65–74	92	2	0	42	776
75+	213	1	0	38	906

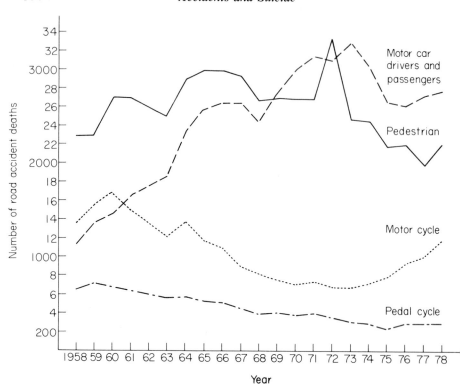

Fig. 30.2. Deaths from road accidents, England & Wales.

increased each year. Deaths of drivers and passengers of motor vehicles increased each year until the early 1970s when they began to fall. There was little change in the numbers of deaths between 1975 and 1977. The numbers of vehicle accident deaths correlates well with the sales of petrol in the country[3]. The fall in 1974 was associated with the world oil crisis and the consequent increase in petrol prices which in turn was associated with a decrease in the amount of petrol sold.

In most countries the post war trend is for road accident rates to increase. There are marked international variations both in the prevailing rates and the rate at which they are increasing. In the oil states of the Arabian Gulf the rate of increase reflects their growing wealth, the cheapness of fuel and the number of cars. In countries that have not seen such marked changes in their economic circumstances the rate of injuries to occupants of vehicles tends to correlate with the number of vehicles per head of population. Mortality rates from accidents vary more than injury rates. England and Wales and Sweden have relatively low death rates, the USA is intermediate; high rates occur in Germany, Italy, Portugal and Turkey[4].

Accident rates rise following the ingestion of alcohol. Up to 25% of drivers who are involved in accidents are found to have excessive blood–alcohol levels. The introduction of stringent regulations governing drinking and driving has reduced this problem to some extent. The most restrictive legislation in the Western world appears to be in Sweden, which now has one of the lowest road casualty rates in the world.

It has been shown that there is a correlation between accident rates and traffic density. Speed is associated with increased rates only when it is associated with high traffic density, or with roads not designed for high speed travel. Thus on motorways the number of accidents per mile travelled is relatively small. Factors other than speed and traffic density have been shown to affect the risk of accidents; these include design of roads, condition of the vehicles, the experience of the driver and his ability to react to unexpected circumstances.

Head injuries are the most common type of injury that causes hospital admission and death (Tables 30.2 and 30.3). A substantial majority of the fatal head injuries involve a fracture of the skull. Soft tissue injuries to the chest, pelvis and abdomen are the next most important cause of death. The factors influencing the severity and type of injury following an accident in motor vehicles has been studied extensively. The most important are the presence of sharp objects and protrusions within the vehicle, the effect of being thrown against the windscreen, and indentation of the cabin and consequent bursting of the doors and locks. Modern car design includes careful attention to safety features. In many countries stringent safety regulations have been introduced. The use of the safety belt by drivers and passengers reduces the risk of injury and its severity. Some countries have made the wearing of seat belts compulsory.

Table 30.2. Hospital admissions following road traffic accidents, England and Wales, 1977 (HIPE statistics).

Nature of injury	Estimated number of admissions
Fractures of skull, spine and trunk	9 330
Fractures of upper limb	5 260
Fractures of lower limb	16 740
Intracranial injury without fracture	31 250
Internal injury to chest, abdomen and pelvis	1 400
Open wounds	5 410
Other and unspecified	7 590
Total	76 980

The commonest cause of death in motorcycle accidents is head injuries. The rider or passenger of a motorcycle has little or no protection if an accident occurs; the high incidence of limb and other fractures is, therefore, not unexpected. The

Table 30.3. Causes of death following road accidents, England and Wales, 1978 (OPCS statistics).

Nature of injury	Pedest-rians	Pedal cyclists	Motor cyclists	Vehicle occupation	Total
Fractures of skull	1010	169	478	853	2510
Fractures of spine and trunk	308	32	87	269	696
Fracture of limbs	188	5	23	75	291
Intracranial injury	273	39	108	212	632
Internal injury of chest, abdomen and pelvis	593	56	452	1247	2348
Burns	0	0	2	28	30
Other	36	4	19	100	159
Total	2408	305	1169	2784	6666

use of crash helmets, which is now compulsory in many countries, has the effect of reducing the severity of head injuries.

It is unlikely that road traffic accidents will be eliminated altogether. Their prevention is only possible if road users behave sensibly, encouraged to do so by the presence of legal sanctions. The design of roads, traffic systems and motor vehicles can also lead to a reduction in casualties. The efforts to produce safer cars and safety devices for drivers and cyclists appears to have produced a worthwhile reduction in the severity of injuries.

Domestic accidents

The domestic environment is not without its dangers. In 1980 nearly 6000 people died in England and Wales as the result of accidents that occurred in the home or in residential institutions. Those age groups particularly liable to injury at home are, the very young and the very old (Table 30.4).

The child is most at risk when he begins to be independently mobile, wishes to explore his environment and is totally unaware of its hazards. The commonest injuries both in terms of mortality and morbidity arise from falls. Although these cause less than 20 deaths each year, fractures and intracranial injuries result in about 7000 hospital admissions in the under-fives. There are over 1000 hospital admissions but only 10 deaths each year from burns in the under-5s. Boys have higher injury rates than girls.

Drowning is the next most common type of fatal accident in the young. Its incidence increases as the child explores its environment beyond his immediate home surroundings. Appropriate preventive strategies must be a compromise between unreasonable supervision that allows the child no space in which to grow and learn and giving the child a degree of freedom that borders on neglect.

Table 30.4. Numbers of deaths from accidents in the home and residential institutions, England and Wales, 1980.

	Male						Female						Total
	All ages	Age (years)					All ages	Age (years)					
		0–4	5–14	15–44	45–64	65+		0–4	5–14	15–44	45–64	65+	
Accidents													
Poisoning	325	10	2	158	105	50	341	6	8	116	130	81	666
Falls	897	16	7	62	155	657	2266	12	1	24	123	2106	3163
Fire and flames	254	21	22	38	51	122	336	26	22	34	42	212	590
Drowning	27	10	1	8	4	4	49	10	6	11	11	17	76
Mechanical suffocation	213	58	4	40	61	50	186	41	2	24	41	78	399
Explosive material, hot substances and corrosives	15	3	0	0	2	10	31	4	0	1	3	23	45
Electric current	40	1	1	23	10	5	11	2	0	4	3	2	51
Other accidents	200	18	18	63	42	59	178	9	6	9	23	131	378
All accidents	1971	137	55	392	430	957	3398	110	39	223	376	2650	5379
Undetermined													
Poisoning	170	0	1	87	59	23	254	1	1	89	94	69	424
Drowning	4	0	0	3	1	0	18	2	0	5	3	8	22
Fall	25	0	0	10	4	11	11	0	0	2	1	8	36
Other	80	5	7	31	19	18	39	3	0	11	10	18	119
All undetermined	279	5	8	131	83	52	322	3	1	107	108	103	601
All accidents and undetermined	2250	142	63	523	513	1009	3720	113	40	330	484	2753	5980

Within the home, improvements in the design of certain common items will reduce danger without necessarily restricting activity. For example, inflammable clothing could be made illegal, and window locks could be child-proofed as are some poison containers.

The aged are at special risk for accidents even within environments that would normally be considered safe. Because of deteriorations in vision, hearing, co-ordination and mobility many old people fail to notice dangers or are unable to respond to them. Neurological defects such as vertigo, which is quite common amongst the elderly, may lead to unexpected falls which, in a group of people with oesteoporosis, result in fractures. The most frequent type of fatal injury is a fall (Table 30.5). There is a substantial increase in fatal falls with increasing age, but little difference in rates between the sexes.

Table 30.5. Mortality rates from accidents in the home and residential institutions, England and Wales, 1978 (per million population).

Type of accident	Male Age (years)		Female Age (years)	
	65–74	75 +	65–74	75 +
Poisonings by solids and liquids	9	16	8	14
Poisoning by gas	7	15	4	7
Falls	124	615	107	932
Fire	26	101	28	80
Drowning	3	11	5	4
Suffocation	11	35	12	33
Other	15	50	25	74

Accidental death rates from poisoning by domestic gas are now a fraction of what they were during the 1950s and early 1960s. This fall correlates with the withdrawal of toxic gas from the domestic grid and its replacement with natural gas. Natural gas is lighter than air. It does not contain carbon monoxide and is therefore virtually non-toxic. There are relatively low death rates from poisoning by solid of liquid substances, this category includes medicines. The accuracy of the mortality data is open to question on 2 counts. Many modern poisons leave no obvious signs that would make a doctor suspect that death was from other than natural causes. Patel[5] has suggested that many elderly people with concomitant disease that could be expected to cause death, who actually die from poisoning, are not recognized. They are certified as having died from the other disease. It is also possible that the accidental poisonings may include disguised suicides.

Deaths from burning are high in the elderly. This may reflect the inability of the elderly to react to emergencies with fire and their tendency to use dangerous and defective heating apparatus.

The commonest type of non-fatal injury that results in admission to hospital is a fracture of a lower limb. Rates in females are much higher than in males. Relatively trivial accidents can, because of osteoporosis, cause a major catastrophe in elderly people. Of those who are admitted, some are quite unable to resume an independent life. Because the proportion of the population that is elderly is increasing, there is likely to be an increase in the number of accidents unless effective preventive strategies can be devised. Unfortunately, there is little research in this field. Although attempts are being made to reduce the obvious hazards there is little progress in persuading many elderly people to adjust their lives to take account of their physical limitations.

Industrial accidents

Less than 5 % of all accidental deaths in the United Kingdom occur at work or on industrial premises. This statistic understates what is a major problem in industrial societies. In addition to the 639 fatal accidents that were reported to the health and safety enforcement authorities in 1979, over 340 000 non-fatal accidents that resulted in personal injury were reported. More than 15 million working days were lost. Even this is an underestimate of the impact of industrial accidents as it does not include injuries that resulted in absence for less than 3 working days. However, in recent years there has been a decrease in both fatalities and injuries.

Accident rates vary for different industries (Table 30.6). Both the highest fatality rates and the highest ratio of fatal to non-fatal accidents occur in the construction industry.

The list used in Table 30.6 gives a broad picture only as the groupings used agglomerate a wide range of occupations within an industry. For example, the coal and petroleum products industry covers activities as diverse as working within refineries, distribution and laboratory research. Even within one particular industry there are wide variations in accident rates between factories; even between different factories under the same management.

Industrial accidents and industrial safety has been extensively researched, particularly because of pressure from the trade unions and from the Health and Safety Executive. The principal factors that have been demonstrated to affect rates are summarized below.

Sex

The investigation of sex as a risk factor is complicated by the fact that few occupations exist where both men and women do the same jobs in the same circumstances, and therefore carry the same risk. The few studies that have been undertaken suggest that women do carry a higher risk than men. However, the

Table 30.6. Accident rates in manufacturing injuries per 100 000 persons at risk, England and Wales, 1977.

Industry	Accident rate Fatal	Serious
Food, drink and tobacco	4.0	760
Coal and petroleum products	19.5	960*
Chemical and allied industry	4.6	590
Metal manufacturing	12.2	970
Mechanical engineering	3.4	740
Instrument engineering	†	†
Electrical engineering	1.4	320
Shipbuilding and marine engineering	10.4	770
Vehicles	0.9	390
Metal goods not elsewhere specified	2.9	750
Textiles	2.3	530
Leather, leather goods and fur	†	†
Clothing and footwear	†	170
Bricks, pottery, glass and cement	3.4	740
Timber and furniture	3.5	760
Paper printing and publishing	2.2	420
Other manufacturing industry	2.4	660
Agriculture	14.1‡	NA
Mining coal	19.6‡	228
Mining quarries	32.6‡	NA

* 1975 figure.
† Less than 5 fatal or 10 serious accidents.
NA Not available.
‡ 1976 figure.

extent to which the findings from workers in a limited range of occupations such as munitions factories and taxi drivers can be extrapolated to all occupations is limited. It has been demonstrated that some women are more at risk in the premenstrual phase than at other times in the menstrual cycle.

Age

Industrial accident rates are high in the teens and early 20s. They begin to rise again from the mid-60s onwards. How much of the excess in the younger age group, which is often during the period of apprenticeship, is due to lack of training or experience, and how much is due to personality factors such as lack of discipline, carelessness or impatience is difficult to determine. There is an association between accident rates and duration of employment in a particular job. This effect appears to be independent of the age of the worker.

Health

Workers who are involved in accidents tend to have more absence from work due to sickness unconnected with accidents than the general population of workers. This may be because their threshold for sickness absence is lower or because they are less fit. Studies of certain specific aspects of general health tend to support the latter hypothesis. Thus workers with hypertension and with definable serious disease have been shown to be more prone to accidents than fit workers.

Specific sensory defects affect accident rates in specific jobs but not generally. The implication of this finding is that specific lower limits of sensory ability (hearing, vision) have to be defined in relation to a particular job.

Personality and intellectual factors

Reaction times, coordination and motor control, have been investigated in relation to accidents. Studies have shown that all are relevant but that the correlations are not particularly strong.

Both alcoholism and consumption of alcohol before or during work increase accident rates. Similarly there is an increased risk in workers taking certain psycho-active drugs.

Above the intelligence levels usually regarded as educationally subnormal there is no correlation between accident rates and intelligence. Other factors that may be confused with intellectual ability, such as concentration, are the important determinants.

Prevention

There is little doubt that the design of the working environment profoundly affects the risk of accidents within it. The Health and Safety at Work Act (1974) defined the responsibilities of employers and laid down regulations for the notification of accidents. It is the responsibility of employers to take all reasonable precautions to ensure the safety of employees and of persons who are on industrial premises. This will include design features of machinery and other apparatus as well as procedures to be followed. Employees do sometimes ignore safety regulations and put themselves at risk of injury or death. There is a particular temptation when the company's safety regulations make a job slower or more difficult, particularly if the worker's earnings are linked to production. A worker cannot be dismissed for such behaviour unless his actions put his fellow workers at risk. However, a worker has to prove negligence by the employer if he is to make a successful claim for damages against him. With the monitoring of accidents by the Health and Safety Executive, few employers would risk high accident rates within their factories or work places.

Clearly progress in accident prevention is more likely to be achieved by education and co-operation in agreed codes of practice than by the application of regulations made without the workers' understanding and agreement.

Accident proneness

Farmer and Chambers[6] introduced the term 'accident prone' to describe individuals whose personal attributes appeared to contribute to the number of accidents they experienced. They believed it to be 'a relatively stable phenomenon manifesting itself in different periods of exposure and in different kinds of accidents'. It was distinguished from accident liability, a term that they used to include features of the environment that affect the probability of accidents. The hypothesis of Farmer and Chambers came from their own studies and from the observations of other research workers. Generally the relevant studies fall into 2 groups, those concerned with the frequency with which accidents occur to individuals and those concerned with the characteristics of individuals who have high accident rates.

One of the earliest systematic studies of the frequency of accidents amongst individuals was amongst female munition workers during the First World War. Greenwood et al.[7] found positive correlations between the numbers of accidents resulting in minor injury experienced by individuals in successive 3 month periods. Thus the number of accidents in one quarter was a good predictor of the number that would occur in the next quarter. A major injury, or death, ended the enhanced risk of accidents as the injury itself affected exposure to situations in which subsequent accidents could have occurred. A later study by Newbold[8] of 16 000 accidents reached a similar conclusion; 'some of the unequal distribution was due to personal tendency'.

Studies of children have also shown that individuals have an unequal distribution of accidents. 29 % of children received medical attention for an accident each year, but only 1.2 % had 3 accidents for which they received medical attention. Mannheimer et al.[9] investigated the accident records of 8874 children (representing 50 000 child years) using records from a pre-paid insurance scheme in California. Children with high accident rates in one 4 year period continued to have up to twice the expected number of accidents in the next 4 year period. This investigation suggests a longer lasting tendency to accidents than is shown in studies of adults. The study can be criticized on the grounds that the consulting patterns are determined by the parent rather than the child himself, it is nevertheless, an important observation.

The second type of study, the investigation of the characteristics of individuals who have high accident rates, is exemplified by the work of Tillman and Hobbs in Ontario (Canada)[10]. They compared the personal characteristics of 20 pairs of taxi drivers. Those with high accident rates significantly more often had divorced parents, had had truancy problems, poor military and work records and were sexually more promiscuous. The same team also compared 96 men who had had more than 4 car accidents with 96 accident-free drivers living in the same district[11]. The courts had records of significantly more men in the high accident group, possibly because of some previous accident. However, people in the high accident group also appeared more frequently in the records of public health agencies, venereal disease clinics, welfare agencies dealing with problem families and local credit bureaux.

The concept of accident proneness was criticised by Haddon, Suchman and Klein[12] who described it as a psychological abstraction based on statistical frequency; they suggested that it could not explain 'any major proportion of accidents . . . . but that as a clinical phenomenon limited to some individuals it may have some validity'. It was demonstrated that a small number of persons could be justly described as accident prone but that their identification in any one time period and elimination from accident situations (for example, driving) would lead to only minute diminution in the number of accidents in a second time period.

In 1974, Reason[13] suggested that 'examination of accident repeaters over a lengthy period indicated that they are members of a club which is constantly changing its membership. New people are added while long standing members cease to qualify'. He did not believe that accident proneness was necessarily a fixed attribute of an individual. The work of Shaw and Sichel[14], based on 17 years' experience in a South African Public Utilities Transport Corporation, strongly supported the hypothesis that accident proneness, though not fixed, was durable enough to be relevant to accident repeating.

Much recent work has been concerned with the identification of factors that may temporarily increase the likelihood of accidents in individuals. It has been shown that accident rates double in the 6 months after a divorce[15]. 28% of drivers responsible for a fatality claimed to have experienced an emotionally disturbing event within 6 hours before the accident[16].

A more formal method of investigating the events in individuals lives uses the schedule of recent experience (SRE)[17]. This measures life change units (LCU). A retrospective study used this schedule to compare patients admitted to hospital for elective surgery and university students with no accident history in the previous 6 months, with individuals who had had an accident. The accident group had a higher life change unit score in the 6 months before the accident. Prospective studies using the SRE to measure the LCU have also shown that a high LCU score correlates with the probability of an accident[18,19].

It is difficult to choose between 2 possible explanations of these observations. One hypothesis is that the individual contributes to his own accident by preoccupation with the bombardment of events in his life. On the other hand, the accident may be simply the latest in a sequence of partially controlled events.

Whatever the explanation there is evidence that accident proneness is a temporary phenomenon. However, there may be permanent features of an individual's personality that predispose him to experience more LCU than the general population.

Appendix: Dangerous occurrences which are notifiable wherever they occur in England & Wales

1   Collapse or overturning of any lift, hoist, crane, excavator or mobile powered access platform, or failure of any load bearing part thereof, which, taking into account the circumstances of the occurrence, might have been liable to cause a major injury to any person; and in this paragraph a 'lift, hoist, crane or mobile powered access platform' does not include a crab, winch, teagle, pulley block, gin wheel, transporter or runway.

2   Explosion, collapse or bursting of any closed vessel including a boiler or boiler tube in which there was any gas (including air) or vapour at a pressure greater than atmospheric which might have been liable to cause major injury to any person or which resulted in significant damage to the plant.

3   Electrical short circuit or overload attended by fire or explosion which resulted in the stoppage of the plant involved for more than 24 hours and which, taking into account the circumstances of the occurrence, might have been liable to cause major injury to any person.

4   An explosion or fire occurring in any plant or place which resulted in the stoppage of that plant or suspension of normal work in that place for more than 24 hours where such explosion or fire was due to the ignition of process materials, their by-products (including waste) or finished products.

5   The sudden, uncontrollable release of 1 tonne or more of highly flammable liquid, within the meaning of Regulation 2(2) of the Highly Flammable Liquids and Liquefied Petroleum Gases Regulations 1972 (a), flammable gas or flammable liquid above its boiling point from any system or plant or pipeline.

6   A collapse or part collapse of any scaffold which is more than 12 metres high which results in a substantial part of the scaffold falling or overturning.

7   At any building or structure under construction, reconstruction, alteration or demolition, a collapse or partial collapse of any part of the building or structure, or of any falsework, involving a fall of more than 10 tonnes of material, except where the manner and extent of the collapse or partial collapse was intentional.

8   The uncontrolled release or escape of any substances or agent in circumstances which, having regard to the nature of the substance or agent and the extent and location of the release or escape, might be liable to cause damage to the health of, or major injury to, any person.

9   Any incident in which any person is affected by the inhalation, ingestion or

other absorption of any substances, or by lack of oxygen, to such an extent as to cause acute ill health requiring medical treatment.

10   Any case of acute ill health where there is reason to believe that this resulted from occupational exposure to isolated pathogens or infected material.

11   Any ignition or explosion of explosives, where the ignition or explosion was not intentional.

12   Failure of any freight container or failure of any load bearing part thereof while it is being raised, lowered or suspended, and in this paragraph a 'freight container' means a freight container as defined in Article II of the International Convention for Safe Containers (CSC) except any container specially designed for air transport or any skip or cage used in a mine or quarry.

13   Either of the following occurrences in relation to a pipeline:

(a)   the bursting, explosion or collapse of a pipeline or any part thereof; or

(b)   the ignition of any thing in a pipeline, or of any thing which immediately before it was ignited was in a pipeline.

14   Any incident in which a road tanker to which the Hazardous Substances (Labelling of Road Tankers) Regulations 1978 (a) applies,

(a)   overturns;

(b)   suffers serious damage to the tank in which a prescribed hazardous substance is being conveyed.

References

1. Arbous AG, Kerrich JE. Accident statistics and the concept of accident proneness. *Biometrics* 1951; **7** (4): 340.
2. Health and Safety Executive. *Health and Safety Statistics 1976.* London: HMSO, 1976.
3. Bull JP. *Accidents and their prevention in theory and practice of public health.* 5th ed. Oxford: Oxford University Press, 1979.
4. Bull JP. International comparisons of road accident statistics. *Accident Analysis and Prevention* 1969; **1**: 293.
5. Patel NS. Pathology of suicide. *Medicine Science and the Law* 1973; **13** (2): 103.
6. Farmer E, Chambers EG. *A Study of personal qualities in accident proneness and proficiency.* Report No 35. London: Industrial Health Research Board, 1929.
7. Greenwood M, Yule GU. An enquiry into the nature of frequency distributions representative of multiple happenings, with particular reference to the occurrence of multiple attacks of disease or repeated accidents. *Journal of the Royal Statistical Society* 1920; **83**: 255–79.
8. Newbold EM. A contribution to the study of the human factor in the causation of accidents. Report No 34. London: Industrial Health Research Board, 1976.
9. Mannheimer DI, Dewey J, *et al.* 50 000 child-years of accidental injuries. *Public Health Records* 1966; **81**: 519.
10. Tillmann WA, Hobbs GE. Accident proneness in automobile drivers. *American Journal of Psychiatry* 1949; **106**: 321–331.
11. Tillman WA, Harris LA, *et al. Group therapy amongst persons involved in frequent automobile accidents.* Report. Washington DC, US Army Research and Development Command: 1965.
12. Haddon W, Suchman EK, Klein D. *Accident research: methods and approaches.* New York: Harper and Row, 1964: 444.

13. Reason J. Style, personality and accidents. *New Society* 1974; **27**: 445–8.
14. Shaw L, Sichel H. *Accident proneness*. Oxford: Pergamon Press, 1971.
15. McMurray AL. Emotional stress and driving performance: the effect of divorce. *Behavioural Research and Highway Safety* 1971; **1**: 100.
16. Conger JJ, *et al*. Psychological and psychophysiological factors in motor vehicle accidents. *JAMA* 1959; **169**: 1581.
17. Holmes TH, Rahe RH. The social readjustment rating scale. *Journal of Psychosomatic Research* 1967; **11**: 213–8.
18. Bramwell ST. *et al*. Psychosocial factors in athletic injuries. *Journal of Human Stress* 1975; **1** (2): 6.
19. Levine JB. *et al*. Recent life changes and accidents aboard an attack carrier. *Military Medicine* 1977; June: 469.

Chapter 31 · Suicide and Attempted Suicide

R D T FARMER

In suicide, death is the result of injuries inflicted by an individual on himself with the intent of ending his life. Although it is not a common cause of death it has been the subject of intensive comment, and more recently investigation, by people from a wide range of backgrounds and disciplines. Until the mid 19th century interest in the subject tended to be limited to philosophers, theologians and legislators. Since then it has been subjected to scientific scrutiny by social scientists, notably Durkheim[1], medical statisticians (including Dr. William Farr) and psychiatrists, the first of whom to engage upon a major investigation was Morselli[2]. It was not until suicide began to be investigated in other than moral terms that some of the punitive legislation relating to people who killed themselves was repealed. In England and Wales until the 1850s magistrates had the power to confiscate all the property of a suicide and this effectively meant that their dependents were disinherited. The Church would not allow the body of a person who had committed suicide to be buried in consecrated ground. Other countries have had a similarly punitive attitude to the victims of suicide.

Strictly speaking, the term 'attempted suicide' refers to survival following a deliberate self injury which was inflicted with the intent of causing death. In England and Wales this was a felony punishable by imprisonment until 1962; until the mid 19th century it was a capital offence!

Since the late 1950s there has been a remarkable rise in the rates of non-fatal self-harm, mainly by poisoning, in most Western countries. Some research workers and many practising psychiatrists believe that a substantial proportion of people who harm themselves do not intend to end their lives[3,4]. It is thought that the majority are using self harm as a 'cry for help' in order to manipulate their environment. The term 'parasuicide' is often used to designate this group. Its use is not universal; other terms that are used as virtual synonyms are 'deliberate self harm' and 'pseudosuicide'.

Ascertainment and classification

The ascertainment of a suicide is a 2 stage process. The death first has to be recognized as having been due to other than natural causes; next it has to be established that it was caused by a deliberate act of the deceased himself with the intention of ending his life.

387

The ease with which a death can be recognized as unnatural depends on the nature of the injury. No real difficulties exist in most of the violent methods used for suicide, for example, hanging, shooting, jumping from high places, cutting and so forth. Even poisoning by carbon monoxide, whether by coal gas or by motor car exhaust fumes, leaves characteristic physical signs and evidence. Poisoning by solid and liquid substances presents particular problems. Many of the modern hypnotic and tranquillizing drugs leave no marks on the body that would lead an investigator to suspect that the death was from other than natural causes. Suspicion is aroused by the circumstances of the death rather than the condition of the body. It has been suggested that some poisonings that occur amongst the elderly and infirm, who are expected to die anyway, are missed because the death follows an expected pattern[5]. The proportion of unnatural deaths that are recognized as such varies with the nature of the injury and the previous state of health of the victim.

In England and Wales, and in many other countries, for example Australia, whose legal systems owe their origins to the English system, a death can only be categorized as suicide by a coroner after a judicial enquiry. Before a coroner may give an inquest verdict of suicide he must have legal proof that the deceased intended to end his life. Admissible evidence at an inquest includes suicide notes or reported statements made by the deceased to others, but suicide cannot be presumed even if the circumstantial evidence would lead an investigator to that conclusion. The relatives may appeal to a High Court to have a suicide verdict reversed if they believe that it was not proven at the inquest. When intent cannot be proven an 'open verdict' is recorded. This is classified in the World Health Organization International Classification of Diseases (ICD) as 'injury undetermined as to whether accidentally or purposely inflicted'. It is thought that this category includes some disguised suicides[6]. In other countries, for example France, Holland, Denmark, Belgium and Sweden, whose legal system is different, suspected suicides are not investigated by the judiciary and presumption of intent is used by the investigators. The certified cause of death is confidential in these systems and is not subject to appeal[7]. These important variations in certification practices mean that international statistics must be interpreted with caution and that even substantial differences in suicide certification rates do not necessarily mean that there are real differences in suicide mortality.

The ascertainment of attempted suicide or parasuicide presents a different series of problems. There is a limited number of methods of suicide from which survival is possible. Most of these are poisonings. All the evidence of a suicide occurs before the event which causes the death. In the case of a suspected attempted suicide the individual is available to discuss his actions and motives with the investigator. The assessment of intent in the case of survivors therefore involves a different set of information. It is impossible to investigate both survivors and the dead in the same way as this would involve discussing the circumstances of the attempt with relatives and friends of both without disclosing whether or not the attempt was successful. From a management point of view there is probably little advantage in ascertaining intent with precision amongst survivors as the task is to make arrangements for the individual's return to normal life. The diagnostic codes used in hospital practice (the 'N' list of the ICD) are concerned only with the nature of the injury and make no judgement on motive. Since 1962, when attempted suicide ceased to be a criminal offence, there has been no statutory obligation to notify suspected suicide attempts, and even before that date it is unlikely that the criminal statistics gave complete data on attempted suicide.

Consequently, there are no routinely collected data on attempted suicide. Episodes of poisoning by medicinal agents in adults are usually used as proxys since most are thought to be deliberate. It is more difficult to find an ICD code within the 'N' list to use as a proxy for attempted suicide by violent methods. Whereas mortality statistics relate to the individual the morbidity data relate to episodes. Repetition of self poisoning does occur. This means that direct comparison of trends in mortality and morbidity must be made with caution, particularly as there has been a change in the lethality of the poisons commonly used. It is essential to use data from special studies to study trends in the number of individuals who have episodes of self poisoning or parasuicide. In the United Kingdom the trends in admissions and individuals admitted to the Regional Poisons Treatment Centre in Edinburgh[8] provide an invaluable source of data. Other special studies have been undertaken elsewhere.

Incidence

The incidence of suicide increases with age and is higher in men than it is in women (Fig. 31.1). However, the contribution of suicide to total mortality is greatest amongst young adults. In the age group 20–24 it accounts for about 10 % of all deaths (Fig. 31.2). At all ages rates are lower amongst married people than amongst unmarried individuals (single, widowed and divorced).

In the 1970–72 occupational mortality survey[9] the 8 occupations with the highest suicide standardized mortality ratios (SMR) were pharmacists (SMR 464), chiropodists (SMR 374), medical practitioners (qualified) (SMR 335), housekeepers, stewards, matrons and housemothers (SMR 320), medical workers not elsewhere classified (SMR 320) and nurses (SMR 297). Most of the suicide deaths in these groups were by poisoning. When occupations are aggregated into social classes, there is a greater mortality by suicide in lower social classes.

Self poisoning rates (attempted suicide or parasuicide) as measured by the proxy of hospital admissions of adults for the treatment of poisoning decrease

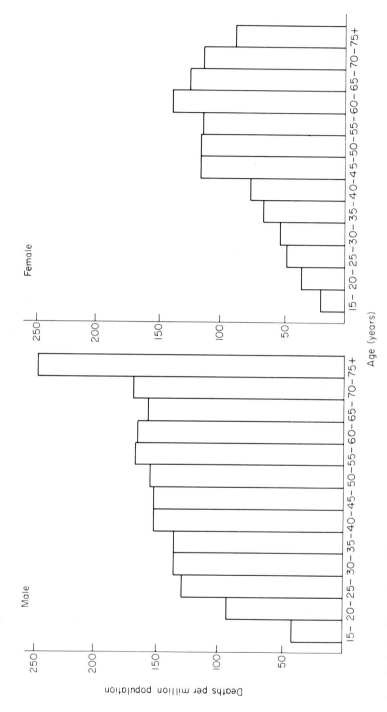

Fig. 31.1. Death rates from suicide at different ages, England and Wales, 1979.

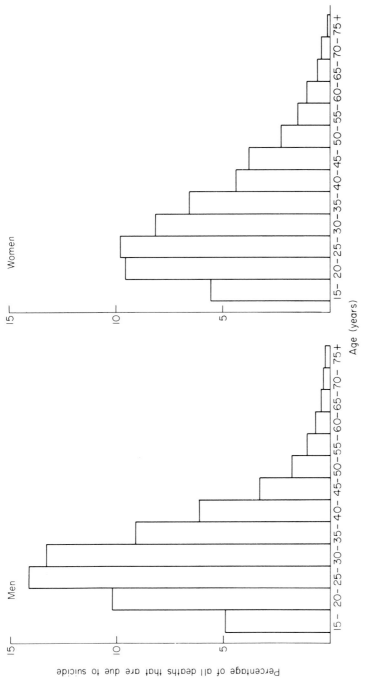

Fig. 31.2. The contribution of suicide to total mortality at different ages, England and Wales, 1979.

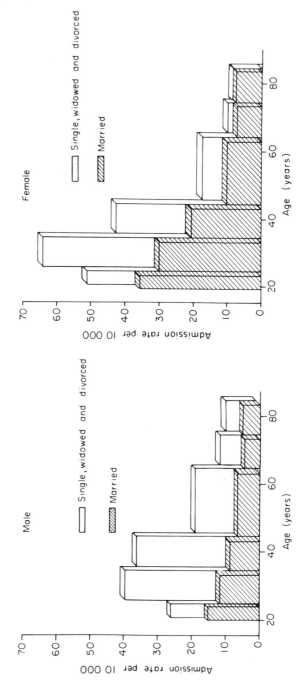

Fig. 31.3. Hospital admission rates for treatment of poisoning by age and marital status, England and Wales, 1973.

with increasing age and are higher amongst women than amongst men. Among both sexes rates are higher in unmarried than in married individuals (Fig. 31.3). Few data exist on variations in the numbers of non-fatal self poisoning by occupation. The proportion of other than first episodes decreases with age.

Secular trends

The suicide rate in England and Wales has shown some major fluctuations during the past 100 years (Fig 31.4). It fell during both of the World Wars, increased during the 1930s and since the 1960s has shown a substantial decline. Similar fluctuations have been noted in other Western countries over similar time periods with a general tendency for rates to decrease during wars and increase during periods of high unemployment. These observations have been interpreted as vindicating the Durkheim hypothesis that the collective sense of belonging (the antithesis of anomie) tends to protect society against suicide[1]. The post-1960 fall in suicide mortality in England and Wales is unique in Western experience. Sainsbury *et al.*[10] believe that this was due to favourable social and economic changes. Others believe that it may be the result of the withdrawal of toxic gas from the domestic supply[11].

　　The secular trends in suicide mortality vary with the method used. The most striking differences are between hanging, domestic gas poisoning, poisoning by solid or liquid substances and all other methods (Fig. 31.5)[12]. The rise in death rates from gas poisoning coincided with the introduction of gas into the domestic environment and the fall was associated with the change to non-toxic gases. The

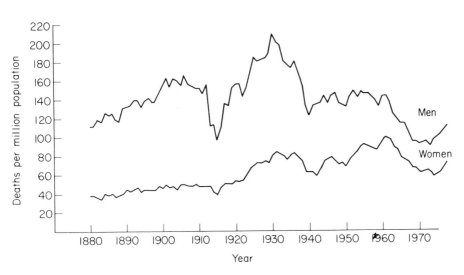

Fig. 31.4. Death rates from suicide, England and Wales, 1880–1979.

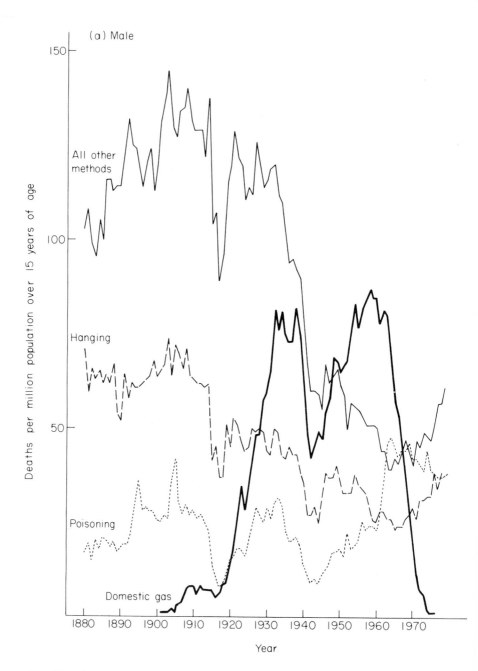

Fig. 31.5.(a) Male death rates for different methods of suicide, England and Wales, 1880–1979.

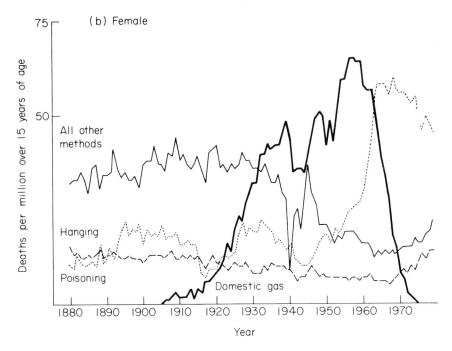

Fig. 31.5.(b) Female death rates for different methods of suicide, England and Wales, 1880–1979.

increase in the rates of poisoning by solid and liquid substances was coincidental with the increase in the number of prescriptions issued for hypnotic and psychoactive drugs.

It is only possible to examine the trends in hospital admission for treatment of the adverse effects of medicinal agents, used here as a proxy for attempted suicide or parasuicide, since 1952. There has been a steady increase since then, principally in the younger age groups (Fig. 31.6). More recently the trend seems to have ceased. It is interesting to note that in the 1950s admission rates were similar in all age and sex groups. The trends in admission rates for different medicinal poisons are dissimilar (Fig. 31.7). They tend to follow the prescribing patterns of those substances quite closely.

Geographical variations

Within England and Wales suicide rates tend to be higher in urban conurbations than in rural areas. Within conurbations the rates tend to be the highest in boroughs with high mobility, high unemployment and a high proportion of single person households[13,14].

There are wide international variations in total suicide mortality and in

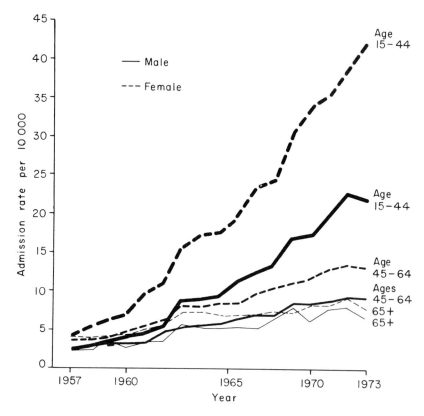

Fig. 31.6. Hospital admission rates for treatment of adverse effects of medicinal agents (used as proxy for attempted suicide), by age and sex, England and Wales, 1958–73.

suicide mortality by different methods. Extremely high rates are recorded in Sweden, West Germany, Denmark and the USA. Spain and Eire have remarkably low rates (Table 31.1). Within the USA suicide by firearms is the most frequent method but in Sweden all methods tend to have a high incidence[15]. Some of the international variations are undoubtedly due to differences in certification practice but even after corrections are made for this artefact, significant differences remain.

International data on non-fatal self poisoning are not widely available and those that that do exist are difficult to interpret as they are affected by admission policies and by the nature of the health information systems available. Those data that are available suggest that most countries have experienced secular trends similar to those in England and Wales but the rates vary considerably between countries.

Male

	All Methods (E950–959)*	Poison (E950)*	Domestic Gas (E951)*	Other Gas (E952)*	Hanging (E953)*	Drowning (E954)*	Firearms (E955)*	Cutting (E956)*	Jumping (E958)*
England and Wales	129	41	14	12	29	9	8	4	4
Belgium	282	20	6	2	175	27	31	3	7
France	304	21	3	5	149	29	58	3	9
Netherlands	132	27	1	2	57	19	3	3	7
German Federal Republic	360	90	7	16	160	13	32	7	12
Denmark	382	97	31	35	132	21	38	6	12
Sweden	382	87	16	38	127	21	62	8	13
Eire	56	11	3	2	21	8	5	3	1
Spain	91	4	0	0	51	11	6	3	9
Australia	236	64	11	29	30	7	79	5	5
USA	239	21	NA	NA	35	NA	143	NA	NA

Female

	All Methods (E950–959)*	Poison (E950)*	Domestic Gas (E951)*	Other Gas (E952)*	Hanging (E953)*	Drowning (E954)*	Firearms (E955)*	Cutting (E956)*	Jumping (E958)*
England and Wales	85	55	7	1	8	7	0	1	2
Belgium	128	24	3	0	56	29	2	2	5
France	110	22	3	2	35	26	4	1	8
Netherlands	87	32	0	0	19	22	0	2	6
German Federal Republic	186	80	4	2	54	18	2	2	14
Denmark	221	112	17	2	43	26	1	4	11
Sweden	154	77	5	2	28	24	2	2	7
Eire	19	8	2	0	2	5	0	1	0
Spain	30	3	0	0	11	7	0	1	6
Australia	113	73	7	3	8	7	6	1	3
USA	90	31	NA	NA	11	NA	28	NA	NA

* ICD Code number.
NA Not available.

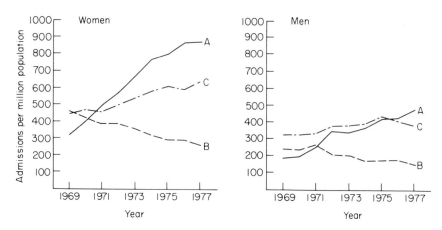

Fig. 31.7. Hospital admissions for treatment of poisoning by different medicines, England and Wales, 1969–77. (A) represents psychotherapeutics; (B) barbiturates and other hypnotics; (C) salicylates and other analgesics.

Special studies

There has been a large number of studies of suicide and attempted suicide (parasuicide) which have sought to identify risk factors and assess prevention. It has been shown that suicide is more common amongst individuals who had previously attempted suicide than it is amongst psychiatric patients. It is also more common amongst psychiatric patients than in the general population[16]. The psychiatric patients most at risk are those suffering from psychotic illnesses and severely depressed patients in the early stages of their recovery.

Attempts have been made to assess the impact in the United Kingdom of the Samaritans emergency counselling service on the prevention of suicide. Although the early studies suggested that they had some impact on the prevention of suicide[17] more recent studies have not confirmed this[18].

Characteristically, survivors of episodes of self-poisoning tend to be young, neurotic individuals who have experienced instability in their early life and are facing a large number of crises in their current life.

Most cases of attempted suicide that are admitted to hospitals in England and Wales are assessed by a psychiatrist. This approach has not been conspicuously successful in secondary prevention. Recent studies have attempted to assess the role of social work in the prevention of repeat episodes, but as yet no conclusive evidence of any benefit has been reported.

Implications

It is unlikely that any single factor determines the incidence of suicide or parasuicide in a community. There is strong evidence that social factors such as unemployment, war and the state of the national economy affect the rates. The epidemiological evidence is consistent with the hypothesis that the availability and acceptability of methods by which people may kill themselves is also a strong determinant. The causes of attempted suicide may or may not overlap with those of suicide. There is evidence to suggest that it is often an impulsive act and its incidence seems to correlate reasonably with the availability of certain medicines. No formal preventive measures have yet been shown to be wholly effective. It is possible that more judicious prescribing to identifiable high risk individuals would reduce the incidence of episodes of parasuicide.

References

1. Durkheim E. *Suicide*. London: Routledge & Kegan Paul, 1957.
2. Morselli H. *Suicide*. 2nd ed. London: Kegan Paul, Trench & Co., 1883.
3. Kessel N. Self poisoning. *British Medical Journal* 1965; **ii**: 1265.
4. Carstairs GM. Characteristics of the suicide prone. *Proceedings of the Royal Society of Medicine* 1968; **61**: 262.
5. Patel NS. Pathology of suicide. *Medicine, Science and the Law* U. **13** (2): 103.
6. Adelstein A, Mardon C. Suicides 1971–74. *Population Trends* 1975. vol. no.
8. Kreitman N, Schreiber M. Parasuicide in young Edinburgh women 1968–75. In: Farmer RDT, Hirsch SR, eds. *The suicide syndrome* New York: Croom Helm, 1980: 54–72.
9. Office of Population Censuses and Surveys. *Occupational Mortality—decennial supplement 1970–72*. London: HMSO.
10. Sainsbury P, Jenkins J, Levey A. Social correlates of suicide in Europe. In: Farmer RDT, Hirsch SR, eds. *The suicide syndrome*. New York: Croom Helm, 1980: 38–53.
11. Low AA, Farmer RDT, *et al.* Suicide in England and Wales: an analysis of 100 years 1876–1975. *Psychological Medicine* 1981; **11**: 359–68.
12. Farmer RDT. Suicide by different methods *Postgraduate Medical Journal* 1979; **55**: 775–9.
13. Sainsbury P. Suicide in London. *Maudsley Monographs No 4*. Oxford: Oxford University Press, 1958.
14. Farmer RDT, Preston TD, O'Brien SEM. Suicide mortality in Greater London. Changes during the past 25 years. *British Journal of Preventive and Social Medicine* 1977; **31** (3).
15. Farmer RDT, Rohde J. Effect of availability and acceptability of lethal instruments on suicide mortality. *Acta Psychiatrica Scandinavica* 1980; **62**: 436–46.
16. Teff BM, Pederson AM, Babigian HM. Patterns of death among suicide attempters: a psychiatric population and a general population. *Archives of General Psychiatry* 1977; **34**, 1155.
17. Bagley C. The evaluation of a suicide prevention scheme by an ecological method. *Social Science and Medicine* 1968; **2**: 1.
18. Jennings C, Barraclough BM, Moss JR. Have the Samaritans lowered the suicide rate? A controlled study. *Psychological Medicine* 1978; **8**: 413.

SECTION 9 · MATERNAL AND FETAL HEALTH

Chapter 32 · Benefits & Risks of Different Methods of Contraception

M P VESSEY

Although a great deal of research has been directed at the development of new methods of fertility control during the last decade[1], the vast majority of couples seeking reliable reversible contraception must still choose between oral contraceptives, an intra-uterine device (IUD) and one of the occlusive methods. This chapter summarizes what is known about the benefits and risks of these contraceptive methods and indicates how this information can be used to help those seeking advice.

Progestogen-only pills have never been in widespread use in any country and, accordingly, have not been the subject of epidemiological investigation. Neither they nor sequential preparations (which have been removed from the market in many countries) will be discussed further in this chapter. The terms 'oral contraceptive' and 'the pill' thus refer in what follows to combined preparations.

Until the mid-1970s, much of the available information about the benefits and risks of different contraceptive methods had been derived from uncontrolled clinical trials and from case–control studies. In 1974, however, the Royal College of General Practitioners (RCGP) in the United Kingdom published the interim results of a large cohort study concerned with the safety of oral contraceptives[2], while 2 years later preliminary data about the effects of the pill, the diaphragm and the IUD became available from another large cohort investigation, the Oxford Family Planning Association (Oxford FPA) contraceptive study[3]. Both these studies began in 1968 and are still in progress. In the first, 23 000 married users of the pill aged 15–49 years, together with a like number of control subjects using other methods or no method of contraception, were brought under observation by 1400 general practitioners. During follow-up, doctors record the diagnoses of episodes of illness, oral contraceptive prescriptions and data about pregnancies and deaths. In the second, 17 000 married women aged 25–39 years using oral contraceptives, the diaphragm or an IUD were recruited at one or other of 17 large family planning clinics. During follow-up, information is collected about changes in contraceptive methods, pregnancies, hospital attendances, deaths and the results of cervical smears. From the 2 studies, morbidity data collected during about 150 000 woman-years of observation, and mortality data collected during about 290 000 woman-years of observation, have now been published.

In the following 3 sections, the benefits and risks of oral contraceptives, IUDs and occlusive methods are briefly outlined. Clearly, any review of the vast amount of published evidence is impossible in a short chapter such as this. In the final section, however, some quantification of the benefits and risks is attempted in a series of simple tables. Most of the findings given in the tables are based on data obtained in the Oxford FPA cohort study.

Oral contraception

Benefits

By far the most important beneficial effect of the pill is its remarkable efficacy which, coupled with a high degree of acceptability (at least among the young), has given many women a new freedom from anxiety about the risk of unplanned pregnancy. Apart from this, the pill also has a number of well established non-contraceptive beneficial effects. First, it tends to suppress some menstrual disorders, notably menorrhagia, leading to a reduction in hospital admissions for dilatation and curettage, and to a lessened risk of iron deficiency anaemia. Secondly, it appears to inhibit the development of benign lesions of the breast (especially chronic cystic disease) thus reducing the need for surgical biopsies. This effect becomes stronger with increasing duration of use and may be particularly associated with the dose of the progestogenic component of the pill. Thirdly, since oral contraceptives act mainly by inhibiting ovulation, it is not surprising that functional ovarian cysts occur less frequently in women on the pill.

A number of other beneficial effects of the pill (e.g. a lessened risk of ovarian cancer, endometrial cancer, thyroid disease, rheumatoid arthritis and peptic ulceration) have been reported in some studies. Further work is necessary, however, before the significance of these observations can be assessed.

Risks

The best known adverse effects of oral contraceptives are the cardiovascular ones. These have recently been reviewed in detail by Vessey and Mann[4]. It is now clear that the pill is a cause of deep vein thrombosis, pulmonary embolism, certain types of acute cerebrovascular disturbance (especially thrombotic stroke) and acute myocardial infarction. There is reasonably convincing evidence that all these hazards are positively associated with the oestrogen content of oral contraceptives, but the progestogenic component is probably of importance too. The increased risk of venous thrombo-embolism seems to be independent of duration of use of the pill and to disappear within a month or two after discontinuation of use. The arterial hazards, however, may become greater with increasing duration of use and may also persist after the pill has been stopped. Oral contraceptives interact in a complex way with other risk factors, especially cigarette smoking, in the production of acute myocardial infarction. The mechanisms underlying the adverse cardiovascular reactions to oral contraceptives are uncertain, but it is known that the preparations have considerable effects on blood pressure levels, serum lipids and the blood coagulation system[5].

Cholelithiasis is an important non-cardiovascular adverse effect of the pill although the increase in risk is small. Hepato-cellular adenoma occurs much more commonly in women using the pill than in other women; the risk is strongly correlated both with the steroidal content and the duration of use of the preparation and with the age of the user[6]. Hepatocellular adenoma, although rare, is a serious condition which demands surgical intervention and may cause fatal haemorrhage.

'Cervical erosion' is an established adverse effect of oral contraception. Although a trivial condition in itself, a diagnosis of cervical erosion often leads to hospital admission for cautery under general anaesthesia. Despite an extensive literature, the prior use of oral contraceptives has not definitely been incriminated as a cause of prolonged secondary amenorrhoea or of prolactinoma of the pituitary which may be associated with this condition. On the other hand, there is usually some temporary impairment of fertility after discontinuation of the pill. It seems unlikely, however, that oral contraceptives are a cause of permanent infertility[7].

As far as malignant disease is concerned, a recent review prepared by a World Health Organization Scientific Group[8] concluded that there was no clear evidence of a relationship, either positive or negative, between the use of combined oral contraceptives and the risk of any form of cancer. It should be noted, however, that a few studies have suggested that oral contraceptives may increase the risk of breast cancer and pre-invasive cervical cancer among certain subgroups of women otherwise predisposed to these diseases. There is also some preliminary evidence that oral contraceptives may increase the risk of malignant melanoma at least in high incidence areas for this disease, like California. The possiblility that the pill might actually decrease the risk of ovarian and endometrial cancer has already been mentioned.

A number of reports have suggested that oral contraceptives taken inadvertently during (or even just before) pregnancy might increase the risk of malformation of the fetus. The evidence to support such claims is, however, uneven and difficult to interpret and the risk certainly cannot be regarded as substantiated[9].

Finally, many other disorders, including migraine, depression, and urinary tract infection have been reported in some studies, but not in others, as possible adverse effects of oral contraception.

Occlusive methods

In general, occlusive methods of contraception are less effective than either the pill or the IUD, but highly motivated users may achieve remarkably good results. There is some evidence that use of the diaphragm (and, presumably the condom) offers protection from the risk of pre-invasive carcinoma of the cervix. Certainly, the wearing of a condom during intercourse will reduce the risk of transmission of venereal disease. The suggestion that women using a diaphragm suffer an increased risk of urinary tract infection remains to be confirmed.

Intra-uterine devices

The IUD is a highly effective method of fertility control which, like the pill, does not detract from the spontaneity of intercourse. The use of an IUD carries no non-contraceptive benefits, but is associated with a number of risks. First, accidental pregnancies in women using an IUD are especially likely to be extra-uterine or to end in spontaneous abortion. Furthermore, there is evidence that spontaneous abortions occurring in women with an IUD *in situ* (especially a Dalkon Shield) are more likely than usual to be complicated by infection which, very rarely, may have a fatal outcome. Secondly, women using an IUD frequently experience pelvic pain and an increase in menstrual flow which sometimes leads to iron deficiency anaemia. Thirdly, pelvic inflammatory disease, which may be severe, is an important complication of IUD use. Finally, insertion of an IUD is occasionally followed by uterine perforation and migration of the device into the peritoneal cavity. Serious complications, such as intestinal obstruction, may then follow, especially if the device is a copper bearing one.

Comparative assessment

In Table 32.1, an attempt has been made to draw together information about non-obstetrical morbidity associated with use of the pill, the diaphragm and the IUD. This 'medical audit' is based very largely on data derived from the Oxford FPA contraceptive study and is limited to a consideration of hospital admissions. It should be noted, however, that a closely similar audit can be drawn up on the basis of data collected about General Practice consultations in the RCGP study. Of the conditions listed, venous thrombo-embolism, stroke, acute myocardial infarction, hepatocellular adenoma, pelvic inflammatory disease and uterine perforation are more serious than the rest, in that they are sometimes fatal and carry a risk of permanent sequelae when they are not. As far as the remaining conditions are concerned, the adverse effects of oral contraceptives (on cholelithiasis and cervical erosion) seem to be fairly closely balanced by their

Table 32.1. Non-obstetrical morbidity associated with different reversible methods of contraception. Rates of hospital admission per 100 000 women of childbearing age per annum.

Condition	Contraceptive method		
	Pill	Diaphragm	IUD
Menorrhagia	260	300	440
Anaemia	40	60	90
Benign lesions of breast	120	280	
Functional ovarian cysts	85	120	
Venous thromboembolism	90	20	
Stroke	45	10	
Acute myocardial infarction			
(non-fatal) ages 30–39	6	2	
40–44	55	10	
Cholelithiasis	180	120	
Hepatocellular adenoma	3	0	
Cervical erosion	540	250	
Pelvic inflammatory disease	55		200
Uterine perforation	—		50

The data for acute myocardial infarction are derived from Mann *et al.*[10]; for hepatocellular adenoma from Rooks *et al.*[6]; and for uterine perforation from Snowden[11]. All the rest of the data are derived from the Oxford FPA study[3] and are based on 31 000 woman-years of observation in the pill group, 15 000 woman-years of observation in the diaphragm group and 10 000 woman-years of observation in the IUD group.

beneficial effects (on menorrhagia, anaemia, and benign lesions of the breast and ovary).

Table 32.2 provides a comparison between the 3 methods of contraception with regard to the frequency of unplanned pregnancies and their outcome. The failure rates for the pill (0.15 pregnancies per 100 woman-years) and the IUD (2.0 pregnancies per 100 woman-years) are derived from the Oxford FPA contraceptive study. 2 failure rates are shown for the diaphragm. The first (2.4 pregnancies per 100 woman-years) is also taken from the Oxford FPA study. The second (5.0 pregnancies per 100 woman-years) is, perhaps, more typical of the rate which might apply to the general population. Throughout the table, the data on outcome of unplanned pregnancies are based on the findings in the Oxford FPA study.

The rates shown in Table 32.2 underline the importance of the benefit conferred by the high efficacy of the pill. The table also shows the high incidence of ectopic gestation among women using an IUD. This condition is, of course, one of the most serious of the possible outcomes of pregnancy.

Table 32.3 is concerned with mortality among women aged 20–34 years attributable to the use of different methods of contraception and to the accidental pregnancies resulting from their failure. Table 32.4 corresponds exactly to Table 32.3, except that the data relate to women aged 35–44 years. In

Table 32.2. Frequency and outcome of unplanned pregnancies associated with different reversible methods of contraception. Rates per 100 000 women of childbearing age per annum.

Outcome of unplanned pregnancies	Contraceptive method			
	Pill	Diaphragm		IUD
	PI 0.15 per HWY	PI 2.4 per HWY	PI 5.0 per HWY	PI 2.0 per HWY
Term birth	90	1460	3040	500
Spontaneous abortion	19	310	640	770
Ectopic gestation	1	10	20	120
Termination	40	620	1300	610
Total unplanned pregnancies	150	2400	5000	2000

PI   Pearl Index: Failure rate per 100 woman-years (HWY)
The data are derived from the Oxford FPA study[3] and are based on the outcome of 500 accidental pregnancies.

both tables, 2 estimates are provided of the mortality from cardiovascular disease attributable to oral contraceptives. The first is based on the results of case–control studies concerned with pulmonary and cerebral thrombo-embolism[12] and with myocardial infarction[13], while the second is based on the data relating to cardiovascular disorders as a whole obtained in the RCGP cohort study[14]. Although the estimates differ quite markedly, it seems reasonable to conclude that oral contraceptives compare unfavourably with the diaphragm and with the IUD as far as mortality is concerned, especially in women aged 35 years or more. A sense of proportion in assessing the figures is provided by comparing them with the mortality rates from various other causes shown in Table 32.5.

   Simple analyses of the sort presented in Tables 32.1–32.4, while of value in providing crude comparisons between contraceptive methods, are subject to many limitations as the following considerations show:
1   Some of the morbidity estimates and all the mortality estimates are based on small numbers of events and are therefore subject to considerable sampling error.
2   Most of the data accumulated in the RCGP and Oxford FPA studies relate to pills containing 50 μg oestrogen. Lower dose preparations have now captured well over half the market in the United Kingdom and may be associated with smaller risks. Furthermore, as has been indicated, the nature and dose of the progestogen contained in oral contraceptives is likely to be a determinant of risk as well.
3   At least some of the risks and benefits associated with oral contraception are related to duration of use.
4   The risks of oral contraception (and the IUD as well) vary with the

Table 32.3. Mortality rates (per 100 000 per annum) for women aged 20–34 years using different reversible methods of contraception.

Mortality	Contraceptive method				
	Pill PI 0.15 per HWY		Diaphragm		IUD
	Estimate A	Estimate B	PI 2.4 per HWY	PI 5.0 per HWY	PI 2.0 per HWY
Attributable to method					
Cardiovascular disease	2.4*	4.4†	—	—	—
Pelvic inflammatory disease and uterine perforation	—	—	—	—	0.2‡
Attributable to accidental pregnancies§	0.0	0.0	0.2	0.5	0.2
'Loading' for IUD	—	—	—	—	0.5**
Total	2.4	4.4	0.2	0.5	0.9

* Based on data from case–control studies – Inman & Vessey[12], Mann *et al.*[13].
† Based on data from RCGP study[14].
‡ Based on data from Kahn & Tyler[15].
§ Based on maternal mortality rate for year 1977.
** The case fatality rate for ectopic pregnancy is about 1 in 250. There is also evidence that fatal septic abortion may rarely complicate pregnancy with an IUD *in situ*. A 'loading factor' has therefore been added in to take account of the unfavourable outcome of accidental pregnancy in IUD users.

Table 32.4. Mortality rates (per 100 000 per annum) for women aged 35–44 years using different reversible methods of contraception.

Mortality	Contraceptive method				
	Pill PI 0.15 per HWY		Diaphragm		IUD
	Estimate A	Estimate B	PI 2.4 per HWY	PI 5.0 per HWY	PI 2.0 per HWY
Attributable to method					
Cardiovascular disease	11.5*	33.0†	—	—	—
Pelvic inflammatory disease and uterine perforation	—	—	—	—	0.2‡
Attributable to accidental pregnancies§	0.1	0.1	1.1	2.3	0.9
'Loading' for IUD	—	—	—	—	0.5**
Total	11.6	33.1	1.1	2.3	1.6

All footnotes as for Table 32.3.

Table 32.5. Death rates from various causes per 100 000 women of childbearing age in England & Wales in 1977.

Cause of death	Age (years)	
	20–34	35–44
Breast cancer	2.8	22.2
Cervical cancer	1.4	6.0
Multiple sclerosis	0.7	1.7
Nephritis & nephrosis	0.6	1.3
Motor vehicle traffic accidents	5.0	4.3
Murder & manslaughter	1.0	0.9
Suicide	5.1	6.7

characteristics of the user. Some account of this has been taken in the mortality analyses by subdividing the data by age, but the interaction between cigarette smoking and the pill in the production of acute myocardial infarction has not been taken into consideration, to give but one important example. Furthermore, most of the estimates of risk relate to healthy women – little is known about the hazards of the pill in those with diabetes, hypertension or cardiac disease.

5   Restriction of the analysis to simple counting of hospital admissions, deaths and obstetric events, is very inadequate. Such an approach cannot, for example, take into account the peace of mind felt by a woman using a highly efficacious contraceptive method.

6   Not all contraceptive methods are acceptable to all women. Furthermore, not all women continue with the contraceptive method they initially choose. Roughly 30 % of women choosing the pill and 15 % choosing an IUD give up in the first year.

7   The analyses presented apply mainly to couples concerned with the problems of birth spacing. For those who have completed their families, male sterilization is the safest method, since vasectomy is associated with little morbidity and virtually no mortality. Female sterilization is preferable to the continued use of reversible methods of contraception, but the procedure is not without hazard. It does, of course, give the best results in terms of morbidity and mortality if carried out at a reasonably young age (say 35 years rather than 45 years).

Although we now have substantial knowledge about the risks and benefits of different methods of contraception, at least in the short and medium term, it is clear from the above that advising the individual couple still requires considerable experience and judgement on the part of the counsellor. It should also be stressed that the data discussed in this chapter have been derived for the most part from British studies. It would be quite incorrect to extrapolate them to other countries with different patterns of disease and different risks associated with childbearing.

References

1. World Health Organization. *Special programme of research, development, and research training in human reproduction.* Seventh Annual Report. Geneva: WHO, 1978.
2. Royal College of General Practitioners. *Oral contraceptives and health.* London: Pitman Medical, 1974.
3. Vessey M, Doll R, *et al.* A long-term follow-up study of women using different methods of contraception – an interim report. *Journal of Biosocial Science* 1976; **8**: 373.
4. Vessey MP, Mann JI. Female sex hormones and thrombosis. Epidemiological aspects. *British Medical Bulletin* 1978; **34**: 157.
5. Briggs MH. Recent biological studies in relation to low dose hormonal contraceptives. *British Journal of Family Planning* 1979; **5**: 25.
6. Rooks JB, Ory HW, *et al.* Epidemiology of hepatocellular adenoma. *JAMA* 1979; **242**: 644.
7. Vessey MP, Wright NH, *et al.* Fertility after stopping different methods of contraception. *British Medical Journal* 1978; **i**: 265.
8. World Health Organization. *Steroid contraception and the risk of neoplasia.* WHO Technical report series No 619. Geneva, 1978.
9. Ambani LM, Joshi NJ, *et al.* Are hormonal contraceptives teratogenic? *Fertility and Sterility* 1977; **28**: 791.
10. Mann JI, Vessey MP, *et al.* Myocardial infarction in young women with special reference to oral contraceptive practice. *British Medical Journal* 1975; **ii**: 241.
11. Snowden R. *Pelvic inflammation, perforation and pregnancy outcome associated with the use of intra-uterine devices.* Family Planning Research Unit. Report No 15. University of Exeter, England, 1974.
12. Inman WHW, Vessey MP. Investigation of deaths from pulmonary, coronary and cerebral thrombosis and embolism in women of childbearing age. *British Medical Journal* 1968; **ii**: 193.
13. Mann JI, Inman WHW. Oral contraceptives and death from myocardial infarction. *British Medical Journal* 1975; **ii**: 245.
14. Royal College of General Practitioners. Mortality among oral contraceptive users. *Lancet* 1977; **ii**: 727.
15. Kahn HS, Tyler CW. Mortality associated with use of IUDs. *JAMA* 1975, **234**: 57.

Chapter 33 · Pregnancy, Childbirth and Perinatal Mortality

C S PECKHAM, E M ROSS AND R D T FARMER

Crude death rates throughout the developed world have fallen dramatically during the past 100 years. This is mainly due to the substantial reduction in mortality in very early life. The causes of this are complex and numerous. There is no doubt that in the late 19th and early 20th centuries the most important factors were the beneficial changes in living conditions that followed the industrial revolution; these included improvements in standards of nutrition, hygiene and housing. More recently, specific interventions such as improved antenatal care with a consequent early recognition of problems, the effective treatment of infections and developments in the management of labour and the new-born infant, have significantly improved the chances of survival of both mothers and their babies.

Until the 1950s, perinatal mortality in Britain was amongst the lowest in the world. In recent years its rate of decline has lagged behind that in many other countries, particularly Japan and the Scandinavian countries (Fig. 33.1). These differences between countries suggest that there is still some room for improvement. Public concern that the perinatal mortality rate in the United Kingdom was higher than in most other European countries prompted a recent enquiry by a Select Committee of the House of Commons[1]. It is frequently said that the perinatal mortality rate of a community is a sensitive indicator of its quality of health and health services available. Such an assertion is probably an over-simplification. Because the mortality rates in early life in most developed countries are now so low, morbidity amongst infants may be a more sensitive index. Unfortunately, there is little morbidity data available from which to make comparisons, therefore most of the investigations rely substantially on neonatal death and stillbirth data.

In this chapter attention is drawn to some of the important maternal, social and environmental factors that influence perinatal mortality and morbidity. There is a risk of over-simplifying the influence of some of these factors as few individual causes of perinatal death act in isolation. It is the interaction of a number of factors that compound risk and make the reduction of mortality a more complex problem than it might at first appear. As the fertility patterns of a community greatly influence perinatal mortality and morbidity the recent relevant changes in reproductive behaviour are discussed.

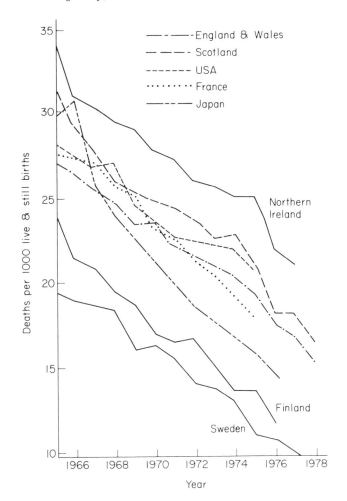

Fig. 33.1. Perinatal mortality in selected nations, 1966–78 (World Health Organization[11].)

Definitions used in perinatal epidemiology

The terms that are used in perinatal epidemiology have precise meanings, although some differ from country to country. The definitions that are given here are those that are currently applied in the United Kingdom, examples of variants used elsewhere are given where appropriate.

An *abortion* is the expulsion from the uterus of a product of conception before it has reached an age when it could be expected to have an independent existence and, which does not breathe or show any other signs of life. The lower limit of fetal viability is defined as the 28th week of pregnancy. Some countries accept a lower limit of 20 weeks. In the USA it varies from state to state between 20 and 28 weeks.

A *stillbirth* is the expulsion of a fetus which does not breathe or show any signs of life after the lower age limit of viability is reached – 28 weeks in England and Wales. Some countries impose a minimum birth weight as well as a presumed gestational age on the definition of a stillbirth. The stillbirth rate is the number of stillbirths per 1000 total births (live and still) that occur during the same period.

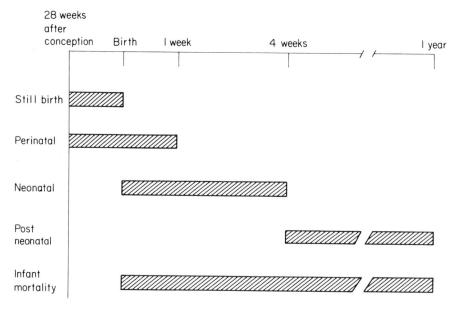

Fig. 33.2. Rates for stillbirths, perinatal, neonatal, post neonatal and infant mortality are calculated thus: stillbirths per 1000 live and stillbirths; perinatal mortality per 1000 live and stillbirths; neonatal mortality per 1000 live births; infant mortality per 1000 live births.

There are 4 important periods of early life defined in Fig. 33.2. The *perinatal* period extends from the presumed 28th week of pregnancy to the end of the first week of life. The perinatal mortality rate is the number of deaths during the perinatal period per 1000 total births (live and still). The aggregation of stillbirths and first week deaths as perinatal deaths is useful because they have similar causes. It is also one of the most satisfactory indices for making international comparisons, as it takes account of the different ways in which countries handle the problem of registering deaths that occur within the first week of life. For example, some countries regard as a stillbirth a baby who dies before its birth is registered. In France, live-born infants who die before registration are coded as a separate category: 'died before registration'.

The *neonatal* period extends from birth to the 28th day. The *early neonatal* (the first 7 days) period is sometimes considered separately. The neonatal mortality rates all use the number of live births as the denominator.

The *post-neonatal* period extends from 28 days to the end of the first year of life. Infancy is defined as the whole of the first year of life (i.e. the neonatal plus the post-neonatal periods).

Sources of data

Routine sources

Since the middle of the 19th century, registration of births occurring in the United Kingdom has been obligatory. Over the years the information that is recorded at registration has been extended. Under the current regulations the person registering the birth is required to disclose the following information:

1   child's name, place of birth, sex and legitimacy;
2   mother's name, place of birth, marital status, date of birth, place of usual residence and occupation;
3   father's name, place and date of birth, occupation (if known).

Additional data are required in respect of legitimate births only. These are: date of present marriage, number of previous marriages, number of previous legitimate children (distinguishing those born dead from those born alive). In the United Kingdom birth weight does not form part of the registration data set. It is included in many other Western countries e.g. Sweden, and it is expected to be included in the United Kingdom in the future.

Stillbirths have been registered since 1927 in England and Wales and since 1939 in Scotland. The data registered are similar to that for births but the cause of stillbirth was not recorded until 1960 in England and Wales and 1939 in Scotland. Most developed countries routinely register both the fact and cause of stillbirth at the present time.

All deaths are registered, together with cause. The death registration data provide sufficient information to link birth and death records. Tabulations of birth and death analyses are prepared and published annually by the Office of Population Censuses and Surveys (OPCS) as Birth Statistics (Series FM1) and Mortality Statistics, childhood and maternity (Series DH3).

The quality of reporting and the accuracy of information recorded varies widely from country to country and it is often more revealing to study trends within a country and to compare trends between countries than to compare rates between countries. The developing countries present particular problems for study. Few have comprehensive systems of registration.

British perinatal studies

There have been 3 major national perinatal surveys in Britain. These were undertaken in 1946, 1958 and 1970. As well as providing a unique overview of the obstetric, economic and social aspects of childbirth, they have provided the epidemiological basis for far reaching changes in medical practice.

1946 survey[2]

The initial aim of the first survey was to assess the quality of maternity services in Britain. Every woman delivered during 1 week in March in England, Scotland and Wales, was interviewed by a health visitor who asked a standard set of questions. The interviews took place at the woman's home 6 weeks after the delivery. Sub-samples of this cohort are still being followed up.

1958 Survey[3,4]

This survey was undertaken to investigate the causes of perinatal mortality, to relate them to factors connected with social background and biological characteristics of the mother and to assess the quality of obstetric care. The first part of the survey was concerned with all births in the United Kingdom in 1 week in March 1958. For each birth a questionnaire was completed by the midwife shortly after delivery. Information was obtained partly from the obstetric notes and partly by interview with the mother. The second part of the survey included all stillbirths and neonatal deaths which occurred in England and Wales during March, April and May of 1958. For the majority of these, detailed post mortems were carried out. For all deaths a questionnaire on maternal background, pregnancy and delivery was also completed. In all, information was gathered on over 7000 stillbirths and neonatal deaths. These were compared with the 17 000 births that had occurred in the 1 week survey. The surviving infants from the 1 week survey of births have been followed up at the ages of 7, 11, 16 and 23 years.

1970 survey[5,6]

The aim of the third national survey was to look at the obstetric services and socio-biological factors related to neonatal morbidity. All births in the United Kingdom and Northern Ireland in 1 week of April were included. As in the 1958 survey, a questionnaire was completed by the midwife shortly after delivery. The children born in the survey week have been followed up at the ages of 5 and 10 years.

These studies each involved many thousands of births and so make it possible to look at the various factors which relate to perinatal mortality and morbidity as well as to the quality of care during pregnancy, the nature of delivery and the health of the infant during the first week of life. They showed that adverse maternal obstetric factors tend to act in a cumulative manner and rarely as single factors. No other country has performed comparable national studies, although large birth populations have been studied in the USA[7] and Denmark[8].

Spontaneous abortion

It is not possible to estimate the frequency of spontaneous abortion in early pregnancy with any accuracy since many women have not realized by then that they are pregnant. Amongst known conceptions it has been estimated that between 15 and 25% spontaneously abort. Miller *et al.*[9] studied β-human chorionic gonadotrophin levels in the urine to establish the fact of pregnancy at the earliest possible stage. They estimated that the true spontaneous abortion rate in these normal women was over 40%. Of 152 identified conceptions in the 623 menstrual cycles studied the pregnancy loss rate was 43% but only 14 of 64 spontaneous abortions were clinically recognized.

Spontaneous miscarriage may be a safety valve for the elimination of abnormal conceptions. A recent review[10] suggests that at the earliest detectable stage of pregnancy over 60% of spontaneous abortions have abnormal chromosomes. This rate falls to below 5% by the end of the sixth month of intra-uterine life. About half the chromosome abnormalities are autosomal trisomy of which a third are trisomy 16 and the remainder are mostly tetraploids, unbalanced translocations, double trisomies and mosaics. Sex chromosome abnormalities account for about one-fifth of abnormal karotypes but other sex chromosomes are rare in abortuses. Among live births, the rate of chromosome abnormalities is about 6 per 1000 although among perinatal deaths, the rate is 10 times higher with the highest prevalence being among macerated still-births[49].

Other reasons for spontaneous abortion include uterine abnormality and cervical incompetence. In developing countries malnutrition and infections are important causes. However, many spontaneous abortions remain totally unexplained. For every 1000 confirmed pregnancies in the United Kingdom, about 150 abort spontaneously, 10 are stillborn and 840 born alive, 10 of whom die in the first 28 days.

Factors affecting perinatal mortality

In 1979 the perinatal mortality rate in England and Wales was 15 per 1000 births. The lowest rates in the world are in Sweden (9.3 per 1000 births in 1978). Within Sweden even lower rates occur in some counties which suggests that even lower rates are achievable. A reduction in rates depends upon the identification of factors that directly or indirectly influence mortality and that are susceptible to intervention. In this section, the important determinants are discussed.

Table 33.1. Perinatal mortality by maternal age, per 1000 live and still births[11].

Country (year)	Maternal age (years)												
	<15	15	16	17	18	19	All <20	20–24	25–29	30–34	35–39	40+	All ages
England and Wales (1973)	34.6	29.2	28.5	25.1	24.6	21.4	23.9	17.9	17.0	20.7	28.1	43.8	19.6
Sweden (1973)	—	—	22.9	13.2	13.2	15.8	14.8	11.7	11.8	12.6	19.2	35.2	12.6
Japan (1973)	—	—	71.4	70.5	34.8	31.5	36.7	17.5	14.4	18.0	29.3	75.5	17.0
Hungary (1973)	37.0	28.4	35.6	30.7	28.6	25.8	28.1	23.4	30.3	39.6	52.3	55.4	29.1
USA (Part) (1973)	31.1	20.9	20.8	17.5	15.5	15.7	16.9	13.3	13.5	16.1	22.1	36.4	14.9
New Zealand (1972–73)	51.1	23.5	21.6	19.4	23.1	16.7	20.1	16.6	14.7	18.0	23.2	43.1	17.3

Biological factors

Maternal age

Within the wide geographical variations and secular trends in perinatal mortality rates there are consistent differences in maternal age-specific perinatal mortality rates. The lowest rates occur in women in their middle reproductive years (20–29). The highest rates are amongst babies born to women at the end of their reproductive life. Young mothers have intermediate rates (Table 33.1). Clearly some of the international variations in total perinatal mortality are the result of differences in maternal age distribution.

Parity

The variations in perinatal mortality by maternal parity (the number of previous legitimate live and stillbirths) are shown in Table 33.2. For England and Wales, only previous legitimate births are included because of the way data are collected at registration. The lowest rates are in the babies of para one mothers. Rates increase with successive pregnancies. First-born babies have consistently higher rates than those who are second-born. The countries shown have wide variations in total perinatal mortality but the parity-specific rates are more constant. Some of the international variation in rates are due to differences in the proportion of high parity mothers.

Table 33.2. Perinatal mortality rates by parity of mother, per 1000 live and still births[11].

Country	Parity					All
	0	1	2	3	4+	parities
England and Wales (1973)	20.1	15.3	19.0	24.6	32.3	19.6
Sweden (1973)	13.2	10.8	13.1	20.1	21.3	12.6
Japan (1973)	17.9	14.1	16.6	32.6	62.5	17.0
Hungary (1973)	25.8	27.2	40.2	44.3	47.5	29.1
USA (Part) (1973)	12.6	11.1	12.6	14.4	20.0	14.9
New Zealand (1972–73)	18.9	11.8	15.1	16.7	25.1	17.3

Birth interval

The data collected at registration in some countries makes it possible to analyse perinatal mortality by interval between births. Table 33.3 shows that the highest rates occur when this interval is under 12 months. In all countries shown, the lowest mortality rates are observed when the interval is between 18 and 35 months. Thereafter, there is a rise in rates with the highest occurring when the interval is greatest.

Table 33.3. Perinatal mortality rates by birth interval, per 1000 live and still births[11].

Birth interval (months)	Hungary	New Zealand	Sweden	USA (Part)
< 12	80.6	40.7	24.0	34.2
12–17	31.0	14.4	17.9	12.1
18–23	23.0	11.3	12.5	9.7
24–35	24.7	12.4	8.5	8.7
36–47	27.8	12.9	10.4	9.2
48–59	30.1	15.5	13.4	9.8
60 +	41.0	25.3	12.9	9.3

Legitimacy

Unmarried women at all ages are at higher risk than married women of losing their babies at all stages of pregnancy and during the neonatal period. However, a special study of stillbirth death certificates between 1975 and 1976 in England and Wales demonstrated marked differences within illegitimate births. Those registered by the mother only, had a rate of 19.5 per 1000 compared with 5.9 per 1000 amongst those registered by both the mother and the putative father[12]. This latter rate is lower than the legitimate stillbirth rate. This difference between the apparently supported and unsupported mothers requires further study. It is possible that the high mortality of the apparently unsupported illegitimate group may be due to factors such as different patterns of care in pregnancy, stress and poor diet. An equally plausible explanation is that joint registration by both the natural parents is less relevant when the child is stillborn than when it is for a live-born child. Thus single registration may be a poor proxy index of support during the pregnancy.

Interactions between maternal age, parity and legitimacy

Clearly these 3 variables are interrelated. High parity mothers are likely to be older than low parity mothers. Primaparous women are more likely to be single than high parity women. Table 33.4 shows stillbirth rates for England and Wales (1978) by maternal age, parity and legitimacy. Because of registration practices it is not possible to subdivide illegitimate births by maternal parity. The illegitimate stillbirth rates are marginally greater than the legitimate primaparous stillbirth rate at all ages. This suggests that parity is an important component in the excessive stillbirth rates amongst illegitimate pregnancies. At all ages, stillbirth rates in first pregnancies exceed those in second pregnancies and the rates increase with third and subsequent births. At all parities the lowest rates are among babies of women aged 20–24 and the highest rates are in the extreme upper limits of maternal age. This is consistent with age and parity acting additively.

It is not possible to examine perinatal mortality by maternal age and parity in combination in England and Wales from routinely collected data because death registration data are not routinely linked to birth registration data. However, the 1958 national perinatal mortality study data showed the same pattern in perinatal mortality as routine data shows for stillbirths only.

Social class and regional variations within Britain

There is a strong association between perinatal mortality and social class of father. The lowest rates occur in the higher social classes and the highest in children of unskilled manual workers (Table 33.5).

Table 33.4. Stillbirth rates by age, parity and legitimacy, England and Wales 1979, per 1000 live and still births.

Maternal age (years)	Illegitimate All parities	Legitimate Parity						All births
		0	1	2	3	4	Over 4	
< 20	10.1	9.9	7.7	(2.9)*	—	—	—	9.7
20–24	9.5	8.9	5.8	6.2	(7.2)	(13.9)	(39.2)	7.8
25–29	9.4	8.7	5.4	6.1	7.6	(7.3)	(13.3)	7.1
30–34	11.1	8.5	5.8	7.5	10.1	(9.8)	(11.2)	7.6
35–39	(13.6)	13.6	7.2	9.9	(9.9)	(12.0)	(16.9)	10.7
40 +	(27.1)	(20.7)	(7.3)	(21.7)	(17.0)	(36.7)	(18.7)	20.4
All ages	10.2	9.1	5.7	7.1	9.2	12.3	15.1	8.0

* Rates in brackets calculated from less than 50 stillbirths.

Table 33.5. Perinatal mortality by father's social class, England 1977, per 1000 live and still births (OPCS 1979).

	Social Class					No male head	All Classes
	I	II	III	IV	V		
Mortality	11	13	16	19	22	23	17

Some of the differences in the mortality of babies born to women of different social classes can be explained by their differing reproductive behaviour. For example, mothers in the higher social classes tend to have fewer children and are less likely to be in the extremes of reproductive age than mothers in the lower social classes. However, even when these differences are taken into account, the perinatal mortality amongst infants born to parents in the professional and managerial groups is significantly lower than that of babies of parents in semi-skilled and unskilled occupations. The most obvious explanation for these residual differences are environmental and social factors, and variations in the quality of medical care.

The international variations in perinatal mortality rates have already been mentioned. Even within Britain there are substantial regional differences. The highest rates occur in Ulster and in Strathclyde, the lowest in East Anglia and Oxfordshire (Fig. 33.3). These differences are explained in part by the differences in the social class structure of the regions. Other explanations may include differences in the quality of services between the regions.

Perinatal mortality amongst immigrants

It has often been suggested that perinatal mortality rates in Britain are higher than in other countries in Europe because of the high rates among immigrants from the New Commonwealth. This has not been shown to be the case from the 1970 British Births Study data. It showed that the immigrant perinatal mortality rate was 24.7 per 1000, compared with the national rate of 21.4 per 1000. This difference was too small to have made an impact on the national perinatal mortality figures. When immigrant births were excluded the national rate only fell to 21.3. Table 33.6 shows the perinatal mortality rates (1975–77) by country of mother's birth. Although the size of the immigrant population and the differences between its perinatal mortality rate and that of the indigenous population are insufficient to have any great impact on national rates there are important findings from immigrant studies. The Asian immigrant population in Bradford (England) is 19 % of the total population. In 1975–77, 30 % of all births were to this ethnic group and amongst them the perinatal mortality rate was $2\frac{1}{2}$ times that of the non-Asian population of Bradford[14].

These findings contrast markedly with observations from another area with a high immigrant population, Brent (England)[15] where one-third of all deliveries are to Asian mothers. There, the perinatal mortality rates were 15 per 1000 amongst Asians, 31 per 1000 Irish immigrants, 33 per 1000 in West Indians and 24 per 1000 in British-born Whites. The most plausible explanation of the difference between the Bradford and Brent Asian groups is that they differ in social class structure. There is no convincing evidence that immigrants differ from the British indigenous population for any biological reason.

Demographic changes

For many years the birth rates in most developed countries have fluctuated markedly. Because perinatal mortality varies with maternal age, parity, birth

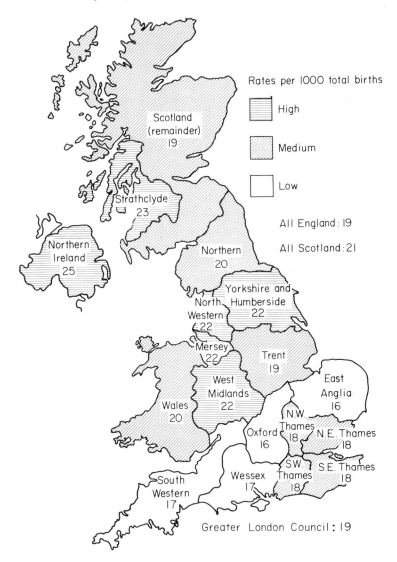

Fig. 33.3. Perinatal mortality in the UK, 1975. Subdivisions of England are regional health authority areas. (*Prevention and health: reducing the risk.* London: HMSO, 1977.)

interval and legitimacy, these fluctuations would have altered the total perinatal mortality rates even if no changes had occurred in specific risk groups. The changes in patterns of fertility can be illustrated by the England and Wales data.

The general fertility rate (i.e. number of births per 1000 women aged 15–44) fell modestly between 1928 and the early years of the Second World War (Fig. 33.4); between 1941 and 1944 it increased. The fall in 1945 was followed by

Table 33.6. Stillbirth and perinatal mortality rates, 1975–77, by country of birth of mother, England and Wales, per 1000 live and still births[13].

Country of birth of mother	Stillbirth rate	Perinatal mortality rate
All countries	9.8	18.2
United Kingdom	9.5	17.7
Irish Republic	10.7	18.1
Australia, Canada and New Zealand	7.5	15.2
New Commonwealth		
India and Bangladesh	14.3	24.0
African Commonwealth	13.6	24.5
West Indies	12.1	23.3
Pakistan	14.7	26.5

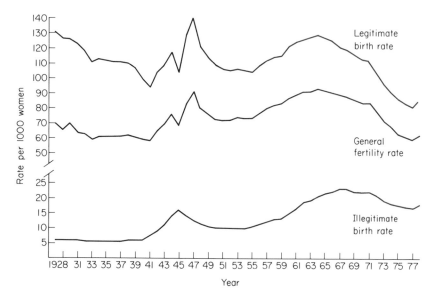

Fig. 33.4. Fertility rate, England and Wales, 1928–77.

a sharp rise that was maintained until 1947. This was followed by a fall between 1955 and 1964 there was a further rise. Since 1964 the general fertility rate has been falling steadily. The changes in the legitimate fertility rate are not dissimilar from those for the general fertility rate. There is some evidence to suggest that the post 1964 fall was influenced by the introduction of efficient oral contraceptives. The trend in the illegitimate fertility rate differs from that of the legitimate rate.

After the post-war fall in the illegitimate birth rate there was a steady rise until 1967–68. Illegitimacy should not be considered in isolation but in conjunction with pre-maritally conceived births, that is, legitimate live births occuring within 8 months of marriage. For example, in both World Wars, the number of illegitimate births rose but the legitimate pre-maritally conceived births fell, presumably because the putative father was absent from home and unable to make the child legitimate. The picture was quite different between 1955 and 1965 when the rise in illegitimate births was accompanied by a rise in pre-marital conceptions (Fig. 33.5).

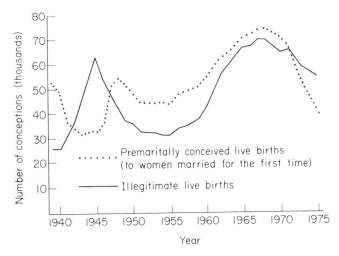

Fig. 33.5. Premaritally conceived live births (to women married once only) and illegitimate live births to women resident in England and Wales, 1939–75 (OPCS).

An increasing proportion of single mothers are keeping their children and more are being registered at birth by both parents. This suggests that an increasing number of illegitimate children are born into stable family units. Illegitimate births are particularly vulnerable and have a high perinatal mortality, currently similar to that of births to women in Social Class V. In the United Kingdom, the rate of birth outside marriage differs markedly from one racial group to another. It ranges from 51 % of births to mothers born in the West Indies to 1 % among mothers born in India, Pakistan and Bangladesh.

Although the birth rates to women aged 20–24 years and those to women aged 25–29 years followed similar trends to each other between 1938 and 1978, those to women at the extremes of reproductive life were different (Fig. 33.6). The rate for 15–19 year old women increased steadily until the early 1970s, then fell. In the older women rates have fallen consistently since the Second World War.

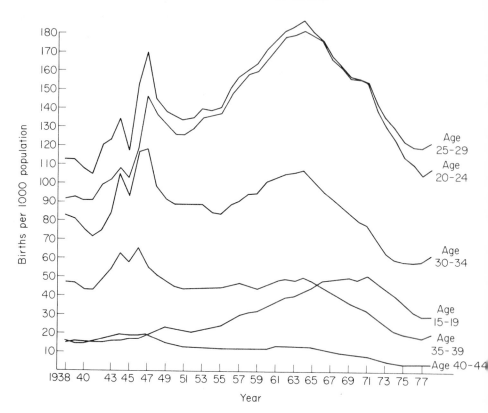

Fig. 33.6. Age-specific birth rates, England and Wales, 1938–77.

The changes in the distribution of maternities by maternal age and legitimacy are shown in Table 33.7. Although there has been a marked increase in the proportion of maternities that were illegitimate – one of the identified risk factors in perinatal mortality – there has been a marked fall in the proportion of maternities occurring to women aged over 35 years. This change in the distribution of births by maternal age accounts for some of the reduction in total perinatal mortality.

The fall in birth rates since the last war was due to a decrease in the number of children born to individual women rather than a reduction in the number of women having children. Therefore, there has been a reduction in the number of high parity women having children (Table 33.8). This change in reproductive behaviour would also reduce total perinatal mortality.

The contribution of maternal age and parity to the decline in perinatal mortality has been estimated[16]. Between 1950 and 1973 the perinatal mortality

Table 33.7 Distribution of maternities by maternal age and legitimacy, England and Wales, 1979.

Age (years)	Maternities Legitimate						All legitimate	Illegitimate						All illegitimate	All maternities
	<20	20–24	25–29	30–34	35–39	40+		<20	20–24	25–29	30–34	35–39	40+		
1949	26 806 (3.6)	191 167 (25.9)	236 264 (32.0)	132 465 (17.9)	84 742 (11.5)	27 118 (3.7)	700 496 (94.9)	5 334 (0.7)	10 859 (1.5)	9 814 (1.3)	5 619 (0.8)	4 014 (0.5)	1 591 (0.2)	37 554 (5.1)	738 050 (100)
1959	38 516 (5.1)	218 551 (28.9)	227 399 (30.1)	139 167 (18.4)	74 421 (9.9)	18 448 (2.4)	716 502 (94.9)	8 121 (1.1)	12 382 (1.6)	7 705 (1.0)	5 372 (0.7)	3 925 (0.5)	1 287 (0.2)	38 792 (5.1)	755 294 (100)
1969	60 403 (7.6)	266 608 (33.3)	227 385 (28.4)	113 996 (14.3)	49 673 (6.2)	14 218 (1.8)	732 283 (91.6)	21 857 (2.7)	23 267 (2.9)	11 165 (1.4)	6 351 (0.8)	3 477 (0.4)	1 363 (0.2)	67 480 (8.4)	799 763 (100)
1978	34 493 (5.8)	162 819 (27.3)	199 487 (33.5)	106 684 (17.9)	25 563 (4.3)	5 656 (0.9)	534 702 (89.8)	21 779 (3.7)	19 741 (3.3)	10 440 (1.8)	5 884 (1.0)	2 322 (0.4)	647 (0.1)	60 813 (10.2)	595 515 (100)

† Figures in brackets are percentages of total maternities in each year.

Table 33.8. Legitimate births by number of previous live-born children, England and Wales, 1979.

Year	Number of previous live-born children							All legitimate births
	0	1	2	3	4	5	Over 5	
1949	286 398	221 205	99 082	42 641	20 401	11 256	17 119	698 102
	(41.7)	(31.7)	(14.2)	(6.1)	(2.9)	(1.6)	(2.5)	(100)
1959	271 264	213 491	108 393	51 650	25 591	13 490	16 002	699 941
	(38.8)	(30.5)	(15.5)	(7.4)	(3.7)	(1.9)	(2.3)	(100)
1969	275 340	233 572	112 433	48 269	21 247	10 592	10 136	711 589
	(38.7)	(32.8)	(15.8)	(6.8)	(3.0)	(1.5)	(1.4)	(100)
1978	226 586	198 088	74 173	23 358	7 684	3 114	2 778	535 781
	(42.3)	(37.0)	(13.8)	(4.4)	(1.4)	(0.6)	(0.5)	(100)

* Figures in brackets are percentages of total legitimate births in each year.

rate in England and Wales fell by 45 %. Changes in the age distribution alone contributed 14.5 % and parity alone contributed 6.5 %. The 2 together accounted for 17.9 % of the overall reduction. The rest of the decline was due to changes in age and parity-specific perinatal mortality rates. This is demonstrated in Tables 33.9 and 33.10.

There are important differences in fertility between groups of differing social or cultural origin. For example, in 1979 13 % of all live births in England and Wales were to mothers born outside the United Kingdom. Mothers born in the Irish Republic accounted for 1.5 % of total live births and mothers from the New Commonwealth and Pakistan for 8.2 %. The high proportion partially reflects

Table 33.9. Comparison of parity distribution and perinatal mortality rates, 1958 and 1970— singleton legitimate births only[6].

Parity	% Distribution		Perinatal mortality rates*		
	1958	1970	1958	1970	
				Rate	% of 1958
0	36.0	35.5	33.6	21.0	63
1	31.2	33.2	23.5	15.1	64
2 & 3	23.8	24.2	33.8	22.6	67
4 +	8.9	7.1	50.5	31.8	63
Total	100.0†	100.0	32.0	20.2	63

* Per 1000 live and still births.
† Parity not known included in the totals.

Table 33.10. Comparison of age distribution and perinatal mortality rates, 1958 and 1970—singleton legitimate births only[6].

Maternal age	% Distribution		Perinatal mortality rates*		
	1958	1970	1958	1970	
				Rate	% of 1958
< 20	5.0	7.7	33.1	25.1	76
20–	28.8	35.4	27.5	16.9	61
25–	32.6	31.9	27.2	18.6	68
30–	20.4	15.7	34.8	20.4	59
> 35	13.1	8.7	48.7	34.6	71
Not known	0.1	0.6	—	21.3	—
Total	100.0	100.0	32.0	20.2	63

* Per 1000 live and still births.
† Age not known included in the totals.

the age structure of women in this population and their birth rate can be expected to fall as immigration decreases and the Asian population in the United Kingdom ages. Married Asian mothers in the United Kingdom have larger families than other racial groups; 40 % had 3 or more children, compared with about 17 % of British-born mothers. In the 1950s, West Indian mothers in the United Kingdom were also having larger families but with the passage of time, their family size has tended to adjust to the norms of the indigenous population. Asian women may follow the same trend.

Within these overall changes in patterns of fertility there are some important social class variations. The reduction in births to high parity women and to women at the upper end of the reproductive age groups occurred in the higher social class before it occurred in Social Classes IV and V. In the period 1970–75 the legitimate birth rate to Social Class I and II women remained stable but it reduced by about one-third in Social Classes IV and V. Despite this, wives of men in manual occupations are still more likely to have 4 or more children (Table 33.11). The improvement in perinatal mortality in Britain in the early 1970s was due in part to these class-specific changes in fertility.

Termination of pregnancy

The termination of an established pregnancy by abortion influences the apparent fertility patterns in a community and may selectively affect age-specific birth rates. It thus can indirectly affect perinatal mortality rates.

Legal termination of pregnancy in England and Wales was introduced in 1968. Legal abortions in England and Wales more than doubled from 5 per 1 000 women between the ages of 15–44 in 1969 to 11 per 1000 in 1978. Since then the

Table 33.11. Percentage of legitimate births, by social class and number of previous children, Great Britain, 1977 (OPCS and Registrar General's Office, Scotland).

Number of previous children	Social class of father (%)				
	Professional	Intermediate	Skilled	Partly skilled	Unskilled
0	45	42	41	40	37
1	39	39	38	35	34
2	12	14	14	15	15
3	2	4	4	6	7
4 +	1	1	3	4	7
Total (%)	100	100	100	100	100
Total legitimate births	47 000	110 000	275 000	90 000	30 000

termination rate has remained fairly constant but the proportion of known conceptions that are aborted has risen. The most marked increase in terminations of pregnancy has been among women under 19 years of age (Table 33.12). About half of all terminations of pregnancy are to single women, with 40% of known conceptions that take place outside marriage being terminated by abortion. In 1970, 19% of extra-marital conceptions were terminated; by 1975 this figure had increased to 39% (Fig. 33.7). This appeared to have reduced the number of births pre-maritally conceived since the percentage of illegitimate live births remained constant.

Table 33.12. Termination of pregnancy (in thousands), by age, England and Wales (OPCS).

Age (years)	1969	1971	1973	1975	1976	1977	1978
< 16	1	2	3	4	3	4	3
16–19	8	18	23	24	24	25	26
20–34	30	56	64	60	58	57	64
35–44	9	16	18	16	15	15	16
45 +	—	—	1	—	—	1	1
Age unknown	1	2	2	2	2	2	2

The United Kingdom Abortion Act (1967) requires that all terminations be notified within 7 days. Reported reasons for terminations being carried out in 1979 are listed in Table 33.13. The vast majority were carried out on the grounds that there was a risk to the mother's health; this includes termination of pregnancy on social grounds. Only a small proportion of terminations were carried out because there was a risk of fetal abnormality. In England and Wales between 1971 and 1977, legal abortions for Down's syndrome increased from 80 to 105 per year, and for central nervous system malformations from 53 to 124 per

(a) 1970 (Total
extramarital conceptions:
172 176)

(b) 1975 (Total
extramarital conceptions:
162 899)

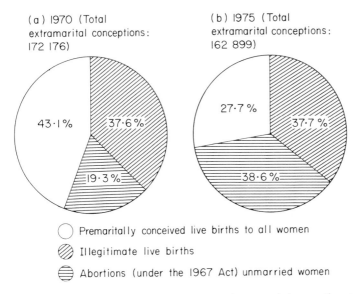

43·1%   37·6%

19·3%

27·7%   37·7%

38·6%

◯ Premaritally conceived live births to all women

▨ Illegitimate live births

⬙ Abortions (under the 1967 Act) unmarried women

Fig. 33.7. Relative importance of the major components of extramarital conceptions to all women resident in England and Wales, 1970–75[17].

Table 33.13. Reasons for induced abortion, England and Wales, 1979 (OPCS).

Reason	Number of abortions
1 Risk to life of woman	574
2 Risk to health of woman	100 733
3 Risk to health of existing children	2 045
4 Substantial risk of abnormal child	1 266
5 To save woman's life or prevent grave permanent injury	13
Other Reasons	14 397
2 with 3	*858*
3 with others	*13 539*
Total	119 028

year. In this time period terminations for 'other malformations' fell markedly from 1295 to 391 per year. The number of terminations carried out because of rubella infection during pregnancy was 222 in 1977 but rose 4-fold to 896 in 1978 at the time of a rubella epidemic. It is obviously important to monitor terminations for rubella in pregnancy as part of the surveillance of rubella vaccine. As more women are vaccinated and a higher proprotion of the pregnant population are immune to rubella, there should be a decline in terminations for this reason.

It has often been argued that as a result of cervical incompetence, induced abortion increases the risk of spontaneous miscarriage and pre-term birth in subsequent pregnancies. In a large follow-up study of 31 917 women seen at their first antenatal visit, Harlap and her colleagues[18] reported an increase in mid-trimester losses among the 2019 nulliparous women with previous induced abortions. Pregnancy loss in the first trimester was not significantly affected by a previous termination, nor was there any change in second trimester losses among the 1493 parous women who reported having induced abortions after a previous pregnancy. This increase in relative risk in nulliparous women increased with previous number of abortions and was not explained by the distribution of demographic or social variables. A more detailed analysis revealed that the risk of subsequent spontaneous abortion in nulliparous women decreased after 1973 when more gentle techniques of cervical dilation were introduced and the authors concluded that there is little or no risk of spontaneous abortion after induced abortions performed by current techniques.

Birth weight

There is a close correlation between maternal factors and birth weight (Table 33.14). Birth weight itself is highly correlated with variations in perinatal mortality (Table 33.15). It appears that the proportion of low birth weight babies within a country largely determines both the perinatal mortality rate and later morbidity. In the United Kingdom babies weighing less than 2500 gms at delivery account for two-thirds of the total perinatal mortality and there are nearly twice as many low birth weight babies in Britain (7%) as in Sweden (3.9%). Within birth weight groups below 2.5 kg the neonatal death rate in Britain is similar to that in Sweden[50]. Since low birth weight accounts for such a high proportion of perinatal mortality, its prevention is important if rates are to be further improved. Fig. 33.8 shows the main causes of low birth weight and

Table 33.14. Relationship between birth weight and some maternal characteristics[11].

Number of previous children	% Babies < 2500 g	Maternal age (years)	% Babies < 2500 g	Birth interval (months)	% Babies < 2500 g
0	4.5	< 20	5.5	< 12	7.6
1	3.2	20–24	4.0	12–17	4.6
2	3.3	25–29	3.3	18–23	3.7
3	4.6	30–34	3.7	23–35	3.0
4 +	4.6	35–39	4.5	35 +	3.2
		40 +	6.2		

Table 33.15. Perinatal mortality rates by birth weight in various countries, per 1000 live and still births[11].

Birth weight (grams)	Austria	Cuba	Hungary	Japan	New Zealand	Sweden	USA (Part)
< 500	954.6	347.8	871.0	—	1,000.0	583.3	906.5
500– 999	891.7	973.3	880.7	932.7	1,000.0	834.2	785.3
1000–1499	656.0	617.6	592.6	636.9	607.2	512.5	400.0
1500–1999	292.6	282.2	257.6	310.6	293.3	242.8	158.8
2000–2499	79.9	63.4	55.5	73.1	69.0	72.1	41.1
2500–2999	16.9	17.3	12.3	11.8	14.6	15.7	9.2
3000–3499	6.3	8.7	6.4	6.8	6.5	4.7	3.5
3500–3999	4.9	9.1	5.7	5.4	4.5	2.9	3.1
4000–4499	6.5	11.2	9.3	11.7	4.6	2.8	4.2
4500 +	22.6	17.3	21.1	57.2	13.3	6.0	54.1
All weights	21.4	26.9	29.1	17.0	17.3	12.6	14.9

perinatal deaths in low birth weight babies. The ultimate weight of a baby is determined both by the length of gestation and by its growth rate *in utero*. Both of these are affected by socio-economic factors, particularly the growth rate. Table 33.16 shows the mean birth weight by social class of babies born in the 1970 perinatal survey.

It is difficult to evaluate the effect of housing standards, mother's work in pregnancy, and social stress on perinatal mortality, but it is known that growth

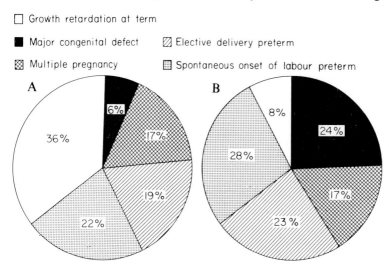

Fig. 33.8. A: Main causes of low birthweight in babies delivered in the United Kingdom. B: Causes of perinatal deaths amongst low birthweight babies in the United Kingdom.

rate is reduced secondary to maternal malnutrition. Short mothers also give rise to an excessive perinatal mortality rate even when allowances are made for other adverse social factors. This may be partly a reflection of the mother's own size at birth and her nutrition and health in childhood which affects the growth rate of her own infant.

Table 33.16. Mean birth weight by social class (singleton births where mothers were sure of their dates), United Kingdom, 1970[6].

Social Class	Mean birth weight (g)
I & II	3377
III	3356
IV & V	3264
Unsupported mothers	3171

Cigarette smoking in pregnancy, which has been shown to increase perinatal mortality by between 10 and 40 % is another important factor which reduces the mean birth weight at a given gestational age, thus contributing to differences in perinatal mortality[20].

Maternal medical complications

Hypertension

Hypertension is the most common and most serious complication of pregnancy. It remains an important cause of maternal mortality, causes intra-uterine growth retardation and, in extreme cases, can cause abruption of the placenta with a consequent high perinatal mortality. The syndrome of hypertension, oedema and proteinuria during pregnancy is conventionally called pre-eclampsia. There is no universally accepted definition of pre-eclampsia for 3 reasons. Firstly, there is no agreed level of blood pressure which is defined as pathological, secondly oedema may be found in healthy women, and finally urine may contain protein in a variety of other conditions. Heavy proteinuria is a late manifestation of pre-eclampsia.

Hypertension of pregnancy was studied in both the 1958[3] and 1970[6] British perinatal surveys. It was shown to affect about 27% of pregnancies in both studies. 3% had essential hypertension, amongst whom 1 in 3 subsequently developed pre-eclampsia. About 15% had mild pre-eclampsia, 4% had moderate pre-eclampsia, 5% had severe pre-eclampsia, 1% had eclampsia. The relative risk of perinatal death in each category fell markedly between the 2 surveys (Table 33.17). In 1958 the infants of a mother with severe pre-eclampsia

Table 33.17. Maternal hypertension and perinatal mortality in the United Kingdom, 1958 and 1970, singletons only.

Degree of hypertension	Perinatal mortality rate (per 1000 live and still births)	
	1958 $n = 16\,994$	1970 $n = 16\,815$
Normotensive	25.5	19.2
Essential hypertension	35.1	15.6
Essential hypertension and pre-eclamptic toxaemia	63.7	30.7
Mild pre-eclamptic toxaemia	28.1	19.5
Moderate pre-eclamptic toxaemia	44.2	18.1
Severe pre-eclamptic toxaemia	73.8	33.7
Remainder	70.0	34.2
Total	33.2	21.4

n Number of observations.

had a 3 times the perinatal mortality rate of those born to normotensive mothers; in 1970 this relative risk in pre-eclampsia fell to 1.5. Women with mild or moderate pre-eclampsia had no increased risk of perinatal death in the second survey.

It is important that blood pressure be monitored regularly during pregnancy. This can be done just as well in the general practitioner's surgery as in the hospital clinic, as long as speedy action is taken when the levels show signs of sustained increase.

Hypertension may occur in one pregnancy but not the next. It is most frequent in first pregnancies, among tall women, in women with multiple pregnancies and among older mothers. There is little association with social class.

In a treatment trial of hypertension in pregnancy[21], surviving children were followed up to age 4 years. The health, birth weight and neurological problems of children born to mothers with hypertension did not differ from controls. However, a slight delay was found in the development of children in the hypertension group and particularly in those whose mothers went untreated.

Diabetes

There has been a steady decline in the rate of perinatal loss associated with maternal diabetes. The definition of high risk patients, co-ordinated medical and antenatal care and improved standards of treatment have all contributed. Despite a lower fertility among diabetic women, 2 per 1000 pregnant women have pre-existing juvenile diabetes, and a further 15 per 1000 become diabetic during pregnancy. This is called gestational diabetes and is usually transient. A study of 18 000 pregnant women[22] showed that the following risk factors were of value in predicting the occurrence of gestational diabetes: close family history of diabetes; a previous baby weighing over 4 kg at birth; glycosuria found on at least 2 occasions, mother's weight over her expected weight-for-height; a previously unexplained fetal or neonatal death; and previous evidence of latent diabetes.

Early recognition and treatment of diabetes is important because if left untreated it is associated both with an increased maternal death rate and with a marked increase in perinatal mortality. In a large study in New York[23], a 10-fold increase in the fetal loss and a $5\frac{1}{2}$ times increase in perinatal mortality was reported among diabetic pregnancies. Much lower loss rates have been reported recently from special centres where very close attention is paid to carbohydrate homeostasis.

Many, but not all studies of diabetic pregnancies have shown excess fetal malformation rates. Among 205 Birmingham (United Kingdom) births[24] to diabetic mothers, 12% had a congenital malformation, twice the rate in the controls. Cardiac malformations were particularly common. The malformation rate was highest in mothers on insulin at the time of conception. Recent evidence[25] suggests that careful control of diabetes in very early pregnancy can reduce this malformation rate.

Renal disease

Asymptomatic bacteriuria can be demonstrated in about 3% of pregnant women[26]. The significance of this observation and its implications for treatment have given rise to much controversy. Because about 30% of women with bacteriuria in early pregnancy develop acute pyelonephritis later in the pregnancy, most antenatal clinics now routinely send urine samples for culture. Short courses of antimicrobial treatment for those found to have bacteriuria are usually effective but care must be taken in the selection of the drug used to avoid those that can harm the fetus.

In addition to the complications to the pregnancy of pyelonephritis, asymptomatic bacteriuria is also associated with low birth weight and increased perinatal mortality[27]. It is difficult to evaluate this finding because infections are more common in women whose pregnancies are at risk for other reasons, including low social class and high parity.

Fertility is decreased if the renal filtration rate falls below 40 mls per minute, but if a mother with renal disease conceives, her pregnancy may continue safely to term if her blood pressure is controlled and her urine kept sterile. In recent years, women with transplanted kidneys have borne healthy babies.

Anaemia

There is a physiological fall in haemoglobin levels during pregnancy caused by haemodilution. It is usual practice to give supplementary iron during the pregnancy in order to maintain the haemoglobin level. Hytten[28] found no evidence that the haemodilution had any adverse effects on healthy women, nor that such women or their babies were at an advantage if they took supplementary iron. The widespread practice of treating all women in this way can be challenged on both medical and financial grounds—a daily proprietary iron tablet prescribed to all pregnant women costs the nation about £1.5 million per year. However, pathological anaemia is associated with an increased risk.

Screening for the haemoglobinopathies such as sickle cell anaemia and thalassaemia are important among women of African descent and those from Mediterranean areas.

Infections

The discovery of hepatitis B virus, both as a cause of disease and also its carrier state, has raised new problems in the management of pregnancy. The carrier rate of hepatitis B antigen in pregnant women in Britain is in the order of 1 per 1000, though it is much higher among women who have migrated from the Far East. There is much discussion about whether it is justifiable to screen pregnant women to identify those few who are antigen-positive when little can be done for those who are so identified. Midwives do not appear to have an excess prevalence of antibodies despite their exposure to maternal blood at delivery[29]. However, positive steps should be taken to protect them from infected blood and contaminated surgical instruments.

For many decades, serological tests for syphilis have played an important part in routine antenatal screening and the efficacy of treatment with penicillin has had a major impact on the problem. Since 1969 the syphilis rate in pregnancy has fallen to such low rates that national (United Kingdom) returns are no longer published. Positive serology among West Indian immigrants may be due to yaws, an innocent condition which can only be distinguished on history and clinical grounds. The relevance of serological tests to detect evidence of past infection to rubella, toxoplasmosis and cytomegalovirus, contracted during pregnancy is discussed in the section on congenital abnormalities.

Maternal behaviour

Nutrition

Although maternal weight is usually recorded throughout pregnancy, few attempts have been made to determine the optimal rate of gain, or decide whether efforts to limit the increase are really justified. Hytten and Leitch[28] reviewed 35 studies on this subject and concluded that some healthy women with clinically normal pregnancies may not increase their weight at all, others may increase by more than twice the average for all women. Within the limits of hospital experience, no extreme of weight gain has been shown to be incompatible with a satisfactory reproductive performance. Massively obese non-diabetic women (more than $1\frac{1}{2}$ times the average weight-for-height before pregnancy) were shown to have a marked increase in the proportion of babies weighing over 4 kg at birth, compared with babies born to moderately obese or non-obese women. However, the risk of having an infant weighing below 2.5 kg at term was similar in all maternal weight groups.

During severe famines when mothers are markedly underweight prior to conception, fertility has been shown to fall and the incidence of low birth weight has been shown to rise. Gopalan and Rao[30] reviewed the role of maternal malnutrition on fetal development. Despite the amount of malnutrition in the world, hard facts based on humans are difficult to come by. Animal experiments do not fully reflect human experience. Although Dutch mothers who were pregnant during the winter famine of 1944 tended to have an increased fetal wastage and undersized live-born babies, survivors grew to normal adult stature. However, the situation is different where mothers are chronically under-nourished prior to pregnancy, as so often happens in India. Children of these mothers are often also underfed. The achievement of full stature requires optimal nutrition both of the mother and throughout the child's growing years, not just during pregnancy. Other factors such as excess work, smoking and chronic infection, should be taken into account when relating weight gain to perinatal outcome as they interact to further reduce birth weight. These issues are particularly relevant to Asian women who have lighter babies than Caucasians. It has proved difficult to determine the optimal weight range for babies of Asian mothers delivering in Britain. Grundy *et al.*[15] showed that for practical purposes Asian babies of similar maturity to Caucasians can be expected to weigh 300 g less at birth.

The effect of excessive maternal weight gain depends on its cause. Fat may not be harmful in itself, but weight gain due to excess fluid secondary to severe pre-eclampsia, carries an increased risk of perinatal mortality (Fig. 33.9)[31].

The main vitamin deficiency found in Britain is hypovitaminosis D which frequently affects Asian mothers, particularly, but not exclusively, those who are

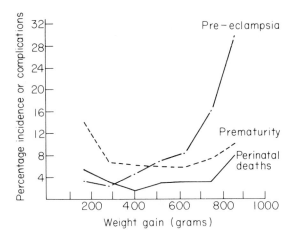

Fig. 33.9. Incidence of obstetric complications in relation to weight gain between the 20th week of pregnancy and term[28].

vegetarians. It is associated with low birth weight and hypocalcaemia in infants[32]. Routine screening for low levels of 25 hydroxycholecalciferol and appropriate treatment with vitamin D has been advocated for Asian mothers. The possible role of multiple vitamin deficiency and neural tube defect is discussed elsewhere.

Smoking

Women who smoke during pregnancy give birth to babies which on average weigh 170 g less at term than the babies of non-smokers. The perinatal mortality amongst babies whose mothers smoked during pregnancy is between 10–40% higher than in non-smokers[20].

Alcohol

Heavy drinking has been associated with a fetal syndrome which includes intra-uterine growth retardation and developmental delay. More recently, it has been shown that the consumption of even moderate amounts of alcohol during pregnancy is associated with an increased risk of spontaneous abortion[33]. Harlap and Shiono[34] showed that this increased risk of abortion among drinkers was particularly marked in the second trimester of pregnancy and that it was not explained by age, parity, race, marital status, smoking or the number of previous spontaneous or induced abortions.

Risk associated with delivery

Place of delivery

Until the advent of antibiotics and an understanding of the prevention of cross-infection within maternity units, it was safer to have babies at home than in hospital. The development of hospital obstetrics only became possible following the control of hospital infection.

In the belief that delivery in obstetric hospitals must be safest because expert care is always immediately available, together with blood banks and, more recently, sophisticated fetal monitoring equipment, the current British policy is to provide sufficient facilities for all births to take place in a hospital. Consequently, the obstetric domiciliary service has been reduced to a bare minimum, and at the same time general practitioner maternity units have been greatly contracted. In 1946 the proportion of babies born at home in England and Wales was 46%. In the decade 1967–77 it has fallen from 25% to less than 2%. This shift to hospital delivery was largely accommodated by decreasing the average length of stay in hospital rather than increasing the number of maternity beds.

Some women prefer a home confinement to avoid separation from the family, or because they are critical of hospitals as a result of their previous experience. When explained that it is safer to give birth in hospital, the majority will choose a hospital confinement. Some have seen this profound social change to hospital delivery as needless medicalization and stressed the safety of home deliveries for women selected as being at low risk. Recent figures have undermined this argument. The perinatal mortality of babies delivered at home in England and Wales in 1977 was 22.9 compared with 17.7 per 1000 among those born in hospitals (Fig. 33.10)[13]. Because all women identified as having 1 or more risk

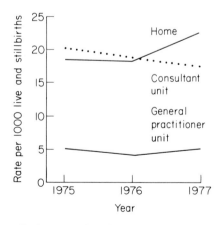

Fig. 33.10. Perinatal mortality by place of confinement, England & Wales, 1975–7[13].

factors in their social or obstetric history normally have planned deliveries in properly equipped hospital units, the perinatal mortality rate for babies born at home should be very low.

The Netherlands appears to be an example of a country where safe home delivery is common practice. There, sophisticated mobile obstetric services are taken to the home. This practice developed because the Dutch medical insurance system did not facilitate the development of intensively equipped hospital maternity units. However, in recent years the proportion of hospital deliveries in Holland has risen. More capital is being invested in hospital maternity units, because the Dutch now think that this is both safer and cheaper. If the average British general practitioner with a list of 2500 were to deliver the 12 mothers per year with a medical and social history potentially suitable for home delivery, he would not gain enough experience to make him a skilled obstetrician.

In recent years, it has become possible to monitor fetal as well as maternal health. This has largely eliminated the risks of late unanticipated fetal death. Goodlin[35] encouraged the development of low dependency units within hospital with a more homely environment than has existed in the past. This is the usual approach in Scandinavia where perinatal mortality is very low and should be studied carefully with a view to adoption elsewhere.

Induction of labour

The advent of ultrasound in the 1960s made possible the accurate assessment of fetal growth and presentation. Monitoring of the fetal electrocardiogram (e.c.g.) enables the obstetrician to recognize the fetus at risk of pre-natal asphyxia and to determine when intervention is needed. Despite these advances, there remains no concensus as to reasonable induction rates. Equivalent perinatal mortality rates can be achieved in hospitals with markedly different induction policies[36]. A re-appraisal of 'interference in obstetrics' has followed the introduction of these techniques and led to the concept of 'the new obstetrics' where closely reasoned and enquiring approaches to the active management of pregnancy have been encouraged, coinciding with more knowledge of the psychological needs of the pregnant mother and her newly born infant.

Births have become increasingly concentrated between Mondays and Fridays with only 80 % of the expected number born on a Sunday. The number born on public holidays falls to even lower proportions[37]. This can be explained, in part, by the trend for induction of labour and for elective Caesarean section to be carried out on week days. The hour of delivery has also changed from the small hours of the morning to working hours. Since perinatal mortality is higher among babies born at weekends it may be correct policy to encourage elective delivery during working hours. The chances of a woman having a Caesarean section varies markedly from one country to another (Fig. 33.11). The different

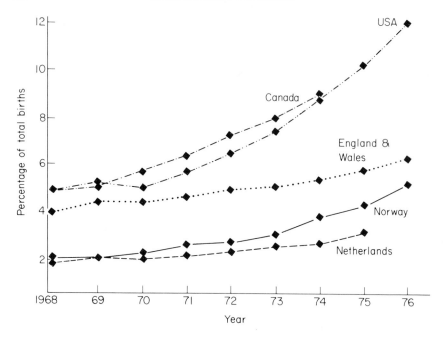

Fig. 33.11. Incidence of birth by Caesarean section in various countries, 1968–76[38].

rates are due to differing opinions about the indications for this operation. For example, the seriousness with which the delivery of immature fetuses, breech presentations and a scarred uterus is viewed, varies. A review of practice in the USA quotes Caesarean section rates ranging from 9 to 23 %. In the New York Cornell Medical Center the rate rose from 4.8 % in 1964 to 18.9 % in 1975[39].

Within the United Kingdom the Caesarean section rate more than doubled from about 3 % to 8 % between 1958 and 1970. Emergency Caesarean sections are more likely to be performed on mothers from the lower social classes, whereas a higher proportion of mothers from the non-manual classes have elective sections. This may reflect higher standards of diagnosis associated with closer antenatal supervision. The management of fetal malpresentation, particularly breech delivery, has attracted considerable attention, since both breech delivery and emergency Caesarean section carry an increased perinatal and maternal mortality risk. Careful interpretation of available evidence is necessary to evaluate the role of Caesarean section in the management of breech presentations.

If the Caesarean section rate in the USA in 1976 had been applied to this country, nearly 35000 additional Caesarean deliveries would have been performed in England and Wales in 1976, at an estimated cost of £18 million.

Furthermore, between 15 and 30 additional maternal deaths associated with this operation and its attendant hazards would have been expected[38].

Multiple pregnancies

Multiple pregnancies have a high risk of stillbirth and birth trauma due to both prematurity and poor intra-uterine growth. The twin rate in Europe is about 1 per 80 pregnancies. Elwood[40] suggested that in Canada, which has a similar twin rate to that in Europe, the twin rates were falling. Twin rates are lower in Japan (1:150 pregnancies) and in other Far Eastern countries. They may be higher in Africa, though community rather than hospital based figures are not available.

The monozygotic twin rate seems to be relatively constant throughout the world. It is the dizygotic which increases within Europe as one goes further north. The rate also rises with increasing maternal age and has been shown to be higher in illegitimate than legitimate births. Mothers who are members of dizygous twin pairs have an increased rate of having twins whereas the rate is not increased where fathers are dizygous twins. The poorly regulated use of drugs that stimulate ovulation puts women treated for subfertility at high risk of multiple pregnancy and accounts for the recent unprecedented spate of quads and quins.

The role of parental height, weight, nutritional status and social class has been shown in some, but not all studies, to influence the twin rate, particularly the dizygous rate. Further analysis of recent British samples are required to clarify this.

The sex ratio

The proportion of males and females at conception is known as the primary sex ratio and the ratio at birth as the secondary ratio (expressed as 100 when similar proportions of boys and girls are born). James[41] entertainingly discussed sex ratios and dismissed a good deal of myth and conflicting evidence. Despite earlier opinions he found that the sex ratio of spontaneous abortions was similar to the sex ratio at birth. He reported that boys were born more frequently to newly weds and after wars and inferred that frequent coitus resulted in a higher proportion of male births due to the cervical mucus favouring the male sperm early in the cycle.

Infant mortality

The infant mortality rate (the number of live born infants per 1000 that die in the first 12 months) has been recorded since 1838. It showed a consistent decline from about 140 in the early years of the 20th century to 12 in 1979. Because the greatest fall occurred long before sophisticated medical intervention became available, this must be largely due to the good effects of improved housing, education and diet. Within the British Isles, two-thirds of the first year deaths occur in the first month of life. The death rate is higher north of the River Severn-Wash line, and is particularly low in East Anglia. Males have an infant mortality one-fifth higher than girls. Babies of Social Class V parents and unmarried mothers have a particularly high neonatal mortality but there is not much difference between Classes I–IV. The British neonatal mortality is a little higher than that of Scandinavia and the Netherlands but this is largely accounted for by the higher British congenital malformation rate and more cot deaths. The reasons for the latter are largely unknown. There is no clear evidence that in other respects health care for British children is inferior to that elsewhere in developed countries. The major causes of infant mortality in England and Wales are shown in Table 33.18. Over a third are due to perinatal causes; other important

Table 33.18. Infant deaths by cause, England and Wales 1978.

International Classification of Diseases (ICD) Code	Cause	Age at death					
		< 1 week		< 4 weeks		< 1 year	
000–136	Infective and parasitic diseases	62	(1.5)*	141	(2.7)	295	(3.7)
140–239	Neoplasms	3	(0.1)	6	(0.1)	42	(0.5)
240–279	Endocrine, nutritional and metabolic diseases	11	(0.3)	18	(0.3)	64	(0.8)
280–289	Diseases of the blood and blood forming organs	4	(0.1)	5	(0.1)	12	(0.2)
320–389	Diseases of the nervous system and sense organs	28	(0.7)	61	(1.2)	165	(2.1)
390–458	Diseases of the circulatory system	4	(0.1)	10	(0.2)	46	(0.6)
460–519	Diseases of the respiratory system	76	(1.8)	166	(3.2)	937	(11.9)
460–466	Acute respiratory infection	0	(0.0)	12	(0.2)	272	(3.5)
480–486	Pneumonia	73	(1.7)	143	(2.8)	546	(6.9)
520–577	Diseases of the digestive system	85	(2.0)	98	(1.9)	135	(1.7)
580–629	Diseases of the genitourinary system	5	(0.1)	10	(0.2)	22	(0.3)
740–759	Congenital abnormalities	1035	(24.4)	1477	(28.5)	2033	(25.8)
740–743	Central nervous system	295	(7.0)	523	(10.1)	617	(7.8)
746–747	Heart and circulatory system	302	(7.1)	474	(9.1)	790	(10.0)
760–779	Perinatal causes	2882	(67.9)	3103	(59.8)	3146	(39.9)
E800–899	Accidents poisoning and violence	33	(0.8)	43	(0.8)	214	(2.7)
	All other causes	14	(0.3)	92	(1.8)	770	(9.8)
	All causes	4242	(100)	5187	(100)	7881	(100)

* Figures in brackets are the percentage of all deaths in that age group.

contributors to infant mortality include congenital abnormalities and diseases of the respiratory system.

Once the first month is past, cot death becomes the single commonest cause of death affecting about 1 in 600 live born infants. At autopsy about one-third have a pathological state, including infectious diseases of sudden onset, others have previously undiagnosed congenital abnormalities, a few have ineffectual parents, but much more commonly they are normal caring parents and the baby at autopsy has no diagnosable lesions.

Maternal mortality

Maternal mortality is the ratio of deaths ascribed to childbirth in 1 year to the total number of live and still births in the same year expressed as a rate per 1000. These deaths exclude those relating to previously existing disease not due to direct obstetric causes, but aggravated by the physiological effects of pregnancy.

Maternal mortality in England and Wales (including deaths associated with abortions), fell dramatically from 43 per 10 000 births in 1935 to 1 per 10 000 births in 1975. Since 1952 a national confidential enquiry into all maternal deaths has been undertaken by obstetricians and findings published every 3 years. This pioneer form of medical monitoring has proved an effective way of establishing cause of death and raising professional awareness. The fact that this has been carried out on a voluntary basis by the profession itself throughout the country led to its acceptance. The 1973–75 report concluded that of 235 deaths directly due to pregnancy, 50 % had 1 or more avoidable factor[42]. Half of these factors occurred in the antenatal period, and 29 % during labour or operative procedure. About a third of deaths in the antenatal period were primarily due to mothers declining or failing to seek medical help.

The maternal mortality rate (excluding abortions) in England and Wales as a whole between 1973 and 1975 was 1.13 per 10 000. The rate varied from 0.43 per 10 000 births in the Oxford region to 1.86 per 10 000 births in the North East Thames region. The current report does not make international comparisons. However, the 1972–73 report showed that when the England and Wales rate was 1.4 per 10 000, the rate in Denmark was 0.51 and the Netherlands 1.21. Britain occupied a mid-place among European countries; Switzerland's level was much higher at 2.39. No other countries adopt the British method of confidential enquiries and it is not possible to be certain whether their figures are gathered in a comparable manner. In the USA this approach would be impossible because their constitution makes the approach illegal, much to the detriment of mothers at risk.

The decline in maternal mortality is due to the interplay of many factors, the most important being improving standards of maternal health related to better housing, diet, working conditions, education and contraception. Medical factors, however, have played their part, particularly the ability to treat infections and the transfer of the majority of deliveries from the home to properly equipped hospitals, where anaesthesia and blood transfusion are readily available.

Beral[43] introduced a concept of 'reproductive mortality' which included all deaths from complications of contraception as well as those associated with pregnancy or abortion. Although this concept has been criticized, it has the virtue of reducing complacency about declining maternal mortality and focussing interest on the whole spectrum of childbirth and contraception. When studied in this way, the reproductive mortality rate shows marked fluctuations. As an example, the reproductive mortality rate has halved since 1960 in the 25–34 age group, but risen from 2.9 to 5 per 100 000 in women aged 35–44.

Promotion of perinatal health

Epidemiology has an important role to play in the promotion of perinatal health. Most of the factors already mentioned operate in conjunction rather than as a single variable, so that multi-variant analysis of data helps to identify the different components of perinatal mortality. Sir Dougal Baird and his colleagues in Aberdeen demonstrated that analysis and interpretations of perinatal data could markedly influence the practice of obstetrics for the better. The 3 national surveys already referred to which were carried out at 12 year intervals in 1946[2], 1958[3], and 1970[5] have increased our knowledge about the relationship between environmental and biological factors and perinatal mortality and morbidity within Britain.

Perinatal mortality statistics have proved a useful measure of the quality of obstetric services for 3 decades but their use can hide explanations of differences in performance between geographically distinct areas. Most perinatal deaths occur in the small group of low birth weight and congenitally deformed babies and it makes interpretation of figures more meaningful if adjustments can be made for this in the analysis of regional data.

Rooth[44] proposed that low birth weight be defined as minus 2 standard deviations of the mean national birth weight, and showed that for most developed countries this would include 3 to 5% of all births. Perinatal mortality rates in England and Wales adjusted for the proportion of infants weighing less than 2 kgs at birth, show that the inter-area variations in perinatal mortality seen in crude data reduce to insignificance. Mallett[45], examining standardized mortality ratios for an area in the Midlands with a high perinatal mortality rate, showed that the local high mortality was not due to inherent social characteristics in the population, but sprang largely from inappropriate allocation of resources. These studies demonstrate the great need for properly standardized perinatal information to be gathered on an international basis. With modern data handling facilities, this should not be an impossible task. The information is already gathered routinely but the results are rarely available in comparable format.

Since perinatal mortality is influenced by the background, health and nutrition of the mother, as well as the quality of obstetric and paediatric care, it seems likely that broad cultural and economic factors which are outside the sphere of direct medical intervention are the key issues in improving safety in childbirth.

A vast literature on the management of the new-born is now emerging. There is a widespread inequality of provision of both special and intensive care baby facilities within the British Isles. The Walker report[46] from Scotland commented that many units were still attempting to provide a range of perinatal care without adequate staff or facilities. The extent to which provision of services influences infant survival is stimulating a great deal of research. However, there is a tendency to introduce new techniques before they have been fully evaluated, thus the practice of neonatal medicine has seen many advances and retreats.

The quality of newborn survival matters more than attainment of the highest possible survival rates. It is clear that good quality care produces the fewest handicapped surviving babies. Studies from major neonatal care centres show that intensively treated survivors have acceptably low rates of handicap and good quality life prospects.

Antenatal screening

Antenatal care was one of the earliest examples of population health screening. In 19th century Paris, in an attempt to reduce the morbidity of unmarried mothers at the Clinique Baudeloque, women were seen by doctors prior to delivery. Although Ballantyne's 'Plea for a Pro-maternity Hospital' in 1901 came from Edinburgh, the first antenatal clinics were set up in the USA and Australia. In 1902 the British Midwives Act resulted in proper professional control of the work of midwives. This was followed in 1918 by an Act of Parliament which required local authorities to establish antenatal clinics. The effectiveness of these measures were soon demonstrated by a decrease in maternal and child mortality.

Antenatal clinics provide an economical and effective method of health surveillance, though even today, there are difficulties in encouraging the poor, the single, and those with large numbers of children to attend, and it is they who have the greatest health problems and the highest perinatal mortality. Scott-Samuel[47] reported in 1980 that only 36% of women presented to a Liverpool Hospital antenatal clinic before 16 weeks, the latest desirable stage of gestation, compared with 91% in Finland and 96% in France, where the payment of generous maternity allowances are linked to antenatal clinic attendance.

Early and regular antenatal care undoubtedly safeguards the health of pregnant women and their babies, but the extent of its benefits are not easy to quantify. The association between early attendance at antenatal clinics and low perinatal mortality[41] could reflect the fact that motivated and healthy women are the most likely to attend early. In a recent study[48], it was found that intra-uterine growth retardation and pre-eclampsia often went undiagnosed despite clinic attendance. Furthermore intra-uterine growth retardation . was sometimes diagnosed, though not present when the baby was delivered. Although there is no question that early booking should be encouraged, frequent visits in uncomplicated pregnancies may divert time and attention away from those pregnancies with the greatest obstetric needs. Table 33.19 shows the frequency with which certain risk factors occur and the relative perinatal mortality risk associated with them.

Improved obstetric care has enabled women with health problems, who in previous generations would have been denied the chance, to deliver live babies. Thus it is important to recognize early conditions such as diabetes mellitus or

Table 33.19. Frequency of some adverse social, maternal and fetal conditions and perinatal risk[3].

Conditions	Frequency %	Perinatal mortality risk*
Maternal factors		
Age 40 +	2.5	200
Parity 4 +	8.9	154
Unmarried mother	2.9	140
Unskilled father	9.3	128
Height < 155 cm	22.0	114
Heavy smoker, cigarettes		
(10 + daily after 4th month)	11.9	128
Problems arising in pregnancy		
Antepartum haemorrhage	3.1	568
Threatened abortion	3.1	237
Severe toxaemia	5.6	226
Problems arising in labour		
Breech	2.6	650
Unattended delivery	2.1	201
Forceps to vertex	4.7	122
Foetal factors		
Low birth weight	6.7	790
Pre-term delivery (< 37 weeks)	4.7	770
Small for dates		
(> 39 weeks and < 2.5 kg)	2.6	520

* Average risk for all deaths in this table is equated to 100.

heart disease which may normally be well controlled, but which can become decompensated during pregnancy and require careful management.

Antenatal screening demands more than following a check-list of disabilities. Potentially serious abnormalities of pregnancy, such as pre-eclampsia and anaemia, can be detected and treated at an early stage. Antenatal clinics also provide an opportunity for education (for both mother and father) about childbirth.

Complications of pregnancy are largely determined by the physical and nutritional state of the mother, acting together with social factors such as parity and extremes of age. Women from higher socio-economic groups tend to begin antenatal care earlier, yet have the best nutritional status, physical health and the lowest mortality. Because of this self-selection, the real value of antenatal care has not been fully assessed and randomized controlled trials of the various elements which make up antenatal care remain to be performed.

Admission to hospital during pregnancy is required most frequently because of chronic health problems such as heart disease or diabetes; or problems detected during antenatal care such as high blood pressure or toxaemia. Women with these conditions are most likely to benefit from antenatal care in terms of detection of physical complications and early treatment. Perinatal death, however, most frequently results from prematurity of unknown cause and it is unlikely that more intensive or earlier antenatal care could eliminate this complication.

References

1. Social Services Committee. *Perinatal and neonatal mortality.* Second report from the Social Services Committee 1979–80. London: HMSO, 1980.
2. Douglas JWB, Blomfield JM. *Children under five.* London: Allen and Unwin, 1958.
3. Butler NR, Alberman ED. *Perinatal problems.* London: Churchill Livingstone, 1969.
4. Butler NR, Bonham DG. *Perinatal mortality.* London: Churchill Livingstone, 1963.
5. Chamberlain R. *British Births 1. The first week of life.* London: Heinemann, 1975.
6. Chamberlain GV, Philip E, *et al. British births Vol 2.* London: Heinemann, 1978.
7. Niswander KR, Gordon M. *The women and their pregnancies.* Philadelphia: Saunders, 1972.
8. Zachau-Christiansen B, Ross EM. *Babies: human development in the first years of life.* Chichester: Wiley, 1975.
9. Miller JF, *et al.* Fetal loss after implantation. *Lancet* 1980; ii: 554–6.
10. Alberman ED, Creasy MR. Frequency of chromosomal abnormalities in miscarriages and perinatal deaths. *Journal of Medical Genetics* 1977; **14**: 313–5.
11. World Health Organization. *Report on the social and biological effects on perinatal mortality.* Geneva: WHO, 1978.
12. Macfarlane A. Social class variations in perinatal mortality. *Journal of Maternal and Child Health* 1979; **4**: 337–40.
13. Davies IM. Perinatal and infant deaths; social and biological factors. *Population Trends* 1980; **19**: 19–21.
14. Barnes J. *The Children's Committee Conference Report. The reduction of perinatal mortality and morbidity.* Department of Health and Social Security. London: HMSO, 1980.

15. Grundy MFB, Hood J, Newman GB. Birth weight standards in a community of mixed racial origin. *British Journal of Obstetrics and Gynaecology* 1978; **85**: 481–6.
16. Hellier J. Perinatal mortality. *Population Trends* 1977; **10**: 13.
17. Edmunds RH, Yarrow A. Newer fashions in illegitimacy. *British Medical Journal* 1977; i: 701–3.
18. Harlap S, *et al.* A prospective study of spontaneous fetal losses after induced abortions. *New England Journal of Medicine* 1979; **301**: 677–81.
19. Golding J. Epidemiology of low birth weight infants 1. *Journal of Maternal and Child Health* 1979; **6**: 218–9.
20. Ball KP, Andrews J, *et al.* Mothers who smoke and their children. *The Practitioner* 1980; **224**: 735–40.
21. Ounsted MK, Moar VA, *et al.* Hypertension during pregnancy with and without specific treatment: the children at the age of 4 years. *British Journal of Obstetrics and Gynaecology* 1980; **87**: 19–24.
22. O'Sullivan JB, *et al.* Screening criteria for high risk gestational diabetic patients. *American Journal of Obstetrics and Gynaecology* 1973; **116**: 895.
23. North AF, Mazumder S, Logrillo VM. Birth weight, gestational age and perinatal deaths in 5471 infants of diabetic mothers. *Journal of Paediatrics* 1977; **90**: 444.
24. Day RE, Insley J. Maternal diabetes and congenital malformations. *Archives of Diseases in Childhood* 1976; **51**: 935–8.
25. Pedersen J, Mølsted-Pedersen L. Congenital malformations; the possible role of diabetes care outside pregnancy. In: Pregnancy metabolism, diabetes and the foetus (CIBA Foundation Symposium 63). *Excerpta Medica* Amsterdam. 1979; 273–82.
26. Kass EH, Brumfitt W. *Urinary tract infections 1978.* Proceedings of the 3rd International Symposium of Pyelonephritis. University of Chicago, USA, 1979.
27. Naeye RL. Causes of the excessive rates of perinatal mortality and pre-maturity in pregnancies complicated by maternal urinary tract infections. *New England Journal of Medicine* 1979; **300**: 819–23.
28. Hytten FE, Leitch I. *The physiology of human pregnancy.* 2nd ed. Oxford: Blackwell Scientific Publications, 1971.
29. Tedder RS. Hepatitis B in hospitals. *British Journal of Hospital Medicine* 1980; **233**: 266–79.
30. Gopalan C, Rao KJ. The problem of malnutrition. In: Falkner F, ed. *Prevention in childhood of health problems in adult life.* Geneva: World Health Organization, 1980.
31. Harrison GG, Udall JN, Morrow G. Maternal obesity, weight gain in pregnancy and infant birth weight. *American Journal of Obstetrics and Gynaecology* 1980; **1363**: 411–12.
32. Brooke OG *et al.* Vitamin D supplements in pregnant Asian women: effects on calcium status and fetal growth. *British Medical Journal* 1980; i: 751–4.
33. Kline J, Stein Z, *et al.* Drinking during pregnancy and spontaneous abortion. *Lancet* 1980; ii: 176–80.
34. Harlap S, Shiono PH. Alcohol, smoking and incidence of spontaneous abortions in the first and second trimester. *Lancet* 1980; ii: 173–6.
35. Goodlin RC. Place of confinement: low risk obstetric care for low risk mothers. *Lancet* 1980; i: 1017–19.
36. Chalmers I, Richards MPM. Intervention and causal inference in obstetric practice. In: Chard T, Richards MPM, eds. *Clinics in developmental medicine No 64.* London: Spastics International Medical Publications/William Heinemann Medical Books, 1977.
37. Macfarlane A. Variations in number of births and perinatal mortality by day of week in England and Wales. *British Medical Journal* 1978; ii: 1670–3.
38. Chalmers I. The epidemiology of perinatal practice. *Journal of Maternal and Child Health* 1980; **5**: 435–7.
39. Jones OH. Caesarean section in present day obstetrics. *American Journal of Obstetrics and Gynaecology* 1976; **126** (2): 521–30.

40. Elwood JM. Maternal and environmental factors affecting twin births in Canadian cities. *British Journal of Obstetrics and Gynaecology* 1978; **85**: 357–8.
41. James WH. Time of fertilization and sex of infants. *Lancet* 1980; **i**: 1124–6.
42. *Report on confidential enquiries into maternal deaths in England and Wales 1973–75*. London: HMSO, 1979.
43. Beral V. Reproductive mortality. *British Medical Journal* 1979; **ii**: 632–4.
44. Rooth G. Low birth weight revised. *Lancet* 1980; **i**: 639–41.
45. Mallett R. Knox EG. Standardized perinatal mortality ratios: technique utility and interpretation. *Community Medicine* 1979; **1**: 6–13.
46. National Medical Consulative Committee. *Report of the Joint Working Party on standards of perinatal care in Scotland*. London: HMSO, 1980.
47. Scott-Samuel A. Delayed booking for antenatal care. *Public Health* 1980; **4**: 246–51.
48. Hall M, Chng PK, MacGillivray I. Is routine antenatal care worthwhile? *Lancet* 1980; **ii**: 78–80.
49. Boué J, Boué A, Lazar P. Retrospective and prospective epidemiological studies of 1500 karyotyped spontaneous human abortions *Teratology* 1975; **12**: 11–26.
50. Pharaoh POD. Present patterns of disease in childhood. *Royal Society of Medicine. Proceedings* 1976; **69**: 335–8.

Chapter 34 · Congenital Malformations

C S PECKHAM, E M ROSS AND R D T FARMER

The relative significance of congenital malformations as a cause of mortality and morbidity in early life has increased as control has been gained over infectious diseases through improvements in the standard of living and medical practice. Although the perinatal mortality rate from congenital malformations has remained relatively constant over many years (about 2.5 per 1000 births[1,2], it now accounts for a quarter of all perinatal deaths compared with 10% in the inter-war years (Fig. 34.1). Malformations remain the commonest cause of death throughout the first year of life (Fig. 34.2) and they are a frequent cause of morbidity in infancy. Some malformations are due to identifiable environmental factors, such as maternal infection of drugs taken during pregnancy, but in the majority of cases, the cause is not known. Constant surveillance of malformations is essential to monitor the appearance of new hazards. Prevention of congenital malformations is limited, at the present time, but new techniques for screening during pregnancy may lead to their early detection and result in termination of an affected pregnancy being offered to the mother.

Sources of Data

The frequency of malformations at birth depends upon the incidence of abnormalities at conception, embryonic damage during pregnancy and fetal loss. The majority of faulty embryos are eliminated and it is estimated that they account for about 40% of all spontaneous abortions. The exact proportion is difficult to estimate, as many pregnancies abort before the woman is aware that she is pregnant and thus material for examination is lacking.

Because the fetal loss rates vary for different abnormalities, the incidence of different types of abnormality at conception cannot easily be inferred from their prevalence at birth. It is preferable to use the term prevalence when discussing congenital abnormalities.

Comprehensive data on congenital abnormalities that cause a stillbirth or death following a live birth are published for most developed countries. In England and Wales, although stillbirths have been registered since 1927, the cause of the stillbirth was not recorded until 1960. In Scotland, causes of stillbirths have been recorded since 1939. Causes of death of live-born infants have been recorded since the mid 18th century. In some cases the cause of a stillbirth or death that is recorded indicates that congenital malformations were

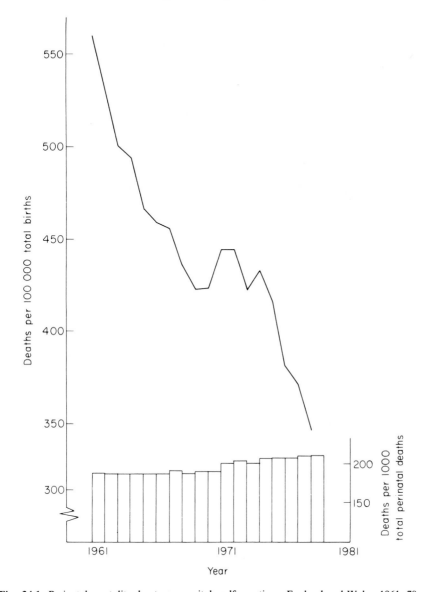

Fig. 34.1. Perinatal mortality due to congenital malformations, England and Wales, 1961–78.

present but does not specify the nature of the abnormality. Such data are not satisfactory for detailed study.

The systematic recording of non-lethal malformations on a national basis in England and Wales was not started until 1964. Its inception was prompted by the Thalidomide tragedy which demonstrated the need to be alert for new

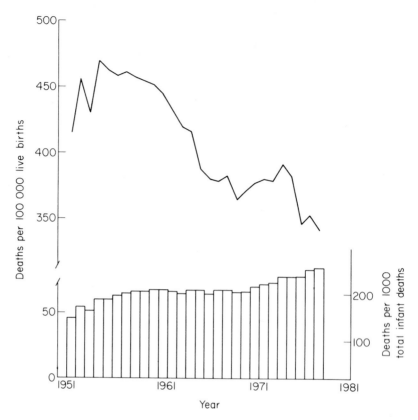

Fig. 34.2. Infant mortality from congenital malformations, England and Wales, 1951–78.

environmental factors which could cause malformations. In this episode, unexpectedly large numbers of children were born with phocomelia but the epidemic went unrecognized because no system existed to collate the experience of the many doctors and midwives involved. Under the present monitoring scheme, babies with malformations that are detected within the first 7 days of life are reported to the District Medical Officer on a voluntary basis. The reports include detailed information about both mother and child and are forwarded to the Office of Population Censuses and Surveys (OPCS) who publish monthly tabulations. The quality of reporting varies, the diagnosis cannot be verified and only malformations that are apparent in the first week of life are notified. This information, therefore, must be interpreted with caution and it does not give accurate prevalence data on malformations. Nevertheless, it does give sufficient data to identify important secular trends.

Survey methods

Strictly, the term 'congenital abnormality' encompasses all structural malformations present at birth, even though they may not be recognized at the time, as well as any irreversible disturbance of function, whether or not it is associated with a recognizable structural abnormality. However, this definition is not used in all epidemiological studies and differences in definition make comparisons between studies difficult. For example, some studies do not include minor abnormalities that have no functional implications. Other studies only include abnormalities that are apparent at birth or within a defined period of birth, both of which will tend to underestimate the prevalence of many conditions.

The effort that is invested in ascertainment of defects also varies. For example, of the babies who die, the proportion who have a post mortem examination differs between centres; even amongst those who do have an autopsy, the quality of the examination is not consistent. Ascertainment of severe malformations such as anencephaly, gross hydrocephaly or spina bifida present no problems, whereas internal defects, particularly when they are not lethal, may go unrecognized. Because of these difficulties, and the additional problems of inconsistent terminology, caution must be exercised in comparing the results from different epidemiological surveys.

The most satisfactory type of study for estimating the prevalence of congenital abnormalities is a prospective investigation in which the population sample is clearly defined and the examination of each infant is standardized. Because of the rarity of many anomalies at birth, this type of study is expensive and large numbers of babies must be included to produce useful results. For example, for conditions such as major malformations of the central nervous system, about 300 births have to be studied in order to find 1 affected baby.

Illingworth[3] stressed the rarity of many conditions and calculated that the general practitioner with 2500 patients could expect to encounter an infant with meningomyelocele in his practice once in every 10 years and 1 with tuberous sclerosis once in 1200 years. This highlights the difficulty of investigating the possible causes of individual defects or syndromes. Although many studies have been undertaken in recent decades, the cause of most malformations remains unknown and new syndromes are still being described.

The 1958 Perinatal Mortality Study[1] was concerned with the analysis of data relating to all births that occurred in England, Scotland and Wales between the 3rd and 9th of March of that year. In addition, detailed post mortem examinations were carried out on two-thirds of perinatal deaths during a 3 month period including that week. This yielded information on 16 000 live births and 7000 perinatal deaths. The study produced invaluable data on the possible origins of fetal abnormality. A comparable 3 month period in Britain now would only contribute 2000 deaths.

Specific malformations

Current estimates suggest that as many as 5 % of live births[4] show some genetic
or developmental anomaly of varying severity. Major malformations resulting in
chronic handicap or necessitating surgery are present in about 2 % of live-born
infants. Known causes of congenital abnormality include chromosomal
abnormalities, genetically inherited disorders and environmental factors such as
drugs or infections in pregnancy, but in the majority of cases, no clear-cut cause
can be found. The most common congenital malformations are of the central
nervous and cardiovascular systems (Table 34.1)[5]. The malformation rate of
individual defects varies, even within small populations. For example, the annual
prevalence of anencephaly is about 1.5 per 1000 births in South East England, 2.5
per 1000 in Northern England, 3 per 1000 in Scotland and Wales, 4 per 1000 in
Northern Ireland and up to 6 per 1000 in Eire. International differences are even
more striking. Deaths from neural tube defects in Ulster are 20 times greater than
in Japan (Fig. 34.3). The high prevalence of neural tube defects in the western
parts of the British Isles led Wynn to describe the condition as 'the curse of the
Celts'[6].

Table 34.1. Approximate frequency and sex ratio of the more common major congenital
malformations in Britain[5].

Malformations	Frequency per 1000 births	Male : Female sex ratio
Spina bifida cystica	2.5	0.6
Anencephaly	2.0	0.3
Congenital heart defects	6.0	1.0
Pyloric stenosis	3.0	4.0
Cleft lip (± cleft palate)	1.0	1.8
Congenital dislocation of the hip (late diagnosis)	1.0	0.14

Most malformations occur only slightly more frequently at extremes of
maternal age and parity, but the risk of Down's Syndrome and other trisomies is
much higher in the babies of older mothers. When an infant has a malformation,
the risk of repetition in subsequent pregnancies is increased; this is greatest where
there is an identified genetic factor.

Congenital abnormalities tend not to relate to social status except for neural
tube defects which are more common in the lower socio-economic groups. For
example, in Scotland, the malformation rate is 2½ times higher in Social Class V
than Social Class I. This difference is largely accounted for by malformations of
the brain and spinal cord.

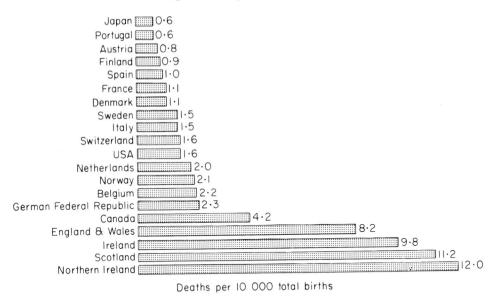

Fig. 34.3. Deaths from neural tube defects in first year, 1973[6].

In Britain there are seasonal fluctuations in the birth of infants with certain abnormalities such as congenital dislocation of the hip and anencephalus, both of which are more common in the winter months. These associations are not consistently found in other countries.

Chromosomal abnormalities

Abnormalities of sex chromosomes and of autosomal chromosomes are each found in about 0.2% of live-born infants. Many more autosomal abnormalities are conceived but a large proportion of these abort spontaneously in the first trimester of pregnancy. Of those with a single X chromosome deletion (Turner's Syndrome), 95% spontaneously abort. Fetuses with sex chromosome trisomies have no increased liability to abort. Sex chromosome trisomies (XXX and XXY) are often difficult to diagnose in the new-born, and may only be recognized in the course of special studies. They are 50% more frequent in males than females (Table 34.2)[5] and become more common with increasing maternal age.

The association between abnormalities of the X chromosome and mental retardation was reviewed by Gerald[8]. A New South Wales study showed a 30% excess of mild mental retardation (intelligence quotient–IQ–in range 50–55) among males. The affected boys had affected brothers more frequently than affected girls had affected sisters. This may be explained by the observation that

Table 34.2. Frequency of sex chromosomal anomalies[5].

Anomaly		Rate per 1000 births
Boys	XYY (extra Y syndrome)	1.0
	XXY (Klinefelter's syndrome)	1.0
Girls	XXX (triple X syndrome)	1.0
Both sexes miscellaneous		0.5
Total both sexes		2.0

many of those affected have a constriction on the marker X chromosome, otherwise known as 'fragile X'. This has been claimed to be the second most common cause of diagnosable mental retardation after trisomy 21. The implication of this observation would be chromosome analysis of mentally retarded children so that carrier families could be detected and counselled.

The most important autosomal abnormalities are shown in Table 34.3[7]. Although the overall risk of giving birth to an infant with Down's syndrome is about 0.15% the risk rises sharply with increasing maternal age, from 0.4% in the age range 35–39 years to 1.2% in the age range 40–44 years and 4% for those aged 45 years and over. Father's age does not influence the risk. The risk of Down's syndrome due to translocation does not alter with age, but this accounts for only about 5% of all cases. In recent years, the number of Down's syndrome births to older mothers has fallen, due largely to a decline in fertility. Accurate information on risk is needed to estimate the most suitable age for prenatal diagnostic screening. An intensive policy for screening older women is clearly desirable, but it would have relatively little impact on the total numbers of Down's Syndrome babies because the birth rate in this high risk group is low. It has been estimated that if all women aged 35 years and over were screened, less than one-third of children with Down's syndrome would be detected antenatally. Genetic counselling for women who have had an affected baby or who have a family history of Down's syndrome is clearly important to prevent the conception of subsequent affected babies.

Table 34.3. Frequency of autosomal anomalies[7].

Anomaly		Rate per 1000 births
Trisomy 21	(Down's syndrome)	1.5
Trisomy 18	(Edward's syndrome)	0.1
Trisomy 13	(Patau's syndrome)	0.1
Miscellaneous	(mainly structural)	0.3
Total		2.0

Down's syndrome is associated with an increased mortality, especially in the first year, but it is compatible with survival to adult life and accounts for about 30% of children with severe mental retardation. A further 2 per 1000 infants are born with a 'balanced' chromosomal anomaly, which, although causing no functional disturbance and rarely diagnosed clinically, can result in a chromosome abnormality in their children. This is the cause of 1 in 20 cases of Down's syndrome. In contrast, the abnormalities associated with the rarer trisomies, particularly 13 and 18, are so serious that few survive infancy.

Inherited disorders

Among congenitally abnormal babies, inherited disorders, presumably due to single gene defects, are much more common than conditions with demonstrable chromosomal abnormalities. They may affect up to 10 per 1000 children. Single gene disorders may be dominant, recessive or sex linked. Examples of dominant conditions include Huntingdon's chorea, neurofibromatosis and polycystic kidney disease. Each child of an affected parent has a 50% chance of inheriting the abnormal gene. Recessive disorders such as thalassaemia, sickle cell disease and cystic fibrosis have a 25% recurrent risk. Many parents find it difficult to understand this fact which must be carefully explained. Sex linked disorders are exemplified by haemophilia which affects 50% of sons and leaves 50% of daughters as carriers.

Abnormalities due to acquired causes

Epidemiological research is gradually clarifying the role that environmental hazards, particularly intra-uterine infection, drugs and irradiation, play in the aetiology of congenital abnormalities (Table 34.4).

Many agents have been reported to be teratogenic but there have also been several false alarms in recent years. For example, the theory, which is now discredited, that consumption of blighted potatoes might predispose to neural tube defect.

Drugs

Since the thalidomide disaster developed countries have required all new drugs to be rigorously tested on a series of different pregnant mammalian species in order to detect any possible damaging effects before the drug is passed for clinical trials in humans. Experimental results of tests in animals, however, may not be reproduced in humans. Although the potential dangers of drugs taken during pregnancy are well appreciated, the assessment of well established drugs, even aspirin, in pregnancy is still required.

Table 34.4. Known causes of congenital abnormalities.

Causal agent	Outcome
Infections	
Rubella	Deafness, heart defects, cataract, etc.
Cytomegalovirus	CNS defects
Toxoplasmosis	CNS defects
Treponema pallidum	Multiple defects
Drugs	
Thalidomide	Phocomelia
Aminopterin, methotrexate	Deformities of skull, bones, cleft palate
Androgens, progesteron	Virilization of female genitalia
Stilboestrol	Adenocarcinoma of vagina
Anticonvulsants	Hairlip $\pm$ cleft palate, heart defects
Iodides	Goitre
Tetracyclines	Discolouration of teeth
Alcohol	Foetal alcohol syndrome
Ionizing radiation	Microcephaly, leukaemia
Diet	? Neural tube defects
Anaesthetics	Abortion, congenital malformation
Heavy metals (lead)	Abortion, mental retardation

CNS Central Nervous System.

Drugs and diagnostic X-rays are given more frequently to mothers who are unwell or whose pregnancies are causing concern. These mothers cannot be directly compared with healthy mothers who do not need medication or require radiography. For example, a higher proportion of babies born to mothers who take anticonvulsant drugs of many types have congenital defects, particularly cleft palate, hare lip, and congenital heart lesions, than babies born to mothers not taking these drugs[9]. The problem is to determine whether the increased deformity rate, which is about twice that of normal controls, is due to the drug, the mother's underlying epileptic condition or the hypoxic convulsive episodes.

Drugs can produce 2 major types of effects on the fetus. Some drugs, such as thalidomide, are teratogenic and cause structural abnormalities by interfering with normal embryogenesis. Other drugs given in late pregnancy produce toxic effects on the fetus or new-born; these include chloroquine and streptomycin, which may cause deafness, and antithyroid drugs, which may produce goitre and hypothyroidism. So far, no other drug has produced such devastating damage as thalidomide.

Androgenic and progestational steroids, when given to the mother in large doses for threatened abortion in early pregnancy, can cause virilizing effects on female foetuses. In his review of environmental teratogens, Smithells[10] concluded that in addition to thalidomide, steroid hormones, folate antagonists, alcohol, anticonvulsants, warfarin and some factors relating to work in operating theatres, possibly anaesthetic gases, should be accepted as teratogens in man.

Forfar and Nelson[11] reported that 97 % of 911 unselected women had been prescribed drugs during pregnancy. Those who had children with congenital defects tended to have taken more medicines during pregnancy than had women who had normal children. This does not necessarily mean that the drugs involved are teratogenic. It took several years before the dangers of thalidomide were appreciated, despite its capacity to produce a wide range of severe but characteristic malformations. Drugs of lower teratogenicity are more difficult to recognize.

More recently, the anti-nausea preparation, Debendox (a mixture of dicylomine hydrochloride, doxylamine and pyridoxine) has been claimed to cause fetal defects. Epidemiological surveys so far have failed to verify these claims but the matter remains under debate. Clearly, the administration of any drug during pregnancy should be avoided unless it is specifically indicated. Pregnant women should be warned against self-medication.

Ionizing radiation

Ionizing radiation is another potential cause of fetal abnormality[12]. Children irradiated *in utero* are more likely to develop malignant conditions than other children. Most studies suggest a 50–100 % increase in risk associated with exposure to diagnostic X-rays *in utero*. Ionizing radiation can also produce congenital malformations, demonstrated by the high incidence of microcephaly among infants irradiated *in utero* by the atomic bomb explosions in Japan.

Dietary factors

The consumption of alcohol during pregnancy has been increasingly discussed as a cause of fetal abnormality, resulting in a syndrome of mental retardation, low birth weight and facial abnormality. However, women who drink heavily tend to have poor diets and to smoke heavily, making the evaluation of the teratogenic effects of alcohol difficult to isolate. There are few convincing reports of the fetal alcohol syndrome from the United Kingdom but many from the USA[13].

The possible role of nutritional deficiencies in the aetiology of neural tube defects has been debated for many years, particularly the role of vitamin deficiency. The Irish and Scots, who have the highest prevalence of neural tube defects in the United Kingdom, eat half the amount of fresh green vegetables that the English eat. Italians and Spaniards, however, who have a very low rate of neural tube defect, consume twice as many fresh green vegetables as the average English person[6]. There is ample evidence from animal work that specific malformations can be produced where vitamin deficient diets or vitamin antagonists are given during pregnancy. The relevance of this work to humans is only just beginning to emerge. Studies have shown that mothers in Social Class IV and V more often have a poor diet in early pregnancy and sometimes suffer from deficiencies of essential dietary constituents[14]. The study of Smithells *et al.*[15], although it was not a controlled trial and used multivitamin supplements, indicated the possible success of dietary improvement. More recently, Laurence and his colleagues [16] concluded that women receiving adequate diets have a lower incidence and recurrence of fetal neural tube defects. They also suggest that dietary counselling was effective in reducing these defects.

Intra-uterine infection

Maternal infections during pregnancy account for only a small proportion of congenital malformations in the United Kingdom each year but are of great practical importance because preventive measures are often possible. Maternal rubella has been the most intensively studied intra-uterine infection. In the first trimester of pregnancy it can result in a wide range of fetal abnormalities varying from severe multisystem disease to sensorineural deafness occurring as a single defect. The damage resulting from congenital infection may be progressive and hearing defects may occur or increase after birth[17]. The risk of an infected mother delivering a damaged infant is about 40–50% when she contracts the illness in the first month of pregnancy, 20% in the second month and 7–8% in the following 8 weeks. Congenital rubella can now be prevented by active immunization before pregnancy with live-attenuated vaccine. British policy is to vaccinate schoolgirls between their 11th and 14th birthdays.

The role of maternal cytomegalovirus (CMV) infection is also attracting interest as a potential cause of mental retardation and microcephaly[18]. The prevalance of CMV infection in live births varies in different parts of the world but is of the order of 0.5% in the United Kingdom. The consequences of primary congenital infection ranges from completely asymptomatic infection to the classical syndrome of neonatal cytomegalic inclusion disease, which accounts for fewer than 2% of the infections. Congenital infection may cause a relatively minor illness with mild transient jaundice or purpura, pneumonitis or hepatosplemomegaly, from which the infant usually recovers. This accounts for about 10% of the infections. It is estimated that 10% of those infants who are asymptomatic at birth may suffer later brain damage resulting in mental retardation and an even larger number may show evidence of sensorineural deafness and perhaps reduced intelligence. Most cases of congential CMV infection in the United Kingdom are thought to result from primary maternal infection during pregnancy, although this is difficult to establish precisely because of the virtual absence of symptoms in the mother.

Congenital toxoplasmosis is associated with severe structural brain abnormalities including microcephaly or hydrocephaly, cerebral palsy and chorio-retinitis[19]. There is great variation between European countries in the prevalence of infection with *Toxoplasma gondii*. Higher rates are reported in areas where uncooked meat is widely eaten. Diagnosis of clinical disease in the neonate is usually delayed because the organism can cause a silent infection in which the development of symptoms may be delayed for many years. British studies suggest that between 1 in 5000 and 1 in 10000 babies are born with congenital infection, although documented cases with neonatal abnormalities are rare. Even lower rates are reported from Scandinavia.

Congenital syphilis was an important cause of neonatal illness and handicap but is now rare, as a result of serological screening in the antinatal period and earlier treatment of the infection (see Chapter 5).

Neural tube defects

Defects of the neural tube are one of the largest single groups of congenital malformations in the United Kingdom. A woman who has had 1 conception with a neural tube defect has a 1 in 20 chance that future pregnancies will be similarly affected. After 2 conceptions with neural tube defects, the risk rises to 1 in 8 in further pregnancies. These mothers can be offered amniocentesis in order to determine the alpha fetoprotein level in the amniotic fluid, which is raised in affected pregnancies. The introduction of a serum alpha fetoprotein (AFP) screening test has made it possible to screen all pregnancies for neural tube defects[20]. The serum AFP reaches its maximum at about 16–18 weeks in affected pregnancies. For this reason, the pregnancy must be accurately dated by ultrasound, which will also exclude multiple pregnancy. A raised serum AFP may have other causes and the diagnosis must be confirmed by amniocentesis, which in itself carries a 0.5–1.0 % risk of dislodging the pregnancy or damaging the fetus. There are too few skilled obstetricians in the country to provide an amniocentesis service for all, and until that time the policy has been to gradually implement the diagnostic service in stages, concentrating particularly on areas where the prevalence of neural tube defect is high. The introduction of this technique imposes new ethical problems and its full implementation would require an increased motivation of mothers to report early in their pregnancies if termination of affected pregnancies are to be performed before the statutory 24 weeks. Unless the screening process is undertaken very carefully, there is a risk of terminating 'false positive' cases.

Conclusion

Routine selective screening of women over the age of 35 for Down's affected fetuses has been widely recommended. In 1977 however, only 16 % of mothers aged 40 and over in the West Midlands were referred for amniocentesis although the figure is higher in the main metropolitan centres[21]. Other chromosomal defects as well as Down's syndrome can now be diagnosed by prenatal amniocentesis. This poses new moral and ethical problems, particularly in the case of XO and XYY fetuses where the defect is compatible with long term survival.

The pattern of handicap will change as increasingly sophisticated antenatal diagnostic methods, including ultrasound and intra-uterine fetal blood sampling, are developed. It seems likely that methods to detect haemo-globinopathies, haemophilia and perhaps cystic fibrosis *in utero* will be developed. These measures will prevent the birth of defective children but are bound to be expensive and depend on their acceptability to parents.

The most effective ways of preventing congenital abnormalities are to provide good living conditions coupled with optimal antenatal care, genetic counselling and prenatal diagnosis. Good antenatal and perinatal care include the monitoring of fetal health as well as the identification of women at high risk. Antenatal diagnosis of fetal abnormality with facilities for early termination of pregnancy are needed in order to avoid the birth of abnormal infants. Until more is known about causal mechanisms, most of the scope for prevention lies in this direction. Emery[22] has estimated that about 1 in 20 children admitted to hospital has a disorder entirely genetic in origin. If partly genetic disorders are included, the proportion rises to 1 in 10 and accounts for over a third of child deaths in hospital.

References

1. Butler NR, Bonham DG. *Perinatal mortality*. London: Churchill Livingstone, 1963.
2. Claireaux A. Stillbirths and first week deaths. In: Chamberlain R, ed. *British births 1970. Vol 1*. London: Heinemann, 1975.
3. Illingworth RS. The incidence of disease in General Practice. *The Practitioner* 1979; **222**: 701–2.
4. Kennedy WP, Epidemiological aspects of the problem of congenital malformations. *Birth Defects. Original Article Series* 1967; **iii** (2): 1–18.
5. Carter CO. Genetics of common single malformations. *British Medical Bulletin* 1976; **32**(1): 21–6.
6. Wynn M, Wynn A. *Prevention of handicap and the health of women*. London: Routledge, Kegan, Paul, 1979.
7. Carter CO, Peel J, eds. The global incidence of genetic illness. *Qualities and inequalities in health*. London: Academic Press, 1976: 1–12.
8. Gerald PS. X-linked mental retardation and an X chromosome marker. *New England Journal of Medicine* 1980; **303** (12): 696.
9. Speidel BD, Meadow SR. Maternal epilepsy and abnormalities of the fetus and newborn. *Lancet* 1972; **ii**: 839–43.
10. Smithells RW. Environmental teratogens of man. *British Medical Bulletin* 1976; **32** (1): 27–33.
11. Forfar JO, Nelson MM. Epidemiology of drugs taken by pregnant women: drugs that may affect the fetus adversely. *Clinical Pharmacology and Therapeutics* 1973; **14**: 632.
12. Stewart A, Webb J, *et al*. Malignant diseases in childhood and diagnostic irradiation *in utero*. *Lancet* 1956; **ii**: 447.

13. Clavren SK, Smith DW. The fetal alcohol syndrome. *New England Journal of Medicine* 1978; **298**: 1063–7.
14. Smithells RW, *et al.* Vitamin deficiencies and neural tube defects *Archives of Diseases in Childhood* 1976; **51**: 944–50.
15. Smithells R, *et al.* Possible prevention of neural tube defects by periconceptual vitamin supplementation. *Lancet* 1980; 339–40.
16. Laurence KM, *et al.* Increased risk of pregnancies complicated by fetal neural tube defects in mothers receiving poor diets, and possible benefit of dietary counselling. *British Medical Journal* 1980; **i**: 1592–4.
17. Peckham CS, Marshall WC. Rubella and other virus infections in pregnancy. *Journal of Antimicrobial Chemotherapy* 1979; **5** (A): 71–80.
18. Stern H. Intrauterine and perinatal cytomegalovirus infections *Journal of Antimicrobial Chemotherapy* 1979; **5** (A): 81–5.
19. Fleck DG. Toxoplasmosis. *Journal of Antimicrobial Chemotherapy* 1979; **5** (A): 87–9.
20. Second collaborative study on alpha–fetoprotein in relation to neural tube defects *Lancet* 1979; **ii**: 651.
21. Edwards JH, Webb T. Amniocentesis rates in older women. *Lancet* 1979; **ii**: 1301.
22. Emery AH. Handicap – prevention of genetic disease. *Health and Hygiene* 1979; **2**: 129–34.

Index

Index